Meet the editor

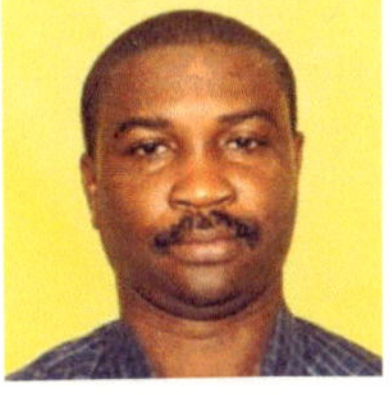

Dr. Hussaini Anthony Makun had his B.Sc. and M.Sc. degrees in Biochemistry from Ahmadu Bello University, Zaria in 1985 and 1991 respectively. He obtained his PhD degree in Biochemistry with specialization in Toxicology from Federal University of Technology, Minna in 2007. He pursued a postdoctoral research with Food, Environment and Health Research Group at University of Johannesburg from 2008 to 2010. He is currently an Associate Professor at the Department of Biochemistry of Federal University of Technology, Minna, Nigeria. His research interests include Food and Environmental Toxicology with focus on detection, health impact, and prevention and control of mycotoxins in foods. He has authored and co-authored 27 journal articles and 2 book chapters. He represents Nigeria on the African Union Codex Committee on Contaminants in Food.

Contents

Preface

The study of fungi and the toxins they secrete in foods and feeds is referred to as mycotoxicology. The subject plays a pivotal role in understanding the origin and pathology of some diseases arising from foods and so has great relevancy to medicine. Food spoilage caused by fungal toxins (mycotoxins) results in the loss of over 25% of world's foods which aggravates the severe food insecurity facing the deeming population of the earth. Mycotoxin contaminated agricultural products are not fit for export and so fungi and mycotoxins impact negatively the international trade with consequent adverse effect on world economy. Mycotoxicology is therefore of immense significance to public health, food safety and security, domestic and international trade, and world economy.

This book provides information on the incidence of fungi and mycotoxins in some African countries, the health implications and possible intervention control strategies for mycotoxins in developing countries and in Africa in particular. It will therefore be of interest to students, educators, researchers and policy makers in the fields of medicine, agriculture, food science and technology, trade and economics. Food regulatory officers also have quite a lot to learn from the book. Although a lot of the generated data in the area of mycotoxicology are available to the developed world, information on the subject area from Africa is scanty and not usually available in a comprehensive form. This book attempts to address the gap. Being an open access book, it will be of great benefit to scientists in developing countries who have limited access to information due to lack of funds to pay or subscribe for high quality journals and data from commercial publishing and database companies.

The book has three sections bordering on incidence of mycotoxins in Africa, health effects and prevention and control strategies of the fungal toxins. The first chapter is devoted to the occurrence of fungi and mycotoxins in foods and feeds in Nigeria, while the second gives a detailed account of the surveys carried out to detect and quantify aflatoxin M_1 in milk in developing countries in the last decade. The second section on health impact of mycotoxins has two chapters; 3 and 4 which address the mechanisms of action of mycotoxins in causing oxidative stress and incidence of diseases induced by mycotoxins (mycotoxicoses) in birds in developing countries respectively.

The six chapters in the section of prevention and control of mycotoxins collectively present the approaches for elimination of the toxins from dietary system. Chapter 5 describes the stratagems for the prevention and reduction of mycotoxins that are practicable in developing countries, while chapter 6 details practical methods towards sustainability and effectiveness of artisanal approaches to control mycotoxins associated with sorghum grains and sorghum based foods in Sahelian zone of Cameroon. Chapter 7 analyses the processes and prospects of Nigerian indigenous fermented foods with a view of eliminating food borne toxicants including fungal toxins. Chapter 8 discusses the prospects and challenges involved in using environment-friendly non-toxic phytochemicals in the control of fungi and mycotoxins as against toxic synthetic chemicals. While chapter 9 deals with the application of antioxidants derived from some African vegetables in alleviating mycotoxin induced oxidative stress and diseases, the last chapter provides practical steps towards regulation and enforcement of legislation on food borne toxicants from the point of view of an experienced Food Regulatory Officer.

Overall, it is our hope that this book will be a valuable addition to mycotoxicology literature and will promote interest in food safety arming researchers, policy makers and regulatory personnel with enough information to reduce the mycotoxin menace. I wish to express my profound gratitude to Dr. Garnett E. Wood of the FDA/Center for Food Safety and Applied Nutrition, USA for suggesting the title of the book, all the authors of the various chapters for their contributions which have made the book a reality and to INTECH Company for publishing it. I am sincerely highly honoured for being the editor of this creative, intellectual and informative project.

Dr. Hussaini Anthony Makun,
Associate Professor,
Department of Biochemistry,
Federal University of Technology,
Minna, Nigeria

Section 1

Occurrence of Mycotoxins

Chapter 1

Fungal and Mycotoxin Contamination of Nigerian Foods and Feeds

Olusegun Atanda, Hussaini Anthony Makun,
Isaac M. Ogara, Mojisola Edema, Kingsley O. Idahor,
Margaret E. Eshiett and Bosede F. Oluwabamiwo

Additional information is available at the end of the chapter

http://dx.doi.org/10.5772/55664

1. Introduction

Fungi are ubiquitous plant pathogens that are major spoilage agents of foods and feedstuffs. The infection of plants by various fungi not only results in reduction in crop yield and quality with significant economic losses but also contamination of grains with poisonous fungal secondary metabolites called mycotoxins. The ingestion of such mycotoxin-contaminated grains by animals and human beings has enormous public health significance, because these toxins are capable of causing diseases in man and animals (Bhat and Vasanthi 2003). Although the involvement of fungi and their toxins in causing diseases to man and animals dates back to the period when the Dead Sea Scrolls were written (Richard, 2007) it seems the evidence of their historic occurrence and impact were not obvious until the Middle Ages, when ergot alkaloids poisoning outbreaks in Europe were responsible for the death of thousands of people. Subsequently, between 1940s and 1950s a lethal human disease caused by *Fusarium* toxins and referred to as 'Alimentary Toxic Aleukia' was reported in Russia (Smith and Moss, 1985). Similarly in 1938 in Japan, *Penicillium* species were responsible for the colouring of rice that erratically led to the fatal human cardiac syndrome called 'yellow rice disease' (Uraguchi and Yamazaki, 1978). The livestock industry was also affected as seen by the devastation of the New Zeland sheep industry by facial eczema a fungal infection caused by *Pithomyces chartarum* in 1822. Other deadly animal syndromes arising from fungal infections and termed differently as equine leukoencephalomalacia (1930 to 1970 in USA), stachybotryotoxicosis (1930 in USSR), red mould diseases (1945-1947 in Japan), and red clover disease, vulvovaginitis and mouldy corn toxicosis (1920 to 1950 in USA) plagued the world (Gbodi and Nwude, 1988). In spite of these episodes little attention was paid to fungal diseases. However, in 1960, when the Turkey X disease killed thousands of poultry animals in Britain (Blount, 1965); the world became fully aware of the potential hazards of mycotoxins and responded to the disaster by a systematic and multidisciplinary approach which led to the discovery of aflatoxins as deadly contaminant of groundnuts.

Following the outbreak of aflatoxicosis and the enormous economic loss in the poultry industry of Britain in 1961, the Federal government of Nigeria, in order to protect her export trade initiated screening studies to determine the extent of aflatoxin contamination of groundnut and groundnut products (Blount, 1961; Darling, 1963, Haliday, 1965, 1966 and Halliday and Kazaure, 1967). McDonald and Harkness (1965) found aflatoxins in groundnut samples from Zaria, Kano and Mokwa, in Northern Nigeria. Bassir and Adekunle (1968) isolated two metabolites of *Aspergillus flavus* from palm wine which were characterized and named palmotoxin Bo and Go. The toxicity of palmotoxin Bo was comparable to that of aflatoxin B_1 in embryonated eggs (Bassir and Adekunle, 1969). Bassir (1969) also isolated aflatoxin B_1 from various mouldy food materials offered for sale in Ibadan markets. Since then, toxigenic fungi and mycotoxins have been found in various foods and feedstuffs in many regions of Nigeria (Tables 1 & 2) thus mycotoxigenic fungi belonging to not less than forty five fungal genera and about twenty different mycotoxins have been detected in Nigerian foods and foodstuffs. Two cases of animal mycotoxicoses (Ikwuegbu , 1984 and Ocholi *et al*. 1992) and two suspected cases of human mycotoxicosis were also reported in the country. The animal mycotoxicosis involved pecking ducklings and horses while the human mycotoxicosis involved primary school pupils that consumed groundnut cake ("kulikuli") in Ibadan (Akano & Atanda, 1990).

The presence of mycotoxins in our food systems and tissues has enormous public health significance because these toxins are nephrotoxic, immunotoxic, teratogenic and mutagenic. They are also capable of causing acute and chronic effects in man and animals ranging from death to disorder of central nervous, cardiovascular, pulmonary systems and intestinal tract (Bhat and Vasanthi, 2003). Of greatest concern is the relevance of these toxins in human hepatoma and oesophageal cancer, increased susceptibility to diseases especially in children and childhood pre-five mortality and reduced life expectancy (Beardall and Miller, 1994, Miller, 1996 and, Marasas, 2001).

Furthermore, Nigeria has experienced high recorded aflatoxin exposure levels in humans and has also reported the highest estimated number of cases of hepatocellular carcinoma (HCC-liver cancer) attributable to aflatoxins (Liu and Wu, 2010) in the whole world.

Due to the insidious nature of mycotoxin production and the resulting disease states which made diagnosis of mycotoxicosis difficult; many cases of both human and animal mycotoxicoses have often not been reported in Nigeria. This suggests that little has been done on mycotoxicosis in Nigeria and there is paucity of information on mycotoxins in the country.

In view of the negative public health and economic impacts of mycotoxins this chapter, written by members of the Mycotoxicology Society of Nigeria, the first of such society in Africa will examine the factors that influence the development of mycotoxin producing fungi and mycotoxin production and provide a current overview of the natural incidence of these toxins in different raw and processed food commodities that serve as principal sources of the toxins. It will also examine the human health hazards of the toxins with particular reference to the Nigerian situation as well as review the control and regulatory strategies possible within the country's technological capacity among others.

2. Factors affecting the incidence of mycotoxigenic fungi and mycotoxins in Nigeria

Various classifications are used in categorizing the factors that affect the incidence of mycotoxigenic fungi and mycotoxins in the food chain. Some classifications categorize these factors as extrinsic and intrinsic, some as physical, chemical and biological factors while others classify them as ecological, environmental and storage factors (D'Mello and MacDonald, 1997; Zain, 2011). Irrespective of the form of classification, Lacey (1986) identified the key elements involved in stating that the type and amount of mycotoxin produced is always determined by the fungi, substrate and environmental factors. In Nigeria, without necessarily sticking with any of the classification systems above, we can group the factors into 15 types as outlined below.

2.1. Climatic conditions

Probably the two most important environmental components favouring mold growth and mycotoxin production are hot and humid conditions. Mycotoxins occur more frequently in areas with a hot and humid climate, favourable for the growth of moulds. Although they can also be found in temperate zones, tropical climates such as those existing in Nigeria have been found to be quite conducive for mould growth and mycotoxin production. Mycotoxigenic fungi are most abundant in the tropics and as such, are major food spoilage agents in these warmer climates (Mclean and Berjak, 1987). Although the optimum temperature and moisture content for growth and toxin production for the various toxigenic fungi vary, many of them achieve best growth and toxin synthesis between 24°C and 28°C and seed moisture content of at least 17.5% (Trenk and Hartman, 1970; Ominski *et al.*, 1994). These conditions approximate the ambient climatic conditions in most parts of Africa and hence also account for the high prevalence of the toxins on the continent. Drought conditions actually constitute stress factors to plants rendering them vulnerable to mould infection with ensuing increase in toxin production. An indelible sign that droughts prop up toxin contamination is the fact that these conditions preceded the fatal outbreak of acute human aflatoxicosis that occurred in Kenya in 2004 (CDC, 2004). Edema and Adebanjo (2000) and Makun *et al* (2009a, b) recorded higher mycotoxigenic fungal contamination during the rainy season than in the dry harmattan season among produce in Nigeria.

2.2. Availability of nutrients and conditions for mould growth

The fact that a strain of mould has the genetic potential to produce a particular mycotoxin is not enough for it to do so. There must be enough nutrients to encourage mould growth and the level of mycotoxin production would in part be influenced by the nutrients available to the mould. Typically, moulds require a source of energy in the form of carbohydrates or vegetable oils in addition to a source of nitrogen either organic or inorganic, trace elements and available moisture for growth and toxin production. Substrate may also play a role in selecting for or against toxin producing strains of a given species, e.g., there is a high proportion of toxin-producing strains of *A. flavus* isolated from peanuts and cottonseed than from rice or sorghum. It has also been found that strains of ochratoxin and citrinin-producing *P. viridicatum* isolated from meat were more unstable than those isolated from grain and rapidly lost toxin-producing ability. Field fungi like *Fusarium* and *Alternaria* contaminate grains before or during harvest. The storage fungi (e.g. *Penicillium* and *Aspergillus*) are capable of growing at lower water content than the field fungi and they tend to contaminate the grains in silos and other storage places. It is known that aflatoxin production is favoured by prolonged end of season drought and associated elevated temperatures (Rachaputi *et al.*, 2002). Moulds can grow and produce mycotoxins under a wide temperature range with optima generally between 20 to 30°C. However, temperatures optimum for toxin production need not correspond to those optimum for growth: *Fusarium tricinctum* grows well at 25°C but produces T-2 toxin best near freezing temperatures. *Penicillium martensii* produces penicillic acid rapidly at 20-30°C, but considerably more toxin eventually accumulates between 4 to 10°C.

2.3. Farming systems and agricultural techniques

A number of farming techniques have been shown in various reports as stimulating mould growth in agricultural produce. For example produce harvested from land on which groundnut has been planted the previous year were infested more by *Aspergillus flavus* and contained more aflatoxin than crops grown on land previously planted with rye, oats, melon or potatoes indicating that crop rotation influences mycotoxigenic mould growth. Likewise, previously fungicide-treated soil has been shown to reduce incidence of A. flavus in groundnuts to very low levels.

2.4. Soil types and soil conditions

Soil is a natural factor that exerts a powerful influence on the incidence of fungi. Crops grown in different soil types may have significantly different levels of mycotoxin contamination. For example, peanuts grown in light sandy soils support rapid growth of the fungi, particularly under dry conditions, while heavier soils result in less contamination of peanuts due to their high water holding capacity which helps the plant to prevent drought stress (Codex Alimentarius Commission, 2004).

2.5. Pre-harvest conditions

Genotypes, drought, soil type, plant density, fertilization level, and insect activities are important components in determining the likelihood of pre-harvest contamination (Cole et al., 1995). However, the most important factor appears to be high night time temperatures, which favour fungal growth and toxin production at a time when the plant is deprived of its usual energy source and thus least able to resist fungal attack (Abbas et al., 2002, 2007; Payne, 1992).

2.6. Time of harvesting

Harvest is the first stage in the production chain where moisture content becomes the most important parameter in terms of the management and protection of the crop. It also marks a shift from problems caused by plant pathogenic fungi, like Fusarium, to problems caused by storage fungi, like *Penicillium verrucosum*. Ideally, grains will always be harvested after a spell of dry weather when it is at a 'safe' moisture content, so that immediate drying is not necessary. However, this is not always possible hence inappropriate harvest time is a risk factor in Nigeria. Another important control measure at harvest will be visual examination of the grain for symptoms of disease, and the segregation of diseased batches from healthy grain. Early harvesting reduces fungal infection of crops in the field and consequent contamination of harvested produce. Even though majority of farmers in Africa are well aware of the need for early harvesting, lack of storage space, unpredictable weather, labour constraint, need for cash, threat of thieves, rodents and other animals compel farmers to harvest at inappropriate time (Bankole and Adebanjo, 2003). Kaaya et al. (2006) observed that aflatoxin levels increased by about 4 times by the third week and more than 7 times when maize harvest was delayed for 4 weeks. However, If products are harvested early, they have to be dried to safe levels to stop fungal growth. Rachaputi *et al.* (2002) reported lower aflatoxin levels and higher gross returns of 27% resulting from early harvesting and threshing of groundnuts.

2.7. Pest infestation

Insects are the chief causes of deterioration and loss of grains and seeds. Their invasion of cereals decreases the quality, grade and market value of these agricultural products which in most instances are rendered unsafe for human and animal consumption. Pest infestation is largely due to improper post-harvest and storage conditions and the level of insect damage influences the extent of mycotoxin contamination. Avantaggio *et al.* (2002) found that insect damage of maize is good predictor of *Fusarium* mycotoxin contamination. Insects carry spores of mycotoxin-producing fungi from plant surfaces to the interior of the stalk or kernels or create infectious wounds through their feeding habits (Munkvold, 2003).

2.8. Post-harvest handling

The post-harvest stages are those stages following harvest and leading up to primary processing such as milling. This will typically involve drying (if required), storage and transportation steps. Post-harvest movement of food/feed commodities can be complex, passing as it may between a number of intermediaries such as traders and intermediate processors, who may be situated at different geographical locations. In the simplest case, produce may remain on-farm in store or buffer storage for short periods of time before being passed directly onto the processor. In more complex cases it may pass through the hands of merchants or third party drying facilities (if harvested wet e.g. grains) and held in storage for periods of time before finally arriving at the processors. At all times the produce can become susceptible to fungal contamination and mycotoxin production if the storage conditions are not strictly controlled.

2.9. Drying conditions and duration

Rapid drying of agricultural products to low moisture level is critical as it creates less favourable conditions for fungal growth, proliferation, and insect infestation. It helps keep products longer (Lanyasunya *et al.*, 2005). Ayodele and Edema (2010, In Press) evaluated the Critical Control Points (CCP) in the production of dried yam chips with a view to reducing mycotoxin contamination and identified the drying stage as a CCP. Aflatoxin contamination can increase 10 fold in a 3-d period, when field harvested maize is stored with high moisture content (Hell et al., 2008). The general recommendation is that harvested commodities should be dried as quickly as possible to safe moisture levels of 10 – 13 %. Achieving this through simple sun-drying under the high humidity conditions of many parts of Africa, such as the humid southern Nigeria is very difficult. Even, when drying is done in the dry season, it is not completed before loading grains into stores as observed by Mestre et al. (2004) and products can be easily contaminated with aflatoxins. During storage, transportation and marketing, low moisture levels should be maintained by avoiding leaking roofs and condensation arising from inadequate ventilation.

2.10. Storage factors

Mycotoxin contamination of foods or feeds may result from inadequate storage and/or handling of harvested products. To preserve quality in storage, it is necessary to prevent biological activity through adequate drying to less than 10% moisture, elimination of insect activity that can increase moisture content through condensation of moisture resulting from respiration, low temperatures, and inert atmospheres (Lanyasunya *et al.*, 2005; Turner *et al.*, 2005). Several field and storage fungi have been reported in Nigeria (Tables 1& 2) and the post-harvest contamination is normally characterized by the activities of the 'storage' fungi, typically *Aspergillus* and *Penicillium* species that are able to grow in relatively dry conditions.

2.11. Sanitation

Basic sanitation measures such as removal and destruction of debris from previous harvest would help in minimizing infection and infestation of produce in the field. Sorting out physically damaged and infected grains (known from colorations, odd shapes and size) from the intact commodity can result in 40-80% reduction in aflatoxins levels

2.12. Traditional processing methods

A study conducted in Benin by Fandohan *et al.* (2005) to determine the fate of aflatoxins and fumonisins through traditional processing of naturally-contaminated maize and maize-based foods, demonstrated that sorting, winnowing, washing, crushing combined with dehulling of maize grains were effective in achieving significant mycotoxins removal. Similar results have been reported by Park (2002) and Lopez-Garcia and Park (1998). This approach is based on separation of contaminated grains from the bulk grains and depends on heavy contamination of only a small fraction of the seeds, so that removing those leaves a much.

Wet and dry milling processes as well as heat in the cooking process have been shown to reduce mycotoxin production in foods. Heating and roasting can significantly decrease aflatoxin content in corn. Grain cleaning and further processing in mills can divert mycotoxins to various mill streams, and further processing such as baking may reduce mycotoxin levels. A review of several studies, however, suggested that processing and pasteurization of milk do not completely destroy mycotoxins (Manorama and Singh, 1995).

2.13. Presence of previous contaminants

The presence of other microorganisms either bacteria or fungi may alter elaboration of mycotoxins on food materials. When *A. parasiticus* was grown in the presence of some bacteria; *Streptococcus lactis* and *Lactobacillius casei*, aflatoxin production was reduced (Ominski *et al.*, 1994). Meanwhile, fungal metabolites such as rubratoxins from *Penicillium purpurogenum;* cerulenin from *Ephalosporium caerulens* and *Acrocylindrium oryzae* enhance aflatoxin production even though they repress growth of aflatoxin-producing fungi (Smith and Moss, 1985). This type of positive interaction between fungi in the same food matrix with regards to aflatoxin synthesis coupled with multi-occurrence of mycotoxins from the different fungi could have additive or synergistic effect on the health of the host (Speijer and Speijer, 2004) and worsen the aflatoxin plight in Nigeria because such simultaneous co-occurrence of fungi and mycotoxins in African agricultural commodities is a very common phenomenon as indicated by many workers such as Makun *et al.* (2007), Makun *et al.* (2009) and Njobeh *et al.* (2009).

2.14. Substrate types and properties

Certain Agricultural produce have been observed to permit the growth of some moulds over others. For example, maize allows the growth of aflatoxins and fumonisins producing moulds above others, while groundnuts have been found to be excellent substrate for aflatoxin contamination (Bankole and Adebanjo, 2003). Other food products for which mycotoxin contamination has been reported in Nigeria are dried yam chips, tiger nut, melon seeds and stored herbal plants. Cereal grains, peanuts, cottonseed and some forages appear to be commongly contaminated with foods and feed substances that may be contaminated with mycotoxins. Similarly, intake of *Fusarium* toxins, such as trichothecenes and fumonisins, is almost solely due to consumption of cereals).

2.15. Lack of awareness

Lack of awareness of the dangers posed by mycotoxin contamination of produce is a major factor responsible for its high incidence in Nigeria. Majority of farmers produce and food handlers and/or processors are illiterate with virtually no knowledge of the implications of toxigenic mould growth. The Mycotoxicology Society of Nigeria has done a lot to reverse this trend. The stake holders believe that the powdery substance can be easily dusted off or rinsed with water before the food material is eaten or processed for consumption with no associated risks. The contaminated, mould infested produce are proudly displayed on market stalls (Figs 1 & 2) for sale.

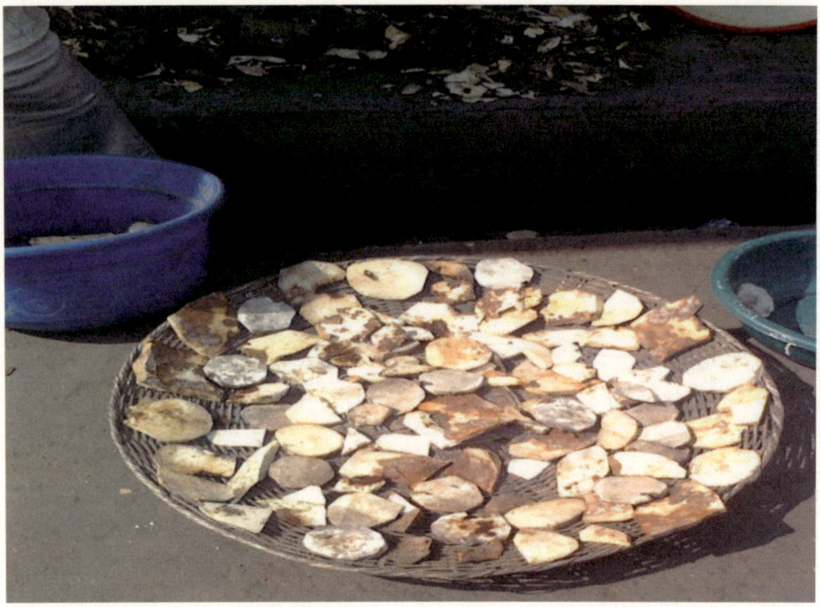

Figure 1. Typical rotten yam slices being dried for processing into yam chips

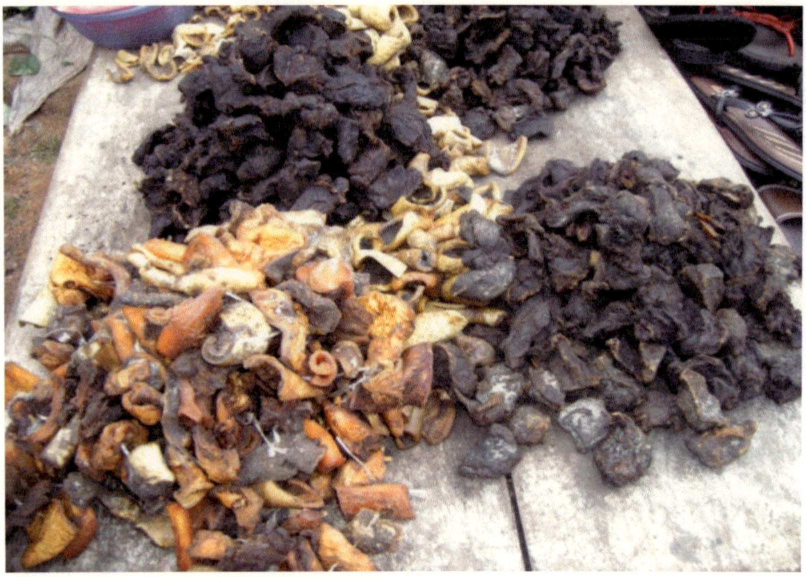

Figure 2. *Aspergillus flavus* contaminated dried meat displayed for sale in an open market in Nigeria

No	Aflatoxin	Crop contaminated	Location	Frequency of contamination	Range of concentration (μg/kg)	Mean concentration (μg/kg)	Author
1.	AFB_1	Groundnut	Northern Nigeria		100-2000		Darling, 1963
2	AFB_1	Stored groundnut	Zaria	35%	100-2000		Peer, 1965
3	AFB_1 & G1	Palm wine	Ibadan				Bassir and Adekunle, (1969)
4	AFB_1	Bitter leaf	Ibadan		>94		Bassir, 1969
5	AFB_1	Groundnut Dried fish Cereals (Millet SorghumRice)	Savannah and Forest regions of Nigeria		>900 600-700 150-300		Okonkwo and Nwokolo, (1978)
6	AFB_1	Sorghum	Northern Nigeria		<20		Dada, 1978
7	AFB_1 AFG_1	Sorghum	Zaria	8/8 8/8	30.32-211.20 2.40-208.00		Uraih and Ogbadu, (1982)
8	AFB_1 AFB_2 AFG_1 AFG_2	Sera of Primary liver cell carcinoma patients	Zaria	20/20 20/20 20/20 20/20	0.009-0.331 0.030-0.278 0.013-0.334 0.005-0.146	0.069 0.095 0.083 0.040	Onyemelukwe *et al.* (1982)
9	AFB_1	Groundnut G/Nut oil Cottonseed oil	Zaria		0-600 >98 >65		Abalaka and Elegbede, 1982
10	AFB_1	Poultry feed made of groundnut cake (aflatoxicosis in pecking ducklings)	Ogun State			3000	Ikwuegbu, (1984)
11	AFB_1	Livestock rations	Vom		4-340		Gbodi *et al.*(1984)
12	AFB_1	Millet beer	Jos				Okoye and Ekpenyong, (1984)
13	AFB_1	Poultry feeds	Southern Nigeria	69/120	0.57-2.55		Oyejide et al. (1987)
14	AFB_1	Maize	Plateau	27/64 21/64	0-960 0-543 0-	0.27-372.49	Gbodi, (1986)

No	Aflatoxin	Crop contaminated	Location	Frequency of contamination	Range of concentration (μg/kg)	Mean concentration (μg/kg)	Author
	AFB_2 AFG_1 AFG_2		State	5/64 3/64	83.33 0-23.53	1.5-113.2 2.0-20 3.92-13.33	
15	AFB_1 AFB_2 AFG_1 AFG_2	Acha	Plateau State	4/24 2/24 0/24 0/24	0-20 0-12		Gbodi, (1986)
16	AFB_1 AFB_2 AFG_1 AFG_2	Cottonseed	Plateau State	3/8 3/8 2/8 1/8	0-271 0-36.6 0-183 0-9.1	52.25 24.85 38.13 1.14	Gbodi, (1986)
17	AFs	Millet beer		10/10	500-5000		Obasi *et al.* (1987)
18	AFB_1	Peanut cake	Nigeria	18/20 29/29	20-455 13-2824	236.69	Akano & Atanda, 1990 Ezekiel *et al.* 2012c
19	AFB_1	Cowpea Maize Millet Rice Sorghum Cottonseed Groundnut Groundnut oil Melon seed Palm kernel	North and South Lagos	3/268 81/281 10/275 13/279 22/318 17/28 414/634 56/57 22/30 41/55	0-48 0-1250 0-160 0-40 0-40 0-8000 0-40 0-53	31.6 74-218 42 5 5 105 151-767 9.5 19	Opadokun, 1992 (Samples collected from 1962-1985)
20	Total AF	Restaurant dishes (gari, bean with soup) Dried okra Dried pepper	Nsukka	17/17	31.20-268.32		Obidoa and Gugnani, (1992)
21	Total AF	Corn Corn cake Corn roll snack	Western Nigeria		25-777 15-1070 10-160	200 233 55	Adebajo *et al.* (1994)
22	AFB_1	Red hot chili pepper	Western Nigeria		>2.2		Adegoke *et al.* (1996)
23	AFB_1 AFB_2	Maize	Niger State	144/288	234-908 234		Tijani, (2005)

No	Aflatoxin	Crop contaminated	Location	Frequency of contamination	Range of concentration (µg/kg)	Mean concentration (µg/kg)	Author
24	AFM_1	Human milk Cow milk Ice cream	Abeokuta &Odeda local Govt. Nigeria	5/28 3/22 2/6		4.00 (µg/l) 3.02 (µg/l) 2.23 (µg/l)	Atanda *et al.*, 2007
25	AFB_1	Mouldy rice	Niger State	97/196	0-1642	200.19	Makun *et al.* (2007)
26	AFB_1	Mouldy sorghum	Niger State	91/168	0-1164	199.51	Makun *et al.* (2009)
27	AFM_1 AFB_1	Powdered milk Bean Wheat	Lagos Minna Minna	7/100 29/50 27/50	0-0.41 0-137.6 0-198.4	0.016-0.325 59.29 85.56	Makun *et al.* (2010)
28	AFB_1 AFB_2 AFG_1 AFG_2 Total AF	Rice	Minna	21/21 21/21 21/21 19/21 21/21	4.1-309 1.3-24.2 5.5-76.8 3.6-44.4 27.7-371.9	37.2 8.3 22.1 14.7 82.5	Makun *et al.* (2011)
29	AFB1	Melon seed	Western Nigeria	30/120	2.3-15.4		Bankole *et al.* 2004
30	Total AF	Maize	Western Nigeria	20/103	3-138		Bankole and Mabekoje, 2004
31	AFB_1 AFB_2 AFG_1	Fonio millet	Plateau State, Nigeria	13/16 4/16 4/16	0.08-1.4 0.07-0.1 0.2-2	0.4 0.08 0.6	Ezekiel *et al*, 2012
32	AFB_1 AFB_2 AFG_1 AFG_2	Commercial poultry feeds	Nigeria	44/58 29/58 35/58 6/58	6-1067 10-114 8-235 10-20	198 34 45 13	Ezekiel *et al.* 2012b
33	AFB_1	Rice Beans Cassava flour Semovita Yam Wheat meal Maize "Gari"	Ogun State, Nigeria	19/21 15/17 3/4 2/6 6/7 2/3 3/3 13/18	*nd - 0.30 nd-0.89 nd-0.07 nd-0.17 nd-0.27 nd-0.06 0.11-0.20 nd-0.69	0.14 0.15 0.05 0.09 0.14 0.04 0.16 0.25	Adejumo et al.,2012. Unpublished. Submitted to Food& Chemical Toxicology

No	Aflatoxin	Crop contaminated	Location	Frequency of contamination	Range of concentration (µg/kg)	Mean concentration (µg/kg)	Author
	AFM_1	Breast milk of lactating mothers	Ogun State, Nigeria	41/50	nd-92.14(ng/l)	15.00(ng/l)	
34	AFB_1 AFB_2 AFG_1 AFG_2 Total AF	Red hot chili pepper	Minna	12/20 12/20 12/20 12/20 12/20	0.05-12.4 0.05-4.95 0.50-10.0 0.55-3.20 0.85-19.45	2.21 0.89 0.58 0.39 5.85	Unpublished. Submitted to Food Control. Makun *et al.* (2012)
35	AFM_1	Fresh milk "Nono" "Kindirmo"	Bida	10/10 10/10 10/10	0.41-0.96 0.25-2.51 015-0.70		Unpublished Okeke, (2012)
36	AFB_1 AFB_2	Maize	Niger State	59/95 67/95	4.0-74.4 8.0-79.2	19.58 30.10	Unpublished Muhammad, 2012
37	AFB_1 AFB_2	Rice	Kaduna State	64/86 41/86	4-292 0.4-27.2	157.34 5.17	Unpublished Olorunmowaju, 2012
38	AFB_1 AFB_2	Groundnut	Niger State	72/82 61/82	4-188 0.40-38.4	53.06 8.08	Unpublished Ifeji, 2012

*nd= Not detected

Table 1. Incidence of Aflatoxins in Nigerian Foods and Feeds

S/No	Fungi	Mycotoxin	Commodity contaminate	Location	Frequency of contami-nation	Concen-tration range (µg/kg)	Mean concentr-ation (µg/kg)	Author
1	*Sphacelia sorghi*	Dihydro-ergosine	Guinea corn	Northern Nigeria				Mantle (1968)
2	*A.flavus*	*Palmotoxin Bo and Go	Palm wine	Ibadan				Bassir and Adekunle, (1969)
3	*Aspergillius, Fusarium, Penicillium, Phoma, Alternaria, Curvularia, Chaetomium* and *Helminthosporium*	ochratoxins A, B and C, sterigmatocystin and zearalenone	Guinea corn	Zaria, Nigeria				Elegbede, (1978),

S/No	Fungi	Mycotoxin	Commodity contaminate	Location	Frequency of contami-nation	Concen-tration range (μg/kg)	Mean concentr-ation (μg/kg)	Author
	Collectotrichum, Pericona, Rhizopus, Mucor, Trichotecium, Cephalosporium							
4	*Collectrotrichum, Curvularia, Fusarium, Mucor, Phoma, Rhizopus, Helminthosporium, Penicillium* and *Trichoderma* apart from the *Aspergillius*	Patulin and Zearalenone	Guinea corn	Northern Nigeria				Salifu 1978
5	*Aspwegillus spp, Phoma sorghina, Fusarium semitectum, Fusarium moniliforme* and *F.equiseti*	two unidentified metabolites	Guinea corn	Bakura, Kano, Samaru and Mokwa.				Dada, (1979)
6		Zearalenone	Native Beer (Burukutu)	Jos, Plateau State				Okoye 1986
7		ochratoxins zearalenone, vomitoxin, T-2 toxin and moniliform	Cocoa, groundnut, palm kernel, maize, yam,	Northern and Southern Nigeria				Okoye (1992)
8		Nivalenol, fusarenon-X and HT-2 toxin, deoxynivalenol and T-2 toxin	Maize	Jos district				Okoye (1993)
9	*Botryodiplodia theobromae Cladosporium herbarum, Diplodia* sp. *Fusarium moniliforme*	Ochratoxin A and zearalenone	Kola nut	South Western Nigeria				Adebajo and Popoola (2003)

S/No	Fungi	Mycotoxin	Commodity contaminate	Location	Frequency of contami-nation	Concen-tration range (μg/kg)	Mean concentr-ation (μg/kg)	Author
	and *F. oxysporum, Aspergillus clavatus, A. flavus* Link, *A. niger, A. ochraceus, A. parasiticus* and *A. tamarii Penicillium digitatum, P. funiculosum, Penicillium sp, Rhizomucor pusillus* and *Rhizopus arrhizus Aspergillus ,Penicillium, Botryodiplodia, Cladosporium* and *Rhizopus* species							
10	*Aspergillus* and *Fusarium* species	Aflatoxins and Fumonisins	Maize	South western Nigeria				Bankole and Mabekoje (2004)
11		Aflatoxins, ochratoxins and fumonisins	Cereals, spices, stockfish and milk and milk products	South western Nigeria				Ogunbanwo (2005)
12		Ochratoxins	Cocoa	South Western Nigeria				Aroyeun and jayeola (2005)
13	*Aspergillus, Penicillium, Fusarium, Alternaria, Mucor, Rhizopus, Trichoderma, Curvularia, Helminthospori um and Cladosporium.* Others include *Arthrinium, Syncephalastru*	Ochratoxin A and zearalenone	Guinea corn and rice		Niger state			Makun (2007)

S/No	Fungi	Mycotoxin	Commodity contaminate	Location	Frequency of contami-nation	Concen-tration range (μg/kg)	Mean concentr-ation (μg/kg)	Author
	m, Geotrichum, Bipolaris, Rhodotorula, Cryptococcus,T orula, Chrysosporium, Collectitrichum, Scopulariopsis, Gilocladium and *Nocardia*							
14		3-Nitropropionic acid Averufanin Averufin Beauvericin Cyclosporin A Emodin Equisetin Kojic acid Nidurufin Norsolorinic acid Ochratoxin A Methlysterigm atocystin Sterigmatocystin Versicolorin A Versicolorin	Peanut cake				20 0.2 1.0 0.02 0.2 1.0 5.0 80 0.4 0.02 4 2 2 0.2 1.0	Ezekiel *et al.*, 2012

Table 2. Fungi and other Mycotoxins in Nigerian Foods

3. Human and animal health implications of mycotoxins in Nigeria

Mycoses and mycotoxicoses are the major ways in which human and animal health is affected due to infection with fungi and contamination with Mycotoxins. When this happens the implications are wide and span from health to economics. Mycosis means fungal infection of man or animals and range in its simplest form from growth that merely annoys the victim to a more complex form of life threatening invasion. Mycotoxicosis on the other hand could be defined as a disease outbreak that is commonly associated with the ingestion of mycotoxins or inhalation of spores produced by fungi. The appearance of mycotoxicoses symptoms depends on the level of contamination, length of exposure, type of mycotoxins, degree of combination with several other mycotoxins, individual differences, species-specific resistance, sex, pre-existing pathological and physiological status of the victim. The synergistic effects associated with several other factors such as genetics, diet, and interactions with other toxins have been poorly studied. Therefore, it is possible that vitamin deficiency, caloric deprivation, alcohol abuse and infectious disease status can all have compounded effects with mycotoxins. Mycotoxins have the potential for both acute and chronic health effects through ingestion, skin contact and inhalation. These toxins can enter the blood stream and lymphatic system and inhibit protein synthesis, damage macrophage systems, particle clearance of the lung and increase sensitivity to opportunistic infections. If symptoms appear within a short period of less than 7 days of contamination, it is termed "acute mycotoxicoses" but if the interval between contamination and appearance of the symptoms persist longer, it is termed "chronic mycotoxicoses". In acute cases, victim may die if adequate treatment measures are not taken whereas in chronic cases, the victim may live longer though with protracted illnesses.

3.1. Human mycotoxicoses

Mycotoxins have been detected in human foods and livestock feeds in Nigeria. Most often these mycotoxins are detected in deleterious levels compounded by synergistic interactions. Whenever these contaminated foods and feeds are ingested, the victim's physiological mechanisms attempt to metabolize the toxins especially the liver, kidneys and some specialized microorganisms in the gastrointestinal tract (Bankole and Adebanjo, 2003). On a world wide scale, relationships between mycotoxins and human illness have been clearly established. Aflatoxins have been shown to be involved with and to aggravate hepatitis B infection (JECFA 2001), while Fumonisins have been shown to be consistently responsible for oesophageal cancer in south Africa (Makaula et al. 1996). In Nigeria, documentation of Mycotoxin related human health problems is not extensive. However the few literature available show evidence of human mycotoxicoses and suspected mycotoxicoses related deaths. The death of some children who consumed mouldy Kulikuli (Groundnut cake) in Ibadan was suspected to be due to aflatoxicosis (Ikeorah and Okoye 2005). Aflatoxins have been found in the urine of liver disease patients in Zaria, in Blood in Southern Nigeria, in organs of children who died of kwashiorkor in Western Nigeria, and in human semen in Benin city (Onyemelukwe 1992, Oluyide 1993, Adegoke et al. 1996 and Oluwafemi 2005). Similarly Aflatoxin M_1 has been found in breast milk and in the blood of umbilical cord of babies in the country (WHO 1997 and Adejumo et al. 2012). Doctors at the National hospital Abuja have reported post mortem examination link between the cause of death from liver cancer to Aflatoxin (Paul Jibrin – personal communication). Some Specialist Hospitals visited, gave reports of several mycological cases suspected to be synonymous with Aflatoxicoses, Ochratoxicoses, Zearalenone and Fumonisin toxicities. However, legislation on Medical Ethics in the country restrained us from accessing individual case files. In some of these hospitals, the cases were documented as fungal infections, mycoses and mycotoxicoses and because this area of study is not yet very popular, many Nigerians are not conversant with the words mycoses and mycotoxicoses (Idahor *et al.*, 2010; Idahor and Ogara, 2010).

3.2. Livestocks

Mycotoxins are known to be consumed by livestock through contaminated feed ingredients. They are probably the causative agents or suspected contributing factors in farm animal diseases that cause great economic losses. Feed ingredients are any of the constituent nutrients of livestock ration. Some of the plants used in ration formulation like cereals, legumes, oil seeds, nuts and root crops are susceptible to mycotoxins contamination yet their deleterious effects are still a grey area. In livestock, mycotoxicoses cases are more severe in monogastric than ruminants due to the detoxifying capabilities of some rumen microorganisms. Young and pregnant animals are generally the most susceptible to mycotoxicoses. Under some conditions, the fungi may produce potent mycotoxins at levels that may adversely affect livestock production. At moderate levels, effects may appear initially with more obvious symptoms within a few days to several weeks of ingestion of the contaminated foods or feeds. Mycotoxins could possibly have pervasive yet subclinical effects on performance and health in ruminants that may be unnoticed. Performance losses of 5 – 10% are typical with consumption of mouldy feeds even in the absence of mycotoxins. On the other hand, mycotoxins contaminations increase production losses even when the mould is not readily visible. In horses, equine leukoencephalomalacia syndrome fatal mycotoxic disease occuring only in horses, donkeys and ponies is is characterized by the presence of liquefactive necrotic lesions in the white matter of the horse cerebrum. Other pathological changes of this disease include lethargy, head pressing, inappetence, convulsion and sudden death. There are few reported suspected cases of aflatoxicoses in horses associated with *Penicillium purpurogenum* in Vom, plateau state (Ocholi et al. 1992) and aflatoxicoses in Pecking ducklings in Ogun state.

Rabbits seem apparently unsusceptible to micro doses of mycotoxins especially when dosed orally for a relatively short period. Idahor *et al.* (2008a) observed gradual decrease in sperm production rates, final live weights, feed consumption and body weight gain concomitantly with increasing Fumonisin B_1 concentration in diet. There were no evidences of mycotoxins (at 1.9mg/kg) diet crossing the placenta to cause developmental abnormalities in the foetuses examined at the first trimester. It was speculated that there might have been some damages on the physiological status of the rabbits and possibly gradual accumulation of the mycotoxins in the carcasses which might in turn pose residual health hazard to humans when consumed (Idahor *et al.* 2008b) . In a similar study, Ogunlade *et al.* (2004) reported sufficient evidences of carcinogenicity and toxicity at micro doses of 1650-1990μg Fumonisin B_1 per kg diet. But there were no negative effects on the rabbit's blood cellular components, serum protein metabolism and serum enzymes activities. On the other hand, Ewuola *et al.* (2003) demonstrated that micro doses of Fumonisin B_1 can induce physiological and pathological damages in rabbits by reducing the feed intake with resultant effects on body weight gain.. Pregnant New Zealand White rabbits are speculated to be very sensitive to the toxic effects of Fumonisin B_1 and that maternal toxicity was observed at daily gavage doses of 0.25mg/kg body weight.

4. Economic impact of mycotoxins in Nigeria

Estimating the economic impact of mycotoxins require good data sets and expertise in the use of various economic impact assessment models. Both of these prerequisites generally are missing in Sub-Saharan Africa. Data which would form the baseline on the effects and related costs of mycotoxin contamination on human health are not available. Cost elements include mortality (the cost of productive capacity lost with premature death), the cost of morbidity(losses resulting from productivity loss, hospitalization and the costs of health care services both for public and private health Institutions). There is also the intangible cost of pain, suffering, anxiety, and reduction in the quality of life (Lubulwa and Davis, 1994). The data on the economic impact of mycotoxins on livestock which should include income losses due to mortality as well as those due to reductions in productivity, weight gain, and the yield of meat, milk and eggs, as well as those due to feed use inefficiency and increased susceptibility to disease are also not available in Nigeria. The economic losses associated with mycotoxin contamination are difficult to assess in a consistent and uniform way. The lack of information on the health costs and other economic losses from mycotoxin induced human illness is partly due to the difficulty of establishing cause-and-effect relationships between mycotoxins and the chronic diseases they are suspected of causing. For Sub-Saharan Africa, capacity building for economic impact assessment is urgent for both impact assessment and trade analysis. Baseline data do not exist in most of the countries including Nigeria, so comparisons often have no basis for normalization.

Even trade data are difficult to obtain. The trade data used in the gravity model by Otsuki *et al.* (2001*a,b*) to establish the baseline put African exports to the European Union in 1998 to be US$ 472 million for dried fruit and nuts and US$ 298 million for cereals, with the bulk of this trade occurring with France. These figures seem implausible, especially for cereals, given Africa's lack of competitiveness in this sector relative to Europe, and statistics from the United Nations COMTRADE database show that European imports from Africa are not large. Africa only exported to Europe approximately US$ 104 million of dried fruit, US$ 45 million of peanuts, US$ 27 million for other edible nuts, and < US$ 14 million for cereals and cereal products in 1998. Thus, the baseline against which economic impacts should be defined is at best fuzzy and often lacking (Leslie et al, 2008)

4.1. Economic losses and impact on international trade

The adverse economic effects attributed to mycotoxin contamination and losses are widely felt in all sectors of food production and particularly in agricultural commodities.

Mycotoxin contamination of agricultural commodities has considerable economic implications. Losses from rejected shipments and lower prices for inferior quality can devastate developing-country export markets.

Produce handlers are affected by restricted storage options, cost of testing produce lots and loss of end market locally. Companies incur higher costs due to higher product losses, monitoring costs and restricted end markets. Consumers who are the primary target in this chain end up paying higher prices due to increased monitoring at all levels of handling, and in extreme cases health problems due to consumption of contaminated products.

Costs to farmers include reduced income from outright food or feed losses and lower selling prices for contaminated commodities. The economic impact on livestock production includes mortality as well as reductions in productivity, weight gain, feed efficiency, fertility, ability to resist diseases and decrease in the quantity and quality of meat, milk and egg production.

Any economic costs must be weighed against the costs of preventing mycotoxins through better production, harvesting and storage practices. The latter costs are likely to be considerable. Member states of the African Groundnut Council (Gambia, Mali, Niger, Nigeria, Senegal, and Sudan) have calculated the annual cost of implementing a program to reduce mycotoxin contamination at US$7.5 million. High levels of mycotoxins have been found in groundnuts and cereal grains in countries such as Gambia, Ghana, Guinea, Nigeria, Senegal, South Africa and indications of the magnitude of the problem.

Contamination of food by microbes and chemicals also has economic consequences due to rejection of exports and loss of credibility as trading partners. Capacity to implement effective food safety controls is of vital importance to agricultural and food exports from developing countries. For example, importing countries frequently require guarantees that minimum standards of hygiene have been applied in the manufacture of a food product and that food do not have excessive mycotoxins contamination. The exporting country must be able to comply with these requirements and demonstrate that compliance has been achieved. While basic scientific and technical infrastructure is clearly vital, administrative structures, management, financing and human capital are also important elements. Indeed, the experiences of many countries suggest that lack of efficient management or sustainable levels of resources can seriously compromise the effectiveness of food safety controls.

In Nigeria, regulatory agencies destroyed mycotoxin-contaminated foods worth more than US$ 200 000 in 2010.

Total aflatoxin (B1, B2, G1 and G2) content in ng/g of product can give an indication of product quality and can be used as a threshold for separating high, medium and low quality produce. This grading is used for pricing a premium (high quality) or a discount (poor quality) crop. The risk of spoilage is a function of factors including: the variety of crop, the time and method of harvest and storage, the storage temperature, the moisture content and the drying method prior to storage. Africa loses an estimate of sixty seven ($67) million dollars annually from export rejects due to high levels of mycotoxins in food and agricultural produce coming from developed countries, including Nigeria. Over the years, Nigeria has received notifications from the European Union Rapid Alert System on export rejects originating from Nigeria.

5. Possible intervention strategies/regulations for mycotoxins in Nigeria

Nigeria is a country of marked ecological diversity and climatic contrasts with biophysical characteristics, agro-ecological zones and socio-economic conditions. (Aregheore 2005). Crop production in the country is dominated by cereal, root and tuber crops (Amujoyegbe 2012) The climatic conditions and agricultural practices therefore affect mycotoxin prevalence greatly in the different parts of Nigeria. Current research in the country shows that the prevalence of mycotoxins is all over Nigeria because they have been identified from various commodities from the various agro ecological zones. The complete elimination of mycotoxin contaminated commodities is not achievable hence good agricultural practices (GAP) represent a primary line of defense against contamination of cereals with mycotoxins, followed by the implementation of good manufacturing practices (GMP) during the handling, storage, processing, and distribution of cereals for human food and animal feed. (Codex alimentarius commissin, 2003). The achievement of mycotoxin reduction and control is dependent on the concerted actions of all actors along the food production and distribution chain. Multidisciplinary approaches are therefore critical (FOS, 2006). Any possible intervention strategies to reduce mycotoxins in Nigeria as elsewhere must begin from good Agricultural practices that involves both pre-harvest and post harvest stages followed by Good manufacturing practices (GMP), Risk Assessment for Mycotoxin Contamination and Good Storage Practices will then follow.

5.1. Good agricultural practices

Good Agricultural Practices is a collection of principles to apply for on-farm production and post-production processes that will result in safe and healthy food and non-food agricultural products. Activities to ensure good agricultural practices must be given a holistic approach to tackle the menace of mycotoxins. Efforts to mitigate mycotoxins contamination will be successful if all good agricultural principles are put in place by farmers in Nigeria.

5.2. Soil

Under good agricultural principles the type of land, soil conditions, soil management must not have any negative effect on the biodiversity. GAP also lead to soil productivity, availability, uptake of water and nutrients through enhanced soil biological activity. The soil organic matter replenished, losses of soil moisture, nutrients, and agrochemicals through erosion are reduced, and runoff and leaching into surrounding environment , sediments, nutrients movement, and mobility of livestock and associated species including predators, pests and biocontrol agents are brought under control.

5.3. Pre-harvest interventions

Crop management at the pre harvest stage is critical to mycotoxin reduction. Planting, pre harvest and postharvest strategies for a particular crop depends on the climatic conditions of that particular year, taking into account the local crops, and traditional production conditions for that particular country or region (CAC RCP 51 2003). Wet weather either during flowering or at harvest is also a major risk factor (Negedu, et al, 2011). In general, pre harvest management must ensure that insect damage and fungal infection in the vicinity of the crop must be minimized by proper use of registered insecticides, fungicides, herbicides and making sure that mechanical injury to plants during cultivation is minimized. Seed varieties that are resistant to insect pest and diseases should be procured. Irrigation is a valuable method of reducing plant stress that is sometimes responsible for mycotoxin development crops in some growing situations. Crop rotation should be developed and maintained but crops identified to be susceptible to toxigenic moulds should not be used in rotation with each other. Grains should be harvested at full maturity, cleaned and infected seeds removed using procedures such as gravity table. They should be promptly dried to low moisture levels (13%) before storage where applicable. Moisture levels of the crop should be determined at several spots during harvest, immediately after harvest, before and during storage in barns or silos. Sampling for such test should be as representative of the lot as possible.

5.4. Storage

Storage is a critical stage where infection and mycotoxin accumulation occur. Care must be taken to store grains that are wholesome and apparently healthy. Prestorage treatment or handling should take care of certain basic issues. Winnowing grains at harvest or later should be done to remove shriveled small grains which may contain more zearalenone than healthy normal grains. Harvesting and storage conditions should be documented with daily temperature and humidity checks. Wet grains provide suitable environment for mould growth and should not be piled up for a long time to reduce the risk of fugal growth. Bagged commodities should be stored on pallets. Storage facilities meant to exclude mold growth should include dry and well-ventilated structures, provide protection from rain, drainage of ground water; prevent entry of rodents and birds, and minimum temperature fluctuations. A temperature rise of 2-3°C may indicate microbial growth and/or insect infestation. Where this happens, the apparently infected portions of the grain should be separated and sent for analysis. Mycotoxin levels in grain should be monitored using appropriate sampling and testing programs.

5.5. Transportation

Transport containers should be dry and free of visible fungal growth, insects and any contaminated material they should be cleaned and disinfected with registered fumigants before use and re-use. Shipment should be covered using airtight containers or tarpaulins, temperature fluctuations that could lead to condensation should be avoided, this could lead to fungal growth and mycotoxin formation.

5.6. Biological control measures

The potential for using microorganisms to detoxify mycotoxins has been reported by Murphy, et.al. (2006) to be promising. One of the management strategies that had been developed is biological control using the competitive exclusion mechanism, which has been successfully implemented In the US, biological control has been used to reduce aflatoxin contamination in various crops such as cotton, maize and groundnut. The Internattional institute for agricultural research IITA,has pioneered this technique in Nigeria, by the development of its product called Aflasafe. Aflasafe has proven successful and is being tried on a number of crops. (Bandyopadhyay and Cardwell, 2003).

5.7. Physical methods of mycotoxin removal

Once a contaminated product has reached a processing facility, clean-up and segregation are the first control options. In some cases, these are the best methods of reducing mycotoxin presence in final products. For example, when peanuts are processed, a significant amount of aflatoxins can be removed by electronic sorting and hand-picking ; separation of mould-damaged maize and/or screening can significantly reduce fumonisin and aflatoxin concentrations. In addition, the removal of rot from apples significantly reduces the patulin content in the final product. Although some contamination may persist, physical removal represents a good alternative for industry (Lopez-Garcia 1999). It is however important for grain handlers to use masks to avoid inhalation and ingestion of spores (as mould spores and mycotoxins are often concentrated in the fines and dust of grains). In general good agricultural practice entails a holistic approach and involves risk assessments throughout the process. These risk assessments can be performed at three points during the season: at the start of the season to assess the agronomic risk, at ear emergence to assess the need for spraying with insecticide and at harvest to assess the overall risk (Mohammed , 2006).

5.8. Hazard Analysis Critical Control Point (HACCP)

HACCP is a food management system designed to prevent safety problems, including food poisoning. It was adopted by the food industry because of its success. The HACCP approach involves conducting a detailed analysis of every step in a food processing operation by following seven clearly defined principles known as the HACCP plan (Adred et al. 2004). HACCP plan is an important aspect of an overall management approach in the control of mycotoxins, and these should include strategies for prevention, control, and quality from farm-to-fork. In the food industry, postharvest control of mycotoxins has been addressed via HACCP plans, which include the use of approved supplier schemes. Implementation at pre harvest stages of the food system through good agricultural practice (GAP) and post harvest stage through good manufacturing practice (GMP) is complementary to HACCP. Following an HACCP plan in mycotoxin control provides a critical front line defense to prevent introduction of contaminants into the food and feed supplies. Preharvest HACCP programs have been documented for controlling aflatoxin in corn and coconuts in Southeast Asia, peanuts and peanut products in Africa, nuts in West Africa, and patulin in apple juice and pistachio nuts in South America (FAO/IAEA2001). A number of HACCP schemes for wheat-based commodities were outlined by Aldred et al. (2004) from preharvest to atmospheric control in storage and Lopez-Garcia et al. (1999) provided guidance for development of an integrated mycotoxin management program.

5.9. Mycotoxin regulations

The framework legislation of a country is to ensure that any food containing a contaminant in an amount that is unacceptable from a public health point of view, particularly, at a toxicological level, cannot be marketed in that country. Contaminant levels are required to be kept as low as can reasonably be achieved by good practice. In most countries, regulations are established to control the contaminants in foodstuffs to protect human health; these regulations may include specific maximum limits for several contaminants for different foods and a reference to the sampling methods and performance criteria of analysis to be used (Mariko Kubo 2012). In 2003 the FAO carried out a worldwide international inquiry of mycotoxin regulations, which indicated that 100 countries had developed specific limits for mycotoxins in foodstuffs and feedstuffs. 99 countries had mycotoxin regulations for food and/or feed, an increase of approximately 30 percent compared to 1995. In 1995, 23 percent of the world's inhabitants were living in a region where no known mycotoxin regulations were in force. Countries with mycotoxin regulations in 2003 have at least regulatory limits for aflatoxin B1 or total aflatoxins (B1, B2, G1 and G2) in foods and/or feeds, specific regulations exist as well for aflatoxin M1; the trichothecenes, deoxynivalenol, diacetoxyscirpenol, T-2 toxin and HT-2 toxins; the fumonisins B1, B2, and B3; agaric acid; the ergot alkaloids; ochratoxin A; patulin; the phomopsins; sterigmatocystin and ochratoxins. The number of countries regulating mycotoxins has significantly increased over the years and more mycotoxins were now being regulated in more products

The inquiry also indicated that, there were 15 nations with known regulation in Africa (i.e. 59% of the inhabitants of Africa). For most African countries, specific mycotoxin regulations probably do not exist. However this does not mean that the problem of mycotoxin is ignored. Several of these countries recognize that they have problems due to

mycotoxins and that regulations should be developed. Aflatoxin has the highest mycotoxin regulations in Africa and Morocco had the most detailed mycotoxin regulations. Nigeria has adopted the European commission mycotoxin regulations which it uses primarily for export commodities, although these are applied in-country whenever there is a need to take a critical look especially on industrially processed food commodities. Consultations are currently on-going among regulatory agencies and other mycotoxin stakeholders in the country on the desirability or otherwise of retaining this status quo or creating a separate standard or set of standards.

6. Challenges of mycotoxin research in Nigeria

Although mycotoxin research started early in Nigeria in relation to the notoriety and worldwide realisation of the significance of aflatoxins, the world's leading mycotoxin, there remain a number of challenges that hinder mycotoxin research in Nigeria. These challenges include limited availability of equipment and kits, economic issues, adequate skills and experience, inadequate government support and inter-agency communications and inadequate funds directed at mycotoxin research among others.

Aflatoxin research in Nigeria began in 1961 after a team from the Tropical Products Research Institute in the United Kingdom visited Nigeria to alert the nation and those concerned with the export and production of groundnuts to the threat posed by aflatoxins. The government of the then Northern Nigeria set up a committee of government Departments and two Nigerian Research Institutes, the Institute of Agricultural Research

(IAR) Samaru Zaria, and the Nigerian Stored Products Research (NSPRI) Ibadan (Blount 1961; Manzo and Misari 1989). Research at NSPRI relied mainly on thin layer chromatography (TLC), which which has been the classical method for mycotoxin analysis in Nigeria for several years and up till today (Arawora, 2010). Early work at IAR from 1961 – 1966 by MacDonald and colleagues relied on methods used in the laboratories of Tropical Products Research Institute London (McDonald Harness and Stone bridge 1965, Harkness et al, 1967). The Department of Crop Protection, IAR, established a mycotoxin research laboratory, in 1980 which has not been functional until recently when a team of researchers within the Department revived mycotoxin work there.

While TLC is a relatively easy technique for analysis, the challenge since the 1980's was the lack of mycotoxin standards which were expensive and not produced in the country. Most University researchers could not afford to carry out studies because standards had to be imported, and the universities barely had enough money to support expensive researches, due to the economic downturn caused by the introduction of the Structural Adjustment Programme (SAP) in 1986. Foreign companies were also sceptical of selling the standards because of the fear of its use for biological warfare. SAP thus resulted into poor funding of National Research Institutes and universities although a few scientists continued to carry out research on mycotoxins. The international institute for tropical agriculture (IITA) remained one of the institutions that continued to carry out mycotoxin research and held workshops to sensitize scientists (Bankole and Adebanjo 2003)

Currently, there is an upsurge of interests in mycotoxin research in Nigeria. New methods of analysis are already in use. These include High performance liquid chromatography (HPLC), Enzyme linked imunosorbent assay (ELIZA)) and more recently liquid chromatography with tandem mass spectroscopy (LC-MS/MS) which provides better quantification, larger and faster sample analysis and multitoxin analysis respectively (Wilson, 1989, Krska *et al*, 2008). Although some organisations and individuals can now afford to buy mycotoxin kits, the new challenge however is that they require the use of high-tech equipment. Most universities and research institutes in Nigeria do not use HPLC. There is no facility for LC-MS/MS analysis in the country at the moment, yet scientists have to ensure their researches are up to date. Researchers have to spend a large chunk of their money for analysis from the few organizations that have equipments, pay representatives of manufacturers of kits at a high cost or send their samples overseas for analysis.

Cooperation between organisations that have to do with mycotoxin research is also below expection. The universities and research institutes on one hand and Government organisations that regulate or formulate policies on mycotoxins need to have a more effective and formal relationship. The Mycotoxicology Society of Nigeria has been trying to fill this lacuna in the past seven years of its existence. The mandates of some of the government agencies such as the National Agency for Food and Drug Administration and Control (NAFDAC) and the standards Organisation of Nigeria (SON) do not allow them to do research. Some other agencies concerned with mycotoxin work are not in contact with the national research network. These agencies need to facilitate research for which they are beneficiary agencies. In Nigeria there is currently no Government agency or Department that specifically provides funds for or promotes mycotoxin research.

Skills for mycotoxin research are currently inadequate. The Mycotoxicological Society of Nigeria is currently the only organization that provides the cheapest training in Mycotoxin analysis through its annual conferences and workshops in collaboration with Mycotoxin kits manufacturers from around the world. The National agency for food and drug control (NAFDAC) and the International institute for tropical Agriculture (IITA) are the other organisations that provide training under certain arrangements. Foreign training such as (MYCORED) has so far come only through the provision of limited opportunities.

For Mycotoxin research to thrive, more capacity building through training, concerted effort of stakeholder organisations and Government to deliberately articulate and work out a mycotoxin research program in view of the importance of mycotoxins to human life and economy, is inevitable. This will immediately remove the constraints of funds and equipment which individual organisations and researchers are confronted with.

7. Conclusion

In many developing countries, the combination of insufficient drying and humid atmospheric conditions encourage mould growth and proliferation which results in unacceptable levels of mycotoxins especially aflatoxins in harvested maize, groundnuts, tree nuts and other agricultural produce.

Several studies in Nigeria have reported toxin levels far above the limits allowed by International regulatory agencies in food and agricultural products. In addition, fatal outbreaks of toxicities resulting particularly from aflatoxins have been widely reported in Nigeria. There is an urgent need to address the food safety and International trade issues associated with mycotoxin contamination in Nigerian consumer goods and agricultural products because there is a huge problem of mycotoxin contamination in developing countries like Nigeria where there exist a dearth of organized scientific information and data on the magnitude of the problem.

Furthermore, no single Governmental or private organization has the resources in personnel, expertise, money or time to mitigate against mycotoxin contamination. Therefore collaboration in projects involving multidisciplinary teams is needed for effective research, documentation, monitoring, evalution and control of mycotoxins in Nigeria.

Some of the suggested solutions to mycotoxin menace in Nigeria include:

1. Collection of a database of predominant fungi and mycotoxins in Nigeria
2. Construction of a Mycotoxin Occurrence Map to know the areas prone to Mycotoxin contamination
3. Establishment of a permanent culture collection centre
4. Good Agricultural practises (early planting and use of recommended crop production practices, irrigation to reduce drought stress, early harvesting, prevention of kernel

damage during harvesting), Storage (adequate drying and proper storage below 13 % moisture, and keeping storage facilities clean and dry) and Good Manufacturing Practices

Author details

Olusegun Atanda *

Mycotoxicology Society of Nigeria . Department of Biological Sciences. McPherson University, Km 96, Lagos- Ibadan Expressway, Seriki-Sotayo, Abeokuta, Ogun State, Nigeria

Hussaini Anthony Makun

Mycotoxicology Society of Nigeria, Department of Biochemistry, Federal University of Technology Minna, Niger State, Nigeria

Isaac M. Ogara

Mycotoxicology society of Nigeria. Department of Agronomy, Faculty of Agriculture, Nasarawa state university, Lafia campus, Lafia, Nigeria

Mojisola Edema

Mycotoxicology society of Nigeria. Department of Food Science & Technology. Federal University of Technology, Akure, Nigeria

Kingsley O. Idahor

Mycotoxicology society of Nigeria. Department of Animal Science, Nasarawa State University, Keffi, Shabu-Lafia Campus, Lafia, Nigeria

Margaret E. Eshiett

Mycotoxicology society of Nigeria. Standards Organisation of Nigeria. Lagos, Nigeria

Bosede F. Oluwabamiwo

Mycotoxicology Society of Nigeria. National Agency for Food and Drug Administration and Control, Central Laboratory, Oshodi, Lagos, Nigeria

8. References

Abbas H. K., Cartwright R. D., Shier W. T., Abouzied M. M., Bird, C. B., Rice, L. G., Ross, P. F., Sciumbato, G .L. and Meredith, F.I. (1998). Natural Occurrence of fumonisins in rice with *Fusarium* sheat rot disease. Plant Disease, 82:22-25.

Abbas H. K., Gelderblom, W. C. A., Cawood, M.E. and Shier W.T. 1993. Biological activities of fumonisins, mycotoxins from *Fusarium moniliforme* in Jimsonweed *(Datura stramonium* L.) and mammalian cell cultures. Toxicon, 31:345-353.

Abbas H. K., Shier W. T. (2010). Mycotoxin contamination of agricultural products in the Southern United States and approaches to reducing it from pre-harvest to final food products.In: Appell M, Kendra D, Trucksess MW, eds. Mycotoxin Prevention and

* Corresponding Author

Control in Agriculture. American Chemical Society Symposium Series. Oxford: Oxford University Press.

Abbas H. K., Shier, W. T., Cartwright, R. D. (2007). Effect of temperature, rainfall and planting date on aflatoxin and fumonisin contamination in commercial Bt and non-Bt corn hybrids inArkansas. Phytoprotection, 88:41–50.

Abalaka J. A. and Elegbede, J. A (1982). Aflatoxin distribution and total microbial count in an edible oil extracting plant 1: preliminary observations. Ed. Chem. Toxic 2:43-46

Abbas H. K., Williams W. P., Windham G. L., Pringle III H. C., Xie. W, Shier, W. T. (2002). Aflatoxin and fumonisin contamination of commercial corn (*Zea mays*) hybrids in Mississippi. Journal of Agriculture, Food and Chemistry, 50:5246–5254.

Adebajo L.O, Idowu A. A, Adesanya O. O. (1994). Mycoflora, and mycotoxins production in Nigerian corn and corn- based snacks. Mycopathologia; 126(3):183-92.

Adebajo, L. O. and Popoola, O. J. (2003) Mycoflora and mycotoxins in kolanuts during storage. African Journal of Biotechnology 2 (10):365-368

Adegoke G. O., Allamu A. E., Akingbala J. O. and Akanni A. O. (1996). Influence of sundrying on the chemical composition, aflatoxin content and fungal counts of two pepper varieties--*Capsicum annum and Capsicum frutescens*. Plant Foods in Human Nutrition. 49(2):113-7

Adejumo, O., Atanda, O. O, Raiola, A., Bandyopadhyay, R., Somorin, Y., Ritieni, A. (2012). Correlation between Aflatoxin M_1 Content of Breast Milk, Dietary Exposure to Aflatoxin B_1 and Socioeconomic Status of Lactating Mothers in Ogun State, Nigeria. Submitted to Food and Chemical Toxicology

Akande, K. E., Abubakar M. M., Adegbola T. A., Bogoro S. E. (2006) Nutritional and health implications of mycotoxins in animal feeds: a review. Pakistan Journal of Nutrition 5 (5): 398-403.

Akano, D. A. and Atanda, O. O. (1990). The present Level of Aflatoxin in Nigeria Groundnut Cake ("Kulikuli"). Letters in Applied Microbiology. 10: 187 – 18

Alberts J. F., Engelbrecht, Y., Steyn P. S., Holzapfel W. H., van Zyl W. H. (2006) . Biological degradation of aflatoxin B_1 by *Rhodococcus erythropolis* cultures. International Journal of Food Microbiology 109, (1–2): 121–126.

Aldred D., N. Magan, and M. Olsen (2004) The use of HACCP in the control of mycotoxins: the case of cereals. In Magan N. and Olsen M(Ed.) Mycotoxins in food: Detection and Control. Woodhead Publishing in Food Science and Technology. pp 139-173.

Amujoyegbe B. M. (2012). Farming systems analysis of two agro-ecological zones of SouthWestern Nigeria. Resjournals .com/ARJ pp1-12

AFRO Food Safety Newsletter Issue No 2. July 2006 World Health Organization Food Safety (FOS)African Society of Toxicological Sciences (ASTS) March 1920, 2009, Baltimore, AST S Satellite Meeting

Aregheore, E. M. (2005) Nigeria Country profile. www.fao.org/ag/AGP/AGPC/doc/Couprofile

Arowora, K. A. and J. N. Ikeorah (2010) Five decades of Aflatoxin research in NSPRI. Fifth annual conference of the Nigeria Mycotoxin awareness research and study network, Nigeria stored products research Institute, Ilorin. 26-28th September 2010.

Aroyeun, S. O. and Adegoke, G. O. (2007) Reduction of Ochratoxin A (OTA) in spiked cocoa powder and beverage using aqueous extracts and essential oils of *Aframomum danielli*. African Journal of Biotechnology. 6(5) :612-616.

Atanda, O. O., Oguntubo, A., Adejumo, A., Ikeorah, H. and Akpan, I. (2007). Aflatoxin M_1 contamination of Milk and Ice-cream in Abeokuta and Odeda Local Governments of Ogun State, Nigeria. Chemosphere. 68: 1455-1458.

Atehnkeng, J., Ojiambo, P.S., Ikotun, T., Sikora, R.A., Cotty, P.J., Bandyopadhyay, R., 2008. Evaluation of atoxigenic isolates of *Aspergillus flavus* as potential biocontrol agents for aflatoxin in maize. Food Additives and contaminants: Part A 25, 1264-1271.

Avantaggio, G., Quaran, F., Desidero, E. and Visconti, A. (2002). Fumonisin contamination of maize hybrid visibly damaged by Sesame. J. Sci. Food Agric. 83:13-18.

Ayodele B. C. and Edema M. O. (2010). Evaluation of the critical control points in the production of dried yam chips for *elubo*. Nigerian Food Journal.

Bacon C. W., Porter J. K. and Norred, W. P. (1995). Toxic interaction of fumonisin B, and fusaric acid measured by injection into fertile chicken egg. Mycopathologia, 129:29-35.

Bankole S. A. and Adebanjo, A. (2003) Mycotoxins in food in West Africa: current situation and possibilities of controlling it. African Journal of Biotechnology. 2(9): 254-263.

Bankole S. A. and Mabekoje, O. O. (2004). Occurrence of aflatoxins and fumonisins in preharvest maize from South-Western Nigeria. Food Addict Contam. (3):251-5.

Bankole S. A, Ogunsanwo, B. M. and Mabekoje O .O. (2004). Natural occurrence of moulds and aflatoxin B_1 in melon seeds from markets in Nigeria. Food and Chemical Toxicology, 42(8):1309-14.

Bankole S. A.,Ogunsanwo, B. M., Eseigbe, D.A., (2005). Aflatoxins in Nigerian dry-roasted groundnuts. Food Chemistry. 89 (4), 503–506

Bassir, O. and Adekunle, A. (1969). Comparative toxicities of Aflatoxin B1 and palmotoxins Bo and Go West African Journal of Biological and Applied Chemistry, 12(1):7-19.

Bassir, O. (1969). Toxic substance in foodstuffs. West African Journal of Biological and Applied Chemistry, 12:4-7

Becker B., Bresch H., Schillinger U. and Thiel P.G. 1997. The effect of fumonisin B_1 on the growth of bacteria. World Journal of Microbiology and Biotechnology, 13:539-543.

Bennett, J.W., Klich, M., (2003). Mycotoxins. Clinical Microbiology Reviews, 16, 497–516.

Bhat, R.V. and S. Vasanthi, (2003). Food Safety in Food Security and Food Trade. Mycotoxin Food Safety Risk in Developing Countries. International Food Policy Research Institute.

Bhat, R., Rai, R. V., & Karim, A. A. (2010). Mycotoxins in Food and Feed: Present Status and Future Concerns. Comprehensive Reviews in Food Science and Food Safety, 9: 57-81

Blount, W. P. (1961). Turkey 'X' Disease. J. Brit. Turkey federation. 9: 52-61.

Bothast R. J., Bennett, G. A., Vancauwenberge, J .E. and Richard J. L. (1992). Fate of fumonisin B in naturally contaminated corn during ethanol fermentation. Applied Environmental Microbiology, 58:233-236.

Boutrif E. (1995). FAO programmes for prevention, regulation, and control of mycotoxins in food. Natural Toxins 3 (4), 322–326.

Brown, D. W., McCoy C. P. and Rottinghaus G. E. 1994. Experimental feeding of *Fusarium moniliforme* culture material containing furnonisin B, to channel catfish (*Ictalurus punctatus).* Journal of Veterinary Diagnostic Investigation, 6:123-124

Bullerman, L. B. (2007). Mycotoxins from Field to Table. International journal of food Microbiology. 119 (1-2) 131-139

Center for Disease Control and Prevention. (2004). Outbreak of aflatoxin poisoning—eastern and central provinces, Kenya, January–July 2004. 53(34):790–793.

Codex Alimentarius Commission (2003). "Proposed Draft Code of Practice for the Prevention (Reduction) of Mycotoxin Contamination in Cereals, Including Annexes on Ochratoxin A, Zearalenone, Fumonisins and Tricothecenes." Codex Committee on Food Additives and Contaminants, Thirty-fourth Session. Codex Alimentarius Commission /RCP 51-2003

Cole R. J., Doner JW, Holbrook CC. (1995). Advances in mycotoxin elimination and resistance. In: Pattee HE, Stalker H.T, (eds). *Advances in Peanut Science*. Stillwater, OK: American Peanut Research and Education Society, pp. 456–474.

Dada. J. D. (1978). Studies of fungi causing grain mould of sorghum varieties in northern Nigeria with special emphasis on species capable of producing mycotoxins. M.Sc. thesis, Ahmadu Bello University, Zaria.

Darling, S. J. (1963).Research on aflatoxin in groundnuts in Nigeria. 13. Institute of Agric. Research, Ahmadu Bello University, Samaru, Zaria.

Diener, U. L., Cole, R. J., Sanders, T. H., Payne, G. A., Lee, L. S., Klich, M. A., (1987). Epidemiology of Aflatoxin, in formation by *Aspergillus flavus*. Annual Review of Phytopathology 25, 240-270.

D'Mello, J. P. F., MacDonald, A. M. C., 1997. Mycotoxins. Animal Feed Science and Technology, 69, 155–166.

Doehlert, D. C., Knutson C.A. and Vesonder R. F. (1994). Phytotoxic effects of fumonisin B, on maize seedling growth.Mycopathologia, 127:117-121.

Dohlman E. (2003). Mycotoxin Hazards and Regulations: Impacts on Food and Animal Feed Crop Trade. In International Trade and Food Safety: Economic Theory and Case Studies. pp 96.

Edema M. O. and Adebanjo, F. (2000) Distribution of Myco-flora of some sun-dried vegetables in South-western Nigeria. Nigerian Journal of Microbiology 14 (2): 119-122.

Elegbede, J. A. (1978). Fungal and Mycotoxin contamination of Sorghum during storage. M.Sc. thesis. Department of Biochemistry, Ahmadu Bello University, Zaria.

Ewuola E. O., Ogunlade J.T., Gbore F. A., Salako A. O., Idahor K. O. and Egbunike G. N. (2003). Performance Evaluation and Organ Histology of Rabbits fed *Fusarium verticillioides* culture Material. Trop. Anim. Prod. Invest., 6:111-119.

Ezekiel, C. N., Sulyok, M., Warth, B and Krska, R (2012a). Multi-microbial metabolites in fonio millet (acha) and sesame seeds in Plateau State, Nigeria. European Food Research Technology, 235: 285-2

Ezekiel, C. N., Bandyopadhyay, R., Sulyok, M., Warth, B and Krska, R (2012b). Fungal and bacterial metabolites in commercial poultry feed from Nigeria. Food Additives and Contaminants: Part A. 29 (8): 1288-1299

Ezekiel, C. N., M. Sulyok, D. A. Babalola, B. Warth, V. C. Ezekiel, Krska, R. (2012c). Incidence and consumer awareness of toxigenic *Aspergillus* section *Flavi* and aflatoxin B1 in peanut cake from Nigeria. Accepted manuscript Food Control.

Ezekiel C. N., M. sulyok, B. warth, A. C. odebode and R. krska (2012). Natural occurrence of Mycotoxins in peanut cake from nigeria. Food control. 27:338-342.

Fandohan, P., Gnonlonfin, B., Hell, K., Marasas, W.F.O., Wingfield, M.J.,(2005). Natural occurrence of Fusarium and subsequent fumonisin contamination in preharvest and stored maize in Benin, West Africa. International Journal of Food Microbiology, 99, 173–183.

Gbodi T.A. Nwude, N, Aliu, Y.O, and Ikediobi, C.O. (1984). Mycotoxins and Mycotoxicoses, the Nigerian situation to Date. National Conference on Disease of Ruminant. 3rd and 6th October, 1984. National Veterinary Research Institute, Vom. pp. 108-115.

Gbodi, T.A. (1986). Studies of mycoflora and mycotoxins in Acha, maize and cotton seed in plateau state,Nigeria. Ph. D. thesis. Department of Physiology and Pharmacology, Faculty of Veterinary Medicine, A.B.U, Zaria, pp 213 .

Goel S., Lenz S. D., Lumlertdacha, S., Lovell R. T., Shelby R. A., Li, M., Riley, R. T. and Kemppainen B., W. (1994). Sphingolipid levels in catfish consuming *Fusaruim moniliforme* corn culture material containing fumonisins. Aquatic Toxicology, 30:285-294.

Gross S. M., Reddy, R. V., Rottinghaus, G.E., Johnson G.and Reddy C.S. (1994). Developmental effects of fumonisin B_1 - containing *Fusarium moniliforme* culture extract in CDI mice. Mycopatholgia, 128:11-118.

Gong Y. Y., K Cardwell, A. Hounsa, S. Egal, P. C. Turner, A. J. Hall, C. P., Wild (2002). Dietary aflatoxin exposure and impaired growth in young children from Benin and Togo: cross sectional study. British Medical Journal. 325:20.

Halliday, D. (1965) the aflatoxin content of Nigeriangroundnuts and cake. Nigerian Stored Products Research Institute, Technical Report, Lagos.

Halliday, D. (1966). Further studies of the aflatoxin content of Nigerian groundnuts and groundnut products. Nigerian Stored Products Research Institute, Technical Report, Lagos.

Halliday, D. & Kazaure, I. (1967). The aflatoxin content of Nigerian Groundnut cake. Nigerian Stored Products Research Institute Technical report No. 8.

Harkness C., D. McDonald, W.C. Stonebridge, J. A'Brook and H. S. Darling (1966) The problem of Aflatoxin in Groundnuts (Peanuts) and other food crops of tropical Africa. Food technology. 20(9): 152-163.

Hussein, H.S., Brasel, J.M.,(2001). Toxicity, metabolism, and impact of mycotoxins on humans and animals. Toxicology 167, 101–134.

IARC. (1993). Toxins derived from *Fusarium moniliforme:* Fumonisms B_1 and B_2 and fusarin C. In: Some naturally occurring substances: Food items and constituents, heterocyclic aromatic amines and mycotoxins. 56:445-466.

Idahor K. O., Adgidzi, E .A. and Usman, E. A. (2010). Awareness of the association of mycotoxins with food and feedstuffs in Nasarawa State. 5th Ann. Conf. Nigeria Mycotoxin Awareness and Study Network, Ilorin. Kwara State. 25pp.

Idahor K. O. (2010). Effects of Fumonisin B_1 on Living Organisms. Production Agriculture and Technology Journal, 6 (1):49-65.

Idahor K. O., Gbore F. A., Salako A. O., Weuola E. O, Ogunlade J. T. and Egbunike G. N. (2008a). Physiologic response of rabbits to fumonisin B_1 dosed orally with maize-based diets. Production Agriculture and Technology Journal, 4(1):91-98.

Idahor K. O., Ewuola E. O., Gbore F. A., Ogunlade J. T., Salako O. A. and Egbunike G. N. (2008b). Reproductive performance of rabbits fed maize-based diets containing FB_1 strain of *Fusarium verticillioides* (Sacc.). Production Agriculture and Technology Journal, 4 (2): 85-92.

Ifeji, E. (2012). Fungi and some mycotoxins found in groundnuts (*Arachis hypogea*)from Niger State, Nigeria. M. Tech Dissertation. Department of Biochemistry. Federal University of Technology, Minna, Nigeria.

Ikwuegbu, O. A. (1984). Two decades of Aflatoxin Research in Vom. National Conference on Diseases of Ruminants 3rd- 6th of October, 1984. National Veterinary Research Institute, Vom. pp100-106.

Jantratail, W., Lovell, R. T. (1990). Subchronic toxicity of dietary aflatoxin B_1 to channel catfish. Journal of Aquatic Animal Health, 2: 248-254.

JECFA (2001). WHO Food additives series 47: Safety Evaluation of certain mycotoxins in foods. Joint FAO/WHO expert committee on food additives. 701pp.

Kaaya, A. N., Kyamuhangire, W., Kyamanywa, S. (2006). Factors affecting aflatoxin contamination of harvested maize in the three agro-ecological zones of Uganda. Journal of Applied Sciences 6, 2401–2407.

Kaneshiro T., Resonder R. F. and Peterson R. E. (1992). Fumonisin-stimulated N-acetyldihydro-sphingosine, N- acelyl- phytosphingosine and phytosphingosine products of *Pichia ciferri* (Hansenula), NRRL Y-1031. Current Microbiology, 24:319-324.

Krska, R., P. Schubert-Ullrich, M. Sulyok, S. MacDonald and C. Crews (2008) Mycotoxin analysis: an update. Food additives and contaminants. 25(2): 152-163.

Kubo, M. (2012) Mycotoxins Legislation Worldwide. European Mycotoxin Nettwork/ Leatherhead Food Research.www.Mycotoxin.com

Kumar V., M. S. Basu, T. P., Rajendran (2008). Mycotoxin research and mycoflora in some commercially important agricultural commodities. Crop Protection. 27 (6), 891–905.

Lacey, T. (1986). Factors affecting mycotoxin production. In: Mycotoxins and phycotoxins edited by Steyn, P.S. and Vlegaar, R. 6th international IUPAC symposium on mycotoxins and phycotoxins, Pretoria, South Africa.

Lamprecht S. C., Marasas W. F. O., Alberts J. F., Cawood M. E., Gelderbcom W. C. A., Shephard G. S., Thiet P. G and Calitz F. J. (1994). Phytotoxicity to fumonisins and TA-toxin to corn and tomate. Phytopathology, 84:383-391.

Lanyasunya, T. P., Wamae, L. W., Musa, H. H., Olowofeso, O., Lokwaleput, I. K., (2005). The risk of mycotoxins contamination of dairy feed and milk on smallholder dairy farms in Kenya. Pakistan Journal of Nutrition, 4, 162–169.

Leslie, J. Bandyopadhyay R. and Visconti A., (2008). Mycotoxins: Detection Methods, Management, Public Health and Agricultural Trade CABI. 464pp.

Liu, Y. and Wu, F. (2010). Global Burden of Aflatoxin-induced Hepatocellular Carcinoma: A Risk Assessment. Environmenral Health Perspectives. 118(6): 818-824

Logrieco A., Doko M.B., Moretti A., Frisullo S. and Visconti A. (1998). Occurrence of fumonisin B_1 and B_2 in *Fusarium proliferation* infected asparagus plants. Journal of Agricultural and Food and Chemistry, 46:5201-5204.

Lopez-Garcia, R., Park, D., (1998). Effectiveness of post-harvest procedures in management of mycotoxin hazards. In: Bhatnagar, D., Sinha, S. (Eds.), Mycotoxins in Agriculture and Food Safety. Marcel Dekker, New York, USA, pp. 407–433.

Lopez-Garcia R., Park D. L. and Phillips T. D. (1999). Integrated mycotoxin management systems. Food Nutrition and Agriculture/ANA 23, (4) 38-48

Lowe D. P. and Arendt, E. K. (2004) The Use and Effects of Lactic Acid Bacteria in Malting and Brewing with Their Relationships to Antifungal Activity, Mycotoxins and Gushing: A Review. Journal of Institute of Brewing, 110(3), 163–180.

Lubulwa, A. S. G. and Davis, J. S. (1994). Estimating the social costs of the impacts of fungi and aflatoxins. In Highley, E., Wright, E.J., Banks, H.J. and Champ, B.R. (eds.) Stored Products protection, Proceedings of the 6th International Working Conference in Stored-product Protection, 17-23 April 1994, Canberra, Australia. CAB International, Wallingford, UK.

McDonald, D. C. Harkness and W. C. Stonebridge (1965). Growth of *Aspergillus flavus* and production of Aflatoxin in groundnuts. Part VI. Samaru research bulletin. Institute of Agricultural research, Ahmadu Bello Universtity, zaria.

Mclean, M. and P., Berjak, (1987). Maize grains and their associated mycoflora: A micro-ecological consideration. Seed Science & Technology, 15: 813-850.

Makaula N. A., Marasas W. F.O., Venter F. S., Badenhorst C.J. Bradshaw D. and Swanevelder, S. (1996). Oesophageal and other cancer patterns in four selected districts of Transkei, Southern Africa: 1985-1990. African Journal of Health Science,3:11-15.

Makun, H. A., Timothy, A. Gbodi, O, H., Akanya, A., Ezekiel, Salako, E.A.and Godwin, H. Ogbadu. (2007). Fungi and some mycotoxins contaminating rice *(Oryza sativa)* in Niger State, Nigeria. African Journal of Biotechnology 6 (2): 99 – 108.

Makun, H. A. , Gbodi T. A., Akanya, H. O. , Sakalo, A. E. and Ogbadu, G. H. (2009a). Health implications of toxigenic fungi found in two Nigerian staples: guinea corn and rice. African Journal of Food Science, 3: 250-256.

Makun, H. A., Gbodi, T. A., Akanya, H. O., Salako, E. A. and Ogbadu, G. H. (2009b). Fungi and some mycotoxins found in mouldy Sorghum in Niger State, Nigeria. World Journal of Agricultural Sciences. 5 (1): 05 – 17.

Makun, H. A. , Anjorin S. T., Moronfoye, B., Adejo, F. O., Afolabi, O. A., Fagbayibo, G., Balogun, B.O. and Surajudeen, A. A. (2010). Fungal and aflatoxin contaminations of some human food commodities in Nigeria. African Journal of Food Sciences. 4 (4): 127 – 135.

Makun H. A., M. F. Dutton, P. B. Njobeh, M. Mwanza and Kabiru, A. Y. (2011). Natural multi- mycotoxin occurrence in rice from Niger State, Nigeria. DOI: 10.1007/s12550-010-0080-5. Mycotoxin Research. 27 (2): 97-104

Makun H. A. , Mailafiya, C. S., Saidi, A. A., Onwuike, B. C. and Onwubiko, M. U. (2012). A preliminary survey of aflatoxin in fresh and dried vegetables in Minna, Nigeria. African Journal of Food Science and Technology 3(10) pp. xxx-xxx,

Manorama, S., Singh, R., (1995). Mycotoxins in milk and milk products. J. Dairying, Foods Home Sci. 14, 101–107.

Mantle, P. G. (1968) Studies on Sphacelia sorghi McRae, an ergot of Sorghum vulgare Pers. Annals of applied Biology. 62(3) 443-449

Manzo, S. K. and S. M. Misari (1989) Status and management of Aflatoxin in Groundnuts in Nigeria. In McDonald, D. And V.K. Mehan (eds.). Aflatoxin contamination of Groundnuts: Proceedings of the international workshop, ICRISAT center, India.77-87.

Marasas, W. F. O., Van Rensburg S. J. and Mirocha C. J. (1979). Incidence of *Fusarium* species and the mycotoxins, deoxynivalenol and zearalenone, in corn produced in oesophageal cancer areas in Transkei, Journal of Agricultural and Food Chemistry, 27:1108-1112.

Meister, U. Symmank, H. and Dahlke, H. (1996). Investigation and Evaluation of the contamination of native and imported cereals with fumonisins.) Z Lebensm Unters Forseh, 203: 528-533.

Meredith, F. I., Riley R. T., Bacon C. W., Williams D. E. and Carlson D. B (1998). Extraction, quantification and biological availability of fumonisin B_1 incorporated into Oregon test diet and fed to rainbow trout. Journal of Food Protection, 61:1034-1038.

Mestres, C., Bassa, S., Fagbohun, E., Nago, M., Hell, K., Vernier, P., Champiat, D., Hounhouigan, J., and Cardwell, K.F. (2004). Yam chip food sub-sector: hazardous practices and presence of aflatoxins in Benin. Journal of Stored Products Research. 40, 575-585.

Milicevic, D., Juric, V., Stefanovic, S., Jovanovic, M., Jankovic, S. (2008). Survey of slaughtered pigs for occurrence of ochratoxin A and porcine nephropathy in Serbia. International Journal of Molecular Science, 9, 2169–2183.

Mohammed H. K. (2012). Fungi and some mycotoxins contaminating maize from Niger State, Nigeria. M. Tech Dissertation. Federal University of Technology, Minna. Nigeria.

Munkvold, G. P. (2003). Cultural and genetic approaches to managing mycotoxins in maize. Annual Review of Phytopathology, 41, 99–116.

Murphy P. A., Hendrich S., Landgren C. and Bryant C.M. (2006). Food Mycotoxins: an Update. A scientific status summary. Journal of Food science 7(5) R51-R65 doi:10.1111/j.1750-3841.2006.00052.x

Naresh Magan and David Aldred International Journal of Food Microbiology, Volume 119: 1-2.

Negedu, A., Atawodi, S. E., Ameh, J. B., Umoh, V.J., and Tanko, H.Y. (2011). Economic and health perspectives of mycotoxins: a review. Continental Journal of Biomedical Sciences, 5 (1): 5 - 26

Obasi O. E, Ogbadu G. H. and Ukoha A. I. (1987). Aflatoxins in Burukutu (Millet Beer). TransTrTransactions of Royal Society of Tropical Medicine and Hygiene, 81: 879

Obidoa, O and Gugnani, H. C. (1990). Mycotoxins in Nigerian foods: causes, Consequences and remedial measures. In: Okoye, Z.S.C Mycotoxins contaminating foods and foodstuffs in Nigeria. First National Workshop on Mycotoxins. 29th November, 1990. University of Jos . pp. 95-114.

Ocholi R. A, Chima, J. C. , Chukwu, C. O. , Irokanulo, E. (1992). Mycotoxicosis associated with *Penicillium purpurogenum* in horses in Nigeria. Veterinary Record, 130(22):495.

Ogunlade, J. T., Gbore F. A., Ewuola E. O., Idahor K. O., Salako A. O. and Egbunike G. N. (2004). Biochemical and haematological response of rabbits fed diets containing micro doses of fumonisin. Tropical Journal of Animal Science, 7(1): 169-176.

Okeke, K. S., Abdullahi, I. O., Makun H. A. and Mailafiya, S. C. (2012). A preliminary survey of aflatoxin M1 in dairy cattle products in Bida, Niger State, Nigeria. African Journal of Food Science and Technology. 3(10) pp. xxx-xxx,

Okonkwo, P. O. and Nwokolo, C. (1978). Aflatoxin B_1: sample procedure to reduce levels in tropical foods. Nutrition Reports International, 17(3): 387-395.

Okoye, Z. S. C. and Ekpenyong, K. I. (1984). Aflatoxins B_1 in native millet beer brewed in Jos suburb. Transactions of Royal Society of Tropical Medicine and Hygiene, 78; 417-418.

Okoye, Z. S. C. (1986). Zearalenone in native cereal beer in Jos Metropolis of Journal of Food safety, 7;233-239.

Okoye, Z. S. C. (1992). An overview of Mycotoxins likely to contaminate Nigerian staple food stuff. First National Workshop on Mycotoxins. 29th November, 1990 . University of Jos. pp. 9-27.

Okoye Z. S. C. (1993) Fusarium mycotoxins nivalenol and 4-acetyl-nivalenol (fusarenon-X) in mouldy maize harvested from farms in Jos district, Nigeria. Food Addit ives and Contaminants;10(4):375-9.

Olorunmowaju, B. Y. (2012). Fungi and mycotoxins contaminating rice (Oryza sativa) from Kaduna State. M. Tech Dissertation. Department of Biochemistry. Federal University of Technology, Minna, Nigeria

Oluwafemi F. and Da-Silva F. A. (2009) Removal of aflatoxins by viable and heat-killed *Lactobacillus* species isolated from fermented maize. Journal of Applied Biosciences 16: 871 – 876.

Oluwafemi, F., and Taiwo, V. O. (2003). Reversal of toxigenic effects of aflatoxin B_1 on cockerels by alcoholic extract of African nutmeg *Monodora myristica.* Journal of the Science of Food and Agriculture, 84: 333-340.

Ominski, K. H. (1994). Ecological aspects of growth and toxin production by storage fungi. In: Miller, J.D., Trenholm, H. S. (Eds.). Mycotoxin in grains: Compounds other than aflatoxin. Eagan press, USA. pp. 287-305.

Onilude A. A, Fagade, O. E, Bello, M. M, Fadahunsi, I. F. (2005). Inhibition of aflatoxin-producing aspergilli by lactic acid bacteria isolates from indigenously fermented cereal gruels. African Journal of Biotechnology, 4(12):1404-1408.

Onyemelukwe, G. C. and Ogbadu, G. H and Salifu, A. (1982). Aflatoxin B, G. and G2 in primary liver cell carcinoma. Toxicology Letters, 10:309-312.

Opadokun, J. S. (1992). Occurrence of Aflatoxin in Nigeria food crops. First National Workshop on Mycotoxins. 29th November, 1990. University of Jos. pp. 50-60

Otsuki, T., Wilson, J. S. and Sewadeh, M. (2001*a*). A Case Study of Food Safety Standards and African Exports. World Bank Policy Research working paper N0. 2563, World Bank, Washington, D.C.

Otsuki, T., Wilson, J. S., and Sewadeh, M. (2001*b*) What price precaution? European harmonisation of aflatoxin regulations and African groundnut exports. European Review of Agricultural Economics, 28: 263-283.

Oyelami O. A., S. M. Maxwell, K. A. Adelusola, T. A. Aladekoma and A. O. Oyelese (1995) Aflatoxins in the autopsy brain tissue of children in Nigeria. Mycopathologia, 132 (1), 35-38.

Oyelami O. A., S. M. Maxwell K. A. Adelusola T. A. Aladekoma A. O. Oyelese (1998) Aflatoxins in autopsy kidney specimens from children in Nigeria. Journal of Toxicology and Environmental Health. 55 (5): 317-323.

Oyejide A, Tewe O. O., Okosum S. E. (1987). Prevalence of aflatoxin B1 in commercial poultry rations in Nigeria. Beitr Trop Landwirtsch Veterinarmed.; 25(3):337-41

Payne, G. A. (1992). Aflatoxins in maize. Critical Rev Plant Sci.10:423–440.

Peers, F. G, (1965). Summary of the work done in Vom (Northern Nigeria) on Aflatoxin levels in groundnut flour. Agric nutr. Document R. 3/Add. P.A.G (WHO/FAO/UNICEF) Rome.

Rachaputi, N. R., Wright G. C., Kroschi, S. (2002). Management practices to minimise pre-harvest aflatoxin contamination in Australian groundnuts. Australian Journal of Experimental Agriculture, 42: 595-605.

Bandyopadhyay, R. , S., Kiewnick , J. Atehnkeng , Donier, M. (2005). Biological control of aflatoxin contamination in maize in Africa International Institute of Tropical Agriculture (IITA), Plant Health Management Program, Ibadan, Nigeria.

Rauber, R. H., Dilkin, P., Giacomini, L. Z., Araujo de Almeida, C. A., Mallmann, C. A. (2007). Performance of Turkey Poults fed different doses of aflatoxins in the diet. Poultry Science, 86: 1620–1624.

Ross P.F, Ledet A. E., Owens D. L., Rice L. G., Nelson H. A., Osweiler G. D. and Wilson T. M. (1993). Experimental equine leukoencephalomalacia, toxic hepatosis and encephalopathy caused by corn naturally contaminated with fumonisins. Journal of Veterinary Diagnostic Investment, 5:69-74. 998.

Rustemeyer, S. M., Lamberson, W. R., Ledoux, D. R., Rottinghaus, G. E., Shaw, D. P., Cockrum, R. R., Kessler, K. L., Austin, K. J., & Cammack, K. M. (2010). Effects of dietary aflatoxin on the health and performance of growing barrows. Journal of Animal Science, Vol. 88, Nov, pp. 3624-3630,0021-8812.

Salifu, A., 1978. Mycotoxins in short season varieties of Sorghum in Northern Nigeria. Samaru Journal of Agriculture Research, 1: 83-87.

Shetty, P. H. and Bhat, R. V. (1997). Natural occurrence of fumonisin B_1 and its co-occurrence with aflatoxin B_1 in Indian sorghum, maize and poultry feeds. Journal of Agriculture, Food and Chemistry, 45:2170-2173.

Shier, W. T., Abbas H. K., Abou-Karam, M., Badria, F. A,, Resch, P.A. (2003). Fumonisins: Abiogenic conversions of an environmental tumor promoter and common food contaminant. Journal of Toxicology-Toxin Reviews, 22:591–616.

Shier, W. T., Abbas H.K , Badria, F. A. (1997). Structure-activity relationships of the corn fungal toxin fumonisin B1: implications for food safety. Journal of Natural Toxins, 6:225–242.

Shier, W. T., Tiefel, P.A. , Abbas, H. K. (1999). Current research on mycotoxins: fumonisins. In: Tu AT, Gaffield W, (eds). Natural and Selected Synthetic Toxins: Biological Implications. American Chemical Society Symposium Series. 745. Oxford, UK: Oxford University Press, pp. 54–66.

Smith, J. S. and Thakur, R. A. (1996). Occurrence and fate of fumonisins in beef. Advances in Experimental Medicine and Biology, 392:39-55.

Sun, T. S. C. and Stahr, H. M. (1993). Evaluation and application of a bioluminescent bacterial genotoxicity test. Journal of the Association of Official Analytical Chemists, 76: 893-898.

Sydenham, E. W., Thiel, P.G., Marasas, W. F. O., Shephard G.S., Van Schalkwyk D.J. and Koch K. R. (1990). Natural Occurrence of some Fusarium mycotoxins in corn from low and high oesephageal cancer prevalence area of the Transkei, Southern AfricaJournal of Agricultural and Food Chemistry, 38:1900-1903.

Teniola, O. D., Addo, P. A., Brost, I. M., Farber, P., Jany, K .D., Albert, J. F., zanZyl, W. H., Steyn, P. S., Holzapfel, W. H., (2006). Degradation of aflatoxin B1 by cell-free extracts of *Rhodococcus erythropolis* and *Mycobacterium fluoranthenivorans* sp. nov. DSM 44556T. International Journal of Food Microbiology, 105:111-117.

Tijani, A. S. (2005). Survey of fungi, aflatoxins and zearalenone contamination of maize in Niger State. M.Sc thesis Department of Biochemistry, Federal University of Technology. Minna.

Trenk, H. L. and Hartman P. A. (1970). Effects of Moisture Content and Temperature on Aflatoxin Production in Corn. Applied Microbiology. 19 (5): 781-784.

Torres, M. R., Sanchis V. and Ramos A. J. (1998). Occurrence of fumonisins in Spanish beers analyzed by an enzyme- linked immunosorbent assay method. International Journal of Food Microbiology, 39:39-143.

Upadhaya, S. D., Park, M. A., & Ha, J. K. (2010). Mycotoxins and Their Biotransformation in the Rumen: A Review. Asian-Australasian Journal of Animal Sciences, 23, 1250-126.

Uriah, N. and Ogbadu, L. (1982). Influence of woodsmoke on aflatoxin production by *Aspergillus flavus*. European Journal of Applied Microbiology and Biotechnology, 14:51-53.

USNTP (1999). Toxicology and carcinogenesis studies of fumonisin B_1 in rats and mice. NTP Technical report. pp. 99-3955.

van Burik J. and Magee P.T. (2001). Aspects of fungal pathogenesis in humans. Annal Review of Microbiology, 55: 743-772.

Vesonder R. F., Labeda D. P. and Peterson R. E. (1992). Phytotoxic activity of selected water-soluble metabolites of Fusarium against Duckweed (*Lemma minor* L.). Mycopathlogia, 118: 185-189.

Voss, K. A., Chamberlam, W. J., Bacon, C. W., Herbert, R. A., Walters, D. B. and Norred, W .l. P. (1995). Subchronic feeding study of the mycotoxin fumonisin B_1 in mice and rats. Fundamentals of Apllied Toxicology, 24:102-110.

Wilson, D. M. (1987). Detection and determination of Aflatoxins in Maize. In zuber, M.s., E.B. Lillehojand B. Reinfro (eds.) Aflatoxins in Maize: A proceedings of the international workshop. CIMMYT, Mexico D.F. 100-109

Wilson, T. M., Ross P. F., Owens, D. L., Rile, L. G., Green, S. A., Jenkins, S. J. and Nelson, H. A. (1992). Experimental reproduction of ELEM-A study to determine the minimum toxic dose in ponies. Mycopathologia, 117:115-120.

Wu W-I, McDonough V. M., Nickels J. T., Ko S. J., Fischl A. S., Vales T. R., Merrill A. H. Jr. and Carman G. M.(1995). Regulation of lipid biosynthesis in *Saccharomyces cerevisiae* by fumonisin B_1. Journal of Biological Chemistry, 270: 13171 – 13178.

Yan, L.-Y., Yan, L.-Y., Jiang, J.-H., Ma, Z.-H. (2008) . Biological control of aflatoxin contamination of crops. Journal of Zhejiang University - Science B 9, 787-792.

Zain, M. E. (2011). Impact of mycotoxins on humans and animals. Journal of Saudi Chemical Society. 15, 129–144.

Chapter 2

A Decade of Aflatoxin M_1 Surveillance in Milk and Dairy Products in Developing Countries (2001-2011): A Review

Mwanza Mulunda, Lubanza Ngoma, Mathew Nyirenda,
Lebohang Motsei and Frank Bakunzi

Additional information is available at the end of the chapter

http://dx.doi.org/10.5772/53286

1. Introduction

Aflatoxin M_1 is the 4-hydroxylated metabolite of aflatoxin B_1 that can be found in animal and human breast milk and dairy products [1]. Aflatoxin M_1 presence in milk is considered as a potential risk for human health because of its carcinogenicity potential and thus a need of regular monitoring in milk and dairy products. Unpredicted climatic and environmental variations as well as poor economic and agriculture practices could easily influence the increase of AFM_1 in milk and dairy products. Aflatoxins are particularly known to be mainly produced in food and feed materials by *Aspergillus flavus* and *A. parasiticus* and at low level by *A. tamarii* and *A. nomius* as well as other emerging fungal *spp.* including *A. ochraceoroseus, A. rambellii, Emericella astellata* and *E. venezuelensis* [2, 3]). *Aspergillus flavus* and *A. parasiticus* (AF producers) mainly contaminate cereals (maize) and nuts (peanuts) and their by-products including animal feeds [4-6]. *Aspergillus* contamination is regarded as a storage problem [7] and may also contaminate plant on the field [4], especially during drought stress and low soil moisture content [3]. Aflatoxin M_1 (AFM_1) was initially classified by the International Agency for Research on Cancer (IARC) as a group 2B agent carcinogenic to humans [1] due to lack of data. However, following further investigations that demonstrated in vivo the genotoxicity and cytotoxicity of AFM_1 [8], the toxin has since been classified as a group 1 human carcinogen [9]. The importance of AFM_1 can be evaluated after considering the quantity of milk and milk products consumed daily; moreover they are of primary importance in infants' diet around the world [10].

The aim of this book chapter therefore was to review the incidence of AFM_1 in milk, dairy products as well as in human breast milk and in addition it was to look into advances of techniques applied for extraction and detection of AFM_1 globally and developing countries in particular during the last decade (2001-2011) and to evaluate extraction and detection methods improvement.

2. Chemistry and metabolism of aflatoxin M_1

Aflatoxin M_1 (Figure 1) is the 4-hydroxy derivative of aflatoxin B_1 (Figure 1) which has a relative molecular mass of 328 Da and has the molecular formula $C_{17}H_{12}O_7$ [28].

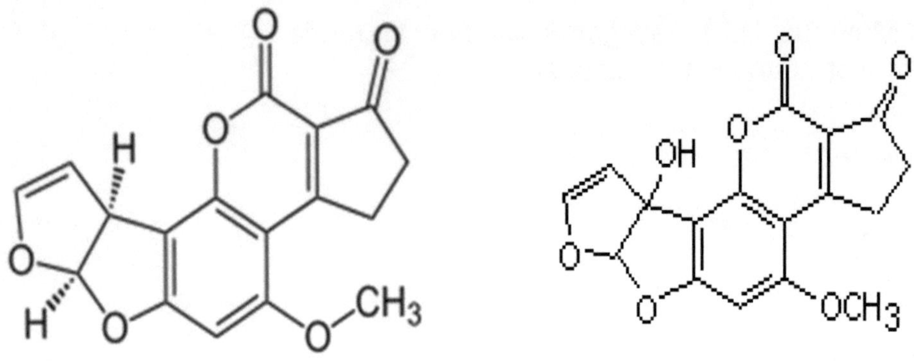

Figure 1. Molecular structures of aflatoxin B1 and M1 (AFM_1)

[28] reviewed extensively on the biochemistry and metabolism of aflatoxins and AFM_1 in particular and it was shown that the metabolism of aflatoxin B_1 was more carcinogenic as compared to AFM_1. It has also been shown that human do not form as much aflatoxin B_1 8, 9-epoxide as rats, but suggested that human do not have glutathione-*S*-transferase (GST) isozymes which have high specific activity towards this epoxide. Significant individual differences in aflatoxin B_1 metabolism and binding suggest the presence of genetic and/or environmental factors that may result in large differences in susceptibility. In a study of the metabolism of aflatoxins M_1 and B_1 in vitro in human liver microsomes, they had a very limited capacity to catalyse epoxidation of aflatoxin M_1 [28]. It is important to mention that the metabolism pathway of AFs is of importance in the determination of toxicity degree [12]. Aflatoxin is metabolized by cytochrome p450 group of enzymes in the liver and converted into different metabolic products like aflatoxicol, aflatoxin Q1, aflatoxin P1, and AFM_1, depending on the genetic predisposition of the species [13]. Along with the above another metabolite called aflatoxin 8, 9 epoxide is also formed. The amount of this metabolite decides the species susceptibility as this can induce mutations by intercalating in to DNA, by forming adduct with guanine moiety in the DNA [14]. The ingested aflatoxin B_1 (AFB_1) through contaminated food and feed by mammals is metabolised to aflatoxin M_1 and excreted mainly into milk and dairy products. Aflatoxin M_1 is also detectable in urine, blood, and internal organs in addition to milk [15]. Aflatoxin B_1 is excreted into milk of lactating dairy cows primarily in the form of aflatoxin M_1 (AFM_1) with residues approximately equal to 1-3% of the dietary concentration [16]. The appearance of AFM1 in

milk have been determined to be within 15 minutes to an hour after consumption and returns to baseline levels within two to three days after removal from the diet [17, 11]. Studies of AFM_1 metabolism have shown that the rate between the amount of AFB_1 ingested by cows and the quantity excreted in milk is usually 0.2 to 4% [11, 18]. Studies have shown that it takes 3-6 days of constant daily ingestion of aflatoxin B_1 before steady-state excretion of AFM_1 in milk can be achieved, whereas AFM_1 becomes undetectable 2-4 days after withdrawal of animals from the contaminated diet [28]. Tolerable limits worldwide including South Africa on AFs vary between 10-20 ppb for AFB_1 and 0.05 ppb for AFM_1 in Europe and South Africa and 0.5 ppb in the United States (US) [19]. Studies done have also demonstrated that concentrations of 20 ppb of AFB_1 in the total mixed ration dry matter of lactating dairy cattle could result in AFM_1 levels in milk below the FDA set up limit of 0.5ppb. European Union and several other countries including South Africa have however, presently set up acceptable level of AFM_1 in milk and milk products at 0.05 ppb [11, 19]. Assumed safe feeding levels may result in milk concentrations above the limited level because absolute concentrations of mycotoxins in the feed are difficult to determine, concentrations may not be uniform throughout a lot of feed and concentrations can change over time [19]. Unfortunately most developing countries and mainly African ones have not yet set tolerable limits on food and feed contamination levels of AFs as well as AFM_1 in milk. This is mostly due to lack of data and information availability in these countries.

3. Stability of aflatoxin M1

Several studies have been done regarding AFs and particularly AFM_1 stability in milk and dairy sub products. Yousef et al [20] extensively reviewed information on the stability of AFM_1. Studies have shown that there was no significant changes of AFM_1 concentration after heat processing (Pasteurisation or boiling) or Ultra-high temperature processing (UHT) technique [21, 11, 22]. The stability measurements on powder milk showed no significant trends for both short- and long-term stability studies [23]. In addition, studies done on AFM_1 concentration changes in cheese showed no significant change of concentration even after 3 months of storage [24]. However, Khoury et al. [25] investigated the binding ability of AFM_1 by Lactic acid bacteria (LAB) such as *Lactobacillus bulgaricus* and *Streptococcus thermophilus* and found that they were effective in reducing the extent of free AFM_1 content in liquid culture medium and during yogurt processing. Therefore, this is a first study showing the capacity which can be played by LAB in AFM_1 removal and could be used as a biological agent for AFM_1 reduction. It is important to mention that the stability of AFM_1 during processing and storage makes it dangerous.

4. Aflatoxins and Aflatoxin M1 contamination

Most of mycotoxins poisoning problems occur in developing countries and particularly in sub-Saharan African region where maize and groundnuts are the staple foods [28]. It is estimated that about 250.000 hepatocellular carcinoma related deaths occur annually in Africa and around the world [28]. Acute aflatoxicosis has been reported in countries such as: Taiwan, Uganda, Kenya and Thailand [29, 30]. Ciegler et al.[31] reported that between 1974 and 1975, there was a disease outbreak affecting humans, killing about 106 among the 397 registered cases caused by the consumption of badly moulded corn contaminated with aflatoxin (between 6.5 and 15.6ppm). In July 2004, over 100 people died in Kenya due to acute aflatoxicosis after eating maize contaminated with aflatoxins [32]. Human aflatoxicosis (acute hepatitis) in Kenya is problematic among 20 hospitalized, 20% mortality was associated with the consumption of maize highly contaminated with AF [33], while during 2004, 125 deaths were recorded from a total of 317 reported cases in an outbreak of acute aflatoxicosis associated with Reye's syndrome [34]. Although such mortalities are viewed as a direct consequence of mycotoxin poisoning, Sharma et al. [35] indicated that these mortalities might have resulted from a predisposition to infectious diseases resulting from immunosuppressive effects probably caused by mycotoxins. In Malaysia, exposure to aflatoxins contaminated foodstuff was strongly implicated in the death of 13 children in 1988 [36]. Contamination occurs through exposure to contaminated AFM_1 milk, milk products such as cheese, yoghurt because as said earlier, AFM_1 is mostly excreted in milk of lactating animals and women exposed to diets previously contaminated with aflatoxin B1 and B2 [26, 27]. Aflatoxin M1 can also be found in the organs, e.g., kidney, liver, and excreta of animals exposed to AFB_1 [11]. Aflatoxin B1 is excreted into milk of lactating dairy cows primarily in the form of AFM_1 with residues approximately equal to 1-3% of the dietary concentration [16]. It has been shown experimentally to present high hepatotoxic and mutagenic risk [11].

5. Health implications of AFM_1

Aflatoxins are classified as mutagen and carcinogen [37] and their exposure and exact effects on human and animals are difficult to determine with precisions due to lack of experimental data, in addition due to co-occurrence with other mycotoxins in food and feed. Aflatoxin M1 has been demonstrated to be cytotoxic on human hepatocytes in vitro and its acute toxicity in several species is similar to that of aflatoxin B1 and liver cancer has been related to dietary intake of aflatoxins [11, 38]. Aflatoxin M1 exhibits a high level of genotoxic activity and certainly represents a health risk because of its possible accumulation and linkage to DNA [39, 38]. Moreover, AFB1 contamination at higher levels has also been correlated with reduced birth weight and jaundice in neonates [40]. The capacity of biotransformation of carcinogens in infants is generally slower than that of adults, this result in a longer circulation time of the chemicals [41].

6. Update on aflatoxin M1 extraction, detection and quantification methods

Several methods of extraction and detection have been used or developed for detection of AFM_1 in milk dairy products during the past decade. It is however important that to consider the type of matrix (fresh, stored, pasteurised milk, liquid or powder milk, cheese) as this can affect the final results [42]. In addition, most of commercial kits or rapid tests are designed for specific matrix. This makes the extraction of mycotoxins and AFM_1 from different matrices a challenge and costly. The detection of AFM_1 in milk or milk products remains a challenge because of the very low concentrations. Therefore there is a need of sensitive methods for extraction and detection. Among screening methods, the enzyme-linked immunosorbent assay (ELISA) has been the most used as a screening method for AFM_1 [43]. The method is invariably based on the competition enzyme-linked immunosorbent assay (competition ELISA). The ELISA microtiter plate is coated with a bound antibody against AFM_1 and the detecting reagent is a covalent complex of this mycotoxin and an enzyme, usually horseradish peroxidase or alkaline phosphatase. The reagent is mixed with a sample of the mycotoxin extract and the mixture is placed in the well. In the control well (absence of mycotoxin in the sample), the mycotoxin-enzyme conjugate can saturate the bound antibody, and addition of a chromogenic substrate results in the development of colour. In the test well, free mycotoxin molecules in the extract compete with the conjugate on the bound antibody [44]. The higher the concentration of mycotoxin, the less the conjugate can react with the bound antibody, leading to fainter colour development [44]. The competition ELISA approaches that of the LC-MS method [44]. However, ELISA has been noticed to be not fully reliable due to cross-reaction interferences, especially at concentrations lower than 0.05 µg/L [44]. Magliulo et al. [45] reported a more specific chemiluminescent assay reaching 0.001µg/L. Another new screening assay using a headspace sensor array obtains results comparable to those of ELISA [119]. While Goryacheva et al. [128] have developed Immunoaffinity pre-concentration combined with on-column visual detection for rapid screening of AFM_1 in milk. This method showed a 2% of false negative results. Kanungo et al. [46] also developed an ultra-sensitive sandwich for the detection of AFM_1 in milk. The assay involved the immobilization of rat monoclonal antibody of AFM_1 in 384 microtiter plate to capture AFM_1 antigen. The miniaturised assay (10µL) enabled ultra-trace analysis of AFM_1 in milk with much improved lower limit of detection at 0.005pg/mL [46]. Sensitive magnetic nanoparticles (MNPs) based ELISA has been also developed and coupled with micro plate ELISA for analysis in milk. The hybrid-assay, by coupling the 1 antibodies (Ab) immobilized MNPs column with microwell plate assay enabled simultaneous measurement of low (0.5 pg/mL) and high AFM_1 contamination (200 pg/mL). The MNPs-ELISA advantages were that it had a small column size, high capture efficiency and lower cost over other reported materials [46].

In addition, commercial portable devices such as Ridascreen ELISA kits (R-Biopharm Germany); ROSA aflatoxin M1 SL, Charm (Charm Sciences Inc. 2009); Lateral Flow Immunoassay (LFIA) or Gold-Colloid Based Immunoassay [47] have since been developed to speed up the detection of AFM_1. Typical lateral flow immunochromatography (LFIA) strip is composed of a loading pad where a sample of the extract is applied; a zone containing coloured particles (e.g., latex, gold) coated with a mouse monoclonal anti-mycotoxin antibody; a zone of nitrocellulose membrane that allows the migration of the particles together with the mycotoxin sample; a test line that contains immobilized mycotoxin; a positive control line that contains a secondary anti-mouse antibody, and an absorbent pad [44]. In principle the LFIA is that AFM_1 extract is applied and migrates along the strip and once the conjugate zone is reached, the mycotoxin binds the anti mycotoxin–particle complex. Free and mycotoxin-containing particles now migrate to the test line. The immobilized mycotoxin captures only the free particles that form a visible coloured line, whereas mycotoxin-containing particles continue to migrate [44].

The presence of a mycotoxin in the sample at higher concentration than the cut-off point of the strip (saturation of the particles with mycotoxin) will fail to bind to the test line, and vice versa. Thus, the intensity of the colour in the test line is inversely proportional to the concentration of the mycotoxin. Upon reaching the positive control line, both free and mycotoxin-containing particles can bind the anti-mouse antibody, thus forming a strongly coloured line regardless of the presence or absence of mycotoxin. The sensitivity of LTF is very high, and is comparable to those of sophisticated methodologies such as LC-MS-MS and surface plasmon resonance (SPR) (see below). The use of fluorescent reagents can bring the LOD to 50–200 ppt, as has been shown with other toxins [49]. The highest sensitivity in the detection of a mycotoxin by LTF was 5 ppb of AFB2 in pig feed, using a commercial immunaffinity column for the purification and concentration of the extract [44].

It is important to mention that the use different of devices available on the market depend on the objectives intended to be achieved by the analysis. It may be screening, confirmatory or both. The most reported methods conventionally used for AFM_1 extraction and detection are liquid-liquid extraction, silica gel, SPE cartridges (C18) cartridges [50] or immunoaffinity column (IAC), [57]. The inconvenience of this method is excessive use of chlorinated solvent in liquid-liquid extraction [21]. recently multifunctional clean-up columns (MFC) have been successfully applied to the clean-up of aflatoxins B_1, B_2, G_1, and G_2 when analysed by LC-FLD. MFC entrap matrix materials of cereal extracts but let the analytes pass through. This is simple, quick, and more stable than IAC [54] will probably be used for AFM_1 in the future as there have been no reports on this. Reports have shown that the detection and quantification of AFM_1 can be done by separation using thin-layer chromatography (TLC) or high-performance liquid chromatography (HPLC) coupled with fluorescence detector [6, 55-57]. The inconvenience of the TLC method is that it is challenging in the determination of mycotoxin concentrations with exactitude. In order to enhance AFM_1 fluorescence, pre or post derivatization with trifluoroacetic acid with detection limits (LOD) (0.01- 0.3 μg/L) or post column derivatization with pyridinium hydrobromide perbromide and lowered the detection limit to 0.001 μg/L on HPLC [50]. The inconvenience of these methods is that they are time consuming as samples are run singularly to ensure the validity of results. In addition, the derivatizing agents (tirfluoroacetic and pyridinium hydrobromide) are corrosive and therefore dangerous for the technician and have corrosive effect on the HPLC column which reduces its longevity.

There are reports on the use of mass spectrophotometer (MS) for AFM_1 detection and quantification [51, 52]. The advantage of this is the low sensitivity. Plattner et al. [52] and Kokkonen [53] also reported on the use of tandem MS (MS/ MS) for AFM_1 detection in dairy products. However, by their sample preparation procedures these two methods did not eliminate matrix effects and must use matrix standards for calibration. Blank matrixes free of the analytes are not easy to obtain, and their storage time is short. As a result, there would be considerable practical benefit from further work on sample preparation and methods for separation prior to MS. Patel et al. [21] reported on AFM_1 detection 1 in milk and milk powder using an LC-MS/MS method and this contrasted the clean-up efficiencies of IAC and MFC. Dutton et al. [57] reported the use of IAC clean-up and HPLC coupled with a fluorometer detector coupled with a Coring cell (Kobra cell) for AFM_1 detection. The advantage of this method is the avoidance the derivatization procedure which is labour cost and health risky for the technician and corrosive for the column. It is important also to mention that data presented in this study cannot be compared because of the use of different extraction and analytical methods. The use of different analytical methods (TLC, HPLC, LC-MS, ELISA) also affected reported concentrations of aflatoxin M1 in milk and therefore may affect intake estimates; therefore there is a need for trained people to give correct estimations of intake or AFM_1 in milk for better evaluation of exposure and anticipation of health problems.

In addition to herein mentioned techniques, Stark [44] in his review on other simple techniques such as the identification of mycotoxins based on molecular techniques for AFs and other mycotoxins detections from fungal strains are being developed and experimented [44]. Bhatnagar et al. [58] mentioned also that the biosynthesis and regulations of AFs involved at least 25 genes. Shapira et al. [59]; Chen et al. [60] used Primers pertaining to sequences of afl-2, aflD, aflM and aflP, (apa-2, nor-2, ver-2, omt-2, respectively) to detect and identify aflatoxigenic strains of *A. flavus* and *A. parasiticus* among isolated colonies or in DNA extracts from food and feedstuff. Differential medium (ADM) as diagnostic medium is another method that enables the identification and enumeration of aflatoxigenic *Aspergillus* [61]. Non-expensive reagents, an autoclave and a simple 365 nm UV lamp [62] allowed the identification of aflatoxigenic fungi. This method can be used by any mycologist in developing countries where the acquisition of expensive equipment or the availability highly trained personnel remains a concern. In this method common media such as czapek, sabouraud dextrose or yeast extract sucrose (YES) can support the growth of *Aspergillus* [44]. Addition of methyl-b-cyclodextrin(Wacker, Munich) [63] or of a combination of methyl-b-cyclodextrin plus bile salts (0.6% Na-deoxycholate) [64] enhances the natural fluorescence of aflatoxins, allowing detection of aflatoxigenic colonies after 3 days [63] or 36 h [64] of incubation.

Rojas-Dura´n et al. [64] also noted that the detection of AFs by studying the fluorescence of fungal colonies remained a challenge because non-aflatoxigenic strains of *Aspergilli,* such as *A. parasiticus* and *A. niger* also fluoresce under UV and erroneous interpretation due to the presence of AFs could happen. Further diagnostic tests done at room temperature and which revealed a phosphorescence of AFs that lasts 0.5 s after switching off the UV light were needed to confirm the presence of AFs in AF-producer aspergilli [64] –aflatoxigenic. In addition to fluorescence and phosphorescence observed during the exposure of AFs to UV light, AFB1 and AFB2 are activated by 365 nm UV light, resulting in AFB2–8,9-oxide [44]. It was also observed that AFB2–8,9-oxide bound to DNA at the N7 position of guanine residues yields 8,9-dihydro-2-(N7-guanyl)-3-hydroxyaflatoxin B2 [44]. It is therefore important to mention that the structure of the AF-DNA photo adduct [65] is identical to the AF-DNA adduct that is formed in vivo from ingested AFB2 by cytochrome P450, mainly in the liver [66]. The formation of AF-DNA adducts is considered as the initiating step of AF-induced carcinogenesis while covalent DNA- and protein adducts are also responsible for acute toxicity [44]. Munkvold et al. [68] exposed AFs contaminated kernel corns to 365 nm UV light and the observation of an intense blue-green fluorescence confirmed the presence of aflatoxin-containing kernel. In this method the presence of more than four fluorescent kernels in a 5-pound sample of corn (approximately 6,000 kernels) was indicative of AFs contamination of at least 20 pp [68}

The use of Polymerase Chain Reaction (PCR) for the detection of mycotoxigenic fungi has been applied recently to prevent contamination of crops by mycotoxigenic fungi [44]. Bhatnagaret al. [58] demonstrated also that at least 25 genes were involved in the biosynthesis of AFs and its regulation. To detect and identify aflatoxigenic strains of *A. flavus* and *A. parasiticus* among isolated colonies, or in DNA extracts from foodstuff and feedstuff primers pertaining to sequences of afl-2, aflD, aflM and aflP, (apa-2, nor-2, ver-2, omt-2, respectively) have been used[59; 60]. In this method, the amplification of genes involved in AF biosynthesis is done using the DNA of *Aspergilli* as template. The identification of AFs biosynthetic genes is confirmed by sequencing of the amplified fragments of the DNA [44]. It is however important to mention that the presence of the genes reflects only AFs productions potential by *Aspergilli* [44]. Several environmental factors such as temperature, humidity, composition of the growth medium, growth phase and age of the culture can influence AFs production. A recent application of reverse transcription polymerase chain reaction (RT–PCR) for the characterization of aflatoxigenic *Aspergilli*, relies on the presence of mRNAs pertaining to AF biosynthesis genes [44]. The RT–PCR has been also used for the confirmation of the presence of aflatoxigenic fungus and of AF biosynthetic enzymes [44]. Multiplex RT–PCR containing 4–5 primer pairs of various combinations of aflD, aflO, aflP, aflQ, aflR and aflS (aflJ) were used to detect toxigenic fungi [69]. The genes, their enzyme products have their functions in the AF biosynthetic pathway while non-aflatoxigenic strains lack one or some AF biosynthetic genes [59) and mRNA products [69].

Other methods used for mycotoxin detection and not yet applied for AFM_1 and will be the future in AFM_1 detection and quantification include Molecular Imprinting (MI) in which a pseudo receptor is formed after polymerization of the surrounding molecules and washout of the mycotoxin. The selective binding of other molecules of the same mycotoxin to the imprinted polymer relies on immuno-competition reactions which are enhanced as compared to binding to a non-imprinted polymer [70]. It is important to mention that frequent production of several mycotoxins by a single fungus or in the same sample [6], and the contamination of crops with several toxigenic fungi are some of the reasons for the development of the arrays [44]. The Arrays biosensors have been developed to perform the simultaneous assays of more than one mycotoxin [71]. Electronic Nose sensors have been developed to identify volatile biomarker compounds such nitrosamines emitted from grains. These volatile biomarkers are dependent also on the types of mycotoxin in the contaminated grains [44]. Solid State SsDNA Odor Sensors with ssDNA 22-mers of ssDNA containing a fluorescent chromophore and dried onto a solid support can interact non-covalently with volatiles resulting in fluorescence increase have been developed. Volatile precursors of AFB_2, ochratoxin A and DON [72] could be used to identify toxigenic fungi by such odour sensors.

Although all the above mentioned methods of evaluating AFs contamination and identification in corn or food are applicable, there is an absolute necessity that the identification and determination of AFs levels with portable kits, and by confirmation of their identity in the laboratory be carried out.

7. Review of a decade survey of AFM_1 in dairy milk

Due to AFs and AFM_1 health hazard potential, it is therefore important to monitor and regulate the level of AFM_1 in milk and milk products through control of animal feed quality for consumer's safety purposes [19]. Aflatoxin M_1 is a metabolite of AFB_1 that can occur in milk and milk products from animals consuming feed contaminated with AFB_1 [73]. Data from this review (Table 1) revealed that not much is done in regard to AFM_1 surveys in many developing countries and particularly in African countries. The list of countries presented in Table 1 is not exhaustive however does represent the trend in AFM_1 survey in developing countries. Numerous epidemiological studies have shown in some areas a correlation between high aflatoxin exposure and high incidence of hepatho carcinoma in several countries in Africa [74]. Data in Table 1 show that only few African countries apart from South Africa [57], Egypt [75] and Morocco [76] and Nigeria [77] were involved in the survey for AFM_1. However the following Middle East, Asian and Latin American countries are implementing controls of the toxin in both dairy and human milk Iran [78] and Kuwait [79] and Pakistan [80-83] India, Argentina [84] and Brazil [18, 85-87]

Data obtained clearly show that ELISA immunoassay technique has been the most used analytical method in the past decade to measure AFM_1. This has also been confirmed in a survey done in Italy on AFM_1 in dairy products by [88] The use of ELISA immunoassay can be justified by the fact that it is affordable, simple and easy, to use and does not need expensive equipment such as liquid chromatography. However, several researchers mostly from developed countries combined Imunoaffinity column and Liquid Chromatography for specificity and confirmation of results [18, 48, and 57].

Survey in developing countries showed high levels of AFM_1 contamination (> 0.05 μg/L) in many milk samples analysed as compared to data obtained from developed countries such as France [89], Italy [90], Portugal and Spain [91] in which the results were mostly low or with very few samples above the European Commission regulation of 0.05 μg/L. The explanation to this might be that, developed countries have imposed strict control on the quality of feed provided to animals which reduces chances for aflatoxin contaminations. Such regulations are not yet implemented or being implemented in developing countries. In addition, climatic conditions mostly tropical; hot and humid conditions favourable for aflatoxin producing fungi contamination in cereals [3] recorded in most developing countries could be the pivotal reason for AFM_1 contamination in milk. In addition, differences noticed between data shown in Table 1 could be also explained by the use of different extraction, and analysis (ELISA, TLC, HPLC, and LC-MS) techniques as said before which could affect significantly the level of mycotoxin detection.

Country	Sample size	Methods of detection	Positive (%)	ranges (μg/L)	References
Argentina	77	ELISA	18(23)	0.012-0.014	[84]
Brazil	107	IAC/HPLC	79 (73.8)	0.010-0.5	[39]
	36	IAC/HPLC	25 (69.4%)	0.001-0.2	[87]
	79	RP-18/HPLC	58(73.4)	0.015-0.5	[85]
	27	IAC/TLC/HPLC	16(59.3)	0.01-0.53	[86]
Croatia	61	ELISA	2(1.6)	0.011-0.058	[106]
Egypt	175	ELISA	86(49)	0.01-0.250	[75]
Libya	49	ELISA	35(71)	0.03–3.13	[114]
Italy	161	ELISA	128(78)	0.015–0.280	[22]
Iran	111	ELISA	85(77)	0.002-0.725	[93]
	126	ELISA	(80)	<0.05	[80]
India	225	ELISA	151(67.1)	0.059-0.515	[78]
Syria	87	ELISA	76(86)	0.028-1.064	[107]
	167	ELISA	81.4	0.007-0.47	[117]
Pakistan	225	ELISA	151(67.1)	0.0056-0.523	[78]
	74	ELISA	70(95)	0.020–0.690	[80]
	168	ELISA	168(100)	0.01–0.70	[81]
	232	ELISA	76 (32.7)	0.002-0.794	[82]
Thailand	40	IAC/ HPLC	15(37.5)	0.008-0.036	[83]
	240	IAC/ HPLC	240(100)	0.014–0.197	[108]
	123	ELISA	103(84)	0.003-0.5	[109]
Turkey	129	IAC/ HPLC	75(58.1)	0.025-0.543	[110]
	90	ELISA	63(63)	0.054-0.065	[111]
Portugal	598	IAC/HPLC	394 (65.8)	0.005-0.08	[91]
South Africa	90	ELISA/IAC/HPLC	85(94.5)	0.02-1.50	[57]
Lebanon	64	ELISA	26(40.62)	0.005-0.05+	[114
Morocco	54	IAC/HPLC	48(88.8)	0.001-0.117	[76]
Nigeria	101	AOAC/TLC	6(5.9)	0.2-0.40	[77]
Indonesia	113	ELISA	65(57.5)	0.005-0.025	[112]
Kuwait	309	ELISA	176(56.9)	0.004-0.083	[79]
Slovenia	60	ELISA	4(10)	0.051-0.223	[116]
South Korea	100	IAC/HPLC	48(48)	0.05–0.10	[48]
Sudan	44	AOAC/HPLC	42(95.45)	0.22-6.90	[113]

+Some samples were above 0.05μg/L

Table 1. Review of aflatoxin M1 survey in dairy products from different countries between 2001 and 2011

The investigation of AFM_1 contamination in milk according to climatic season variations (winter and summer) showed clear effect of seasons on the occurrence and concentration of AFM_1 in milk. Most of the studies showed that higher levels of AFM_1 are obtained in winter milks as compared to summer samples [22; 57, 92]. The reason being that during the summer, animals are fed on pasture, grass, weeds and green fodder while during winter, due to shortage or unavailability of fresh green feed, animals are more on concentrate feeding based on corn, wheat, and cotton seeds which could harbour mycotoxins than the fresh fodder [92]. Moreover, green fodder and hay preserved as silage under inadequate storage conditions which is ideal for toxigenic fungi such as *Aspergillus* contamination and aflatoxins production may occurred under favourable conditions [5, 93-95]). There is also evidence that milk yield is lower in winter, which means that AFM_1 and other components become more concentrated [92].

A comparison study was also carried out between milk samples obtained from rural subsistence and commercial farm in South Africa [96]. Analysed samples revealed the incidence of contamination with AFM_1 of 86.0% in rural subsistence farms samples while in samples from commercial farms, the incidence of contamination was of 100%. The lower frequency of contamination of AFM_1 in rural milk samples, as compared to those from commercial farms was explained by the fact that in subsistence farming animals were not fed with commercial feed on daily basis but mainly with leftovers from harvest season found on poor pastures with very little or no supplementation [6] while in commercial farms animals were fed on concentrates and silage which were also contaminated with toxigenic fungi and aflatoxins. This explaining the presence of AFM_1 in all milk samples analysed [4, 57]. Hence, the low intake of AFs in rural subsistence farm animals as compared to commercial farm animals exposed on feed.

8. Update on Aflatoxin M1 in human breast milk

Human breast milk has nutritional and immunological beneficial components for children and may contain trace amounts of a wide range of contaminants including AFM_1 following maternal dietary exposures [97]. Maternal consumption of aflatoxin contaminated food such as grain products, milk and milk products, legumes, meat, fish, corn oil, cottonseed oil, dried fruits, and nuts during breastfeeding can result in the accumulation of aflatoxins and their metabolites in breast milk [20]. Approximately 95% of AFB1 metabolite is excreted in milk as AFM_1in breast milk [98]. Studies on possible effects of infant exposure to AFs and AFM_1 have revealed growth retardation in human children [98] and foetal growth retardation in some animals exposed to aflatoxins prenatally [98]. In addition, AFs have been detected in blood of pregnant women [100]. A review done by Weidenborner [101] (Table 2) revealed the presence of AFM_1 in breast milk of lactating women in several countries with contamination levels varying according to countries and type of food exposed to. In addition to this, other studies confirmed the presence of AFM_1 in milk of lactating women (Table 2) at varying concentrations with some samples being above accepted limit in the USA and Europe (25ppb) or Australia and Switzerland (10 ppb). Methods used in studies to determine AFM_1 contamination in human breast milk have been mainly ELISA and HPLC as observed in studies done with dairy milk. Similar to the situation of dairy milk, few developing countries and in particular African countries have done investigations regarding AFM_1 contamination in human breast milk. Such investigations would be indicative of human exposure to AFs through food.

Country	Sample size	Positive (%)	ranges (μg/L)	References
Sierra Leone	113	25(23)	0.003-336	[101]
	113	35 (30.9)	0.2-99	"
UAE	140	129(73.8)	≤0.0034	[118]
	64	10(6.4)	0.3-13	
	445	443(99.5)	0.002-3	[101]
Australia	73	13 (69.4%)	0.028-1.031	"
Thailand	11	5(73.4)	0.039-1.736	"
Egypt	10	2(20)	0.5-5	"
	120	66(55)	0.2-2.09	"
	388	138(35.6)	5.6-5.13	"
	443	245(55.3)	0.0042-0.889	[126]
	150	98(65.3)	0.01-0.05	[101]
Gambia	5	5(100)	≤0.0014	[127]
Sudan	99	13(78)	0.005-0.064	[101]
	94	51(54.3)	0.401 - 0.525	"
Sudan/Kenya/	800	12(77)	0.005-1.379	[121]
Ghana	231	1(80)	0.194	[101]
Italy	82	4(4.8)	0.007-0.140	[22]
	75	75(100)	0.006-0.229	[123]
Turkey	61	8 (13.1)	0.0051-0.0069	[122]
	63	63(70)	0.054-0.65	[111]
Iran	160	157(98)	0.0003-0.0267	[20]
	2022	(9)	0.0069	[125]
	80	(1.3)	0.0069	[120]
	132	13(6)	0.007-0.018	[124]

Table 2. Summary of aflatoxin M1 survey in women's breast milk from different countries

9. Worldwide Aflatoxins control and regulations

Tolerable limits worldwide including South Africa for AFs vary between 10-20ppb [19]. Studies done have demonstrated that a concentration of 20 ppb of AFB_1 in the total mixed ration dry matter of lactating dairy cattle will result in AFM_1 levels in milk below the FDA set up limit of 0.5ppb [19]. European Union and several other countries including South Africa have however, presently set up acceptable level of AFM_1 in milk and milk products at 0.05 ppb. It is estimated that safe feed and food is the one in which detection levels may result in mycotoxin concentrations in milk being above limited level because absolute concentrations of mycotoxins in these feed and food are difficult to determine and concentrations may not be uniform throughout a lot of feed and concentrations can change over time [19]. The application of these regulations requires the use of sophisticated, expensive scientific equipment, and highly trained professional personnel commonly not found in developing countries where contamination of cereals by AFs producing fungi are mainly found and observed. To reduce crops contamination by these AFs producing fungi, the trend is the experimentation of molecular enabling detection of their mycotoxins producing potential [44]. In addition, recently researchers are proposing the use of strains of lactic acid bacteria to effectively remove AFB_1 and AFM_1 from contaminated liquid media and milk (102, 103]. In vitro binding ability of AFM_1 by *Lactobacillus bulgaricus* and *Streptococcus thermophilus* was investigated in PBS liquid medium and during yogurt making by Ayoub et al. [104].and obtained positive results with reduction of AFM_1.

Binders or sequestering agents added to feed have been another approach to reduce toxicity of mycotoxins by reducing reactivity of bound mycotoxins and reducing their intestinal absorption. Substances used as mycotoxin binders include indigestible adsorbent materials such as silicates, activated carbons, complex carbohydrates and others. Whitlow [67] extensively reviewed information on mycotoxins binders. The addition of mycotoxin binders to contaminated diets has been considered the most promising dietary approach to reduce effects of mycotoxins [105]. The use of binders offers an approach to salvaging feeds with low levels of mycotoxins and to protecting animals from the background levels of mycotoxins that, although low in concentration, routinely occur and may cause chronic disease problems and losses in performance [67]. Researchers have also noticed that there is no binder product that meets all the desirable characteristics, however, the potential currently exists for practical judicial use of mycotoxins binders for reducing mycotoxin exposure to animals [67]. Aflatoxin and some other mycotoxins which have chemical structure similar to aflatoxin such as sterigmatocystin, can bind to silicate. Silicates vary and bind to mycotoxins depending on the structure of mycotoxins. Chemically modification of silicates can increase binding to mycotoxins such as deoxynivalenol and zearalenone. Activated carbon (charcoal) has produced variable binding results most probably because of differences in physical properties of the test product [105]. Aflatoxin binding by activated charcoal has been variable, but mostly positive [67]. Complex indigestible carbohydrate polymers derived from [44] yeast cell walls are shown effective in binding aflatoxin and restoring performance to animals consuming multiple mycotoxins (generally *Fusarium* produced). Bacterial cell walls also have potential to bind mycotoxins, but limited research has been conducted. Inorganic polymers such as cholestyramine and polyvinylpyrrolidone also have binding potential [67].

There is an excellent potential for binders to help manage the mycotoxin problem. Various materials can bind mycotoxins in feed and thus reduce toxic exposure to consuming animals. No product currently meets all the characteristics for a desirable binder. Mycotoxin control measures may require many approaches [67]. Animals may also be supplemented with antioxidants and other beneficial substances. In addition, the enforcement of legislation against mycotoxins and public enlightenment on hazards and control of mycotoxins should be emphasized by government in developing countries to ensure the control of mycotoxins contamination in food and milk.

10. Conclusion

Aflatoxin M1 remains a mycotoxin that is yet to be investigated in most of developing countries including Africa. As long as conditions favourable for aflatoxin contamination in food and animal feed are present, AFM_1 in milk and milk products will continue to be an issue that needs constant monitoring because of the serious effects it could cause on human health, particularly children. Developing countries compared to developed nations need to develop and implement regulations and control systems that would regulate AFM_1 in milk and its products thus ensuring food quality and safety. The coming decade will definitively focus on development and application of new, quick and low cost technology for aflatoxin detection. This would be key to developing strategies that would improve prevention, promotion awareness with regards to fungi and aflatoxins contamination.

Author details

Mwanza Mulunda, Lubanza Ngoma, Mathew Nyirenda,
Lebohang Motsei and Frank Bakunzi
Department of Animal Health, Faculty of Agriculture and Technology, Mafikeng Campus,
North West University, Private Bag X2046 Mmabatho, South Africa

11. References

[1] International Agency for Research on Cancer (IARC). Monographs on the evaluation of the carcinogenic risk of chemicals to human: Some naturally occurring substances. Food items and constituents, heterocyclic aromatic amines and mycotoxins. IARC, Lyon 1993; 397-444.

[2] Vargas J, Due M, Frisvad JC and Samson RA. Taxonomic revision of Aspergillus section Clavati based on molecular, morphological and physiological data. Studies in Mycology 2007; 59:89-106.

[3] Klich MA. Identification of common Aspergillus spp, Ponson and Looijen, Wageningen. The Netherlands, 2002; 1-107.

[4] Pitt JI and Hocking AD. Fungi and mycotoxins in foods. In Fungi of Australia, vol.1B, Introduction Fungi in the environment, ed. A.E. Orchard. Canberra, Autralia: Australian Biology Research Study 1997; 315-342.

[5] Klich MA. Environmental and developmental factors influencing aflatoxin production by Aspergillus flavus and Aspergillus parasiticus. Mycoscience 2007; 48:71-80.

[6] Mwanza M, 2007. A survey of fungi and mycotoxins with respect to South African domestic animals in Limpopo Province. Dissertation submitted in partial fulfilment for the degree of magister biotechnology. http://152.106.6.200:8080/dspace/bitstream/10210/884/1/Mwanza%20M%20tech%20dissertation.pdf.

[7] Pittet A. Natural occurrence of mycotoxins in foods and feeds: an updated review. Revue de Médecine Vétérinaire 1998; 149: 479-492.

[8] Caloni F; Stammati A, Friggé G and De Angelis I. Aflatoxin M1 absorption and cytotoxicity on human intestinal in vitro model Toxicon 2006; 47: 409-415.

[9] International Agency for Research on Cancer (IARC). Some Traditional Herbal Medicines, Some Mycotoxins, Naphthalene and Styrene. Monograph Volume 82, http:// monographs, 2002.

[10] European Commission. Commission Directive 2002/27/EC of 13 March 2002 amending Directive 98/53/EC laying down the sampling methods and the methods of analysis for the official control of the levels for certain contaminants in foodstuffs. Official Journal of the European Communities L75: 2002; 44-45.

[11] Henry SH, Whitaker T, Rabbani I, Bowers J, Park D, Price W and Bosch FX.. Aflatoxin M1. Joint FAO/WHO Expert Committee on Food Additives (JECFA) 2001; 47.

[12] Eaton DL and Gallagher EP. Mechanisms of aflatoxin carcinogenesis. An Review Pharmacology and Toxicology 1994; 34: 135-172.

[13] Mace K, Gonzalez FJ, McConnell, IR, Garner RC, Avanti O, Harris CC and Pfeifer AM. Activation of promutagens in a human bronchial epithelial cell line stably expressing human cytochrome P450 1A2. Molecular Carcinogens 1994; 11:65–73.

[14] Smela ME, Currier SS and Bailey EA. The chemistry and biology of aflatoxin B1: from mutational spectrometry to carcinogenesis. Carcinogenesis 2001; 22(4): 535-545.

[15] Kuilman ME, Maas M, Judah, RFM and Fink-Gremmels, J. Bovine hepatic metabolism of aflatoxin B1. Journal of Agriculture and Food Chemistry 1998; 46: 2707-2713.

[16] Van Egmond HP. Current situation on regulations for mycotoxins: Overview of tolerances and status of standard methods of sampling and analysis. Food Additives and Contaminants 1989; 6:139-188.

[17] Frobish RA, Bradley DD, Wagner DD, Long-Bradley PE and Hairston H. Aflatoxin residues in milk of dairy cows after ingestion of naturally contaminated grain. Journal of Food and Proteins 1986; 49:781-785.

[18] Sassahara M. Netto PD and Yanaka EKAflatoxin occurrence in foodstuff supplied to dairy cattle and aflatoxin M1 in raw milk in the North of Paraa state. Food Chemistry and Toxicology 2005; 43: 981-984.

[19] Whitlow WM, Hagler Jr and Diaz Mycotoxins in feeds. Quality feed Mycotoxins. Feedstuff. Feedstuffs 83, 2010.

[20] Yousef AE and Marth EH. Stability and degradation of aflatoxin M1. In: van Egmond, H.P, ed, Mycotoxins in Dairy Products, London, Elsevier Applied Sciences 1989; 127-161.

[21] Patel PM, Netke SP, Gupta DS and Dabadghao AK. Note on the effect of processing milk into khoa on aflatoxin M1 content. Indian Journal of Animal Sciences 1981; 51: 791-792.

[22] Galvano F, Galofaro V and Galvano G. Occurrence and stability of aflatoxin M1 in milk and milk products: a worldwide review. Journal of Food Protection 1996; 59: 1079-1090.

[23] Josephs RD, Ulberth F, Van Egmond HP, Emons HAflatoxin M1 in milk powders: processing, homogeneity and stability testing of certified reference materials. Food Additives and Contaminants 2005; 22(9): 864-74.

[24] Doveci O. Changes in the concentration of aflatoxin M1 during manufacture and storage of White Pickled cheese. Food Control 2006; 18: 1103-107.

[25] Khoury A. El, Atoui A, Yaghi J. Analysis of aflatoxin M1 in milk and yogurt and AFM1 reduction by lactic acid bacteria used in Lebanese industry. Food Control 2011; 22: 1695-1699.

[26] Scott PM. Methods for determination of aflatoxin M1 in milk and milk products: a review of performance characteristics. Food Additives and Contaminants 1989; 6 (3): 283-305.

[27] Wild CP, Pionneau FA, Montesano R, Mutiro CF and Chetsanga CJAflatoxin detected in human breast milk by immunoassay. International Journal of Cancer 1987; 40: 328-333.

[28] Wagacha JM. and Muthomi JW. Mycotoxin problem in Africa current status implicationsto food safety and health and possible management strategies. International Journal of Food Microbiology 2008; 124:1-12.

[29] World Health Organization (WHO), A compendium (FAO food Nutrition Paper, 64). FAO, Rome, 6,1995,

[30] Autrup H., SeremetT., Wakhisi J. and Wasuna A. Aflatoxin exposure measured by urinary excretion of aflatoxin B1-guanine adduct and hepatitis B virus infection in areas with different liver cancer incidence in Kenya. Cancer Research 1987; 47: 3430.

[31] Ciegler A., Lee LS. and Dunn JJ. Production of naphthoquinone mycotoxins and taxonomy of Penicillium viridicatum. Applied Environmental Microbiology 1981; 42: 446-449.

[32] Sibanda L, Marovatsanga LT. and Pestka JJ. Review of mycotoxin work in sub-Saharan Africa. Food Control 1997; 8: 21-29.

[33] Ngindu A. Johnson B. and Kenya PR. Outbreak of acute hepatitis by aflatoxin poisoning in Kenya. Lancet, 1982; 319: 1346-1348.

[34] Barrett J. Mycotoxins: of moulds and maladies. Environmental Health Perspective 2000; 108 A: 20-23.

[35] Sharma SL. Kaith DS. and Khan MA. Cultural control of Sclerotinia stalks rot of cauliflower. Indian Phytopathology 1983; 36: 601-603.

[36] Chao TC. Maxwell SM. Wong SY. An outbreak of aflatoxicosis and boric acid poisoning in Malaysia: a clinicopathological study. Journal of Pathology 1991; 164:225-233.

[37] International Agency for Research on Cancer (IARC), Some Traditional Herbal Medicines, Some Mycotoxins, Naphthalene and Styrene. Monograph Volume 82, http://monographs. 2002.

[38] Makun HA, Dutton, MF, Njobeh PB, Gbodi TA and Ogbadu GH, Aflatoxin Contamination in Foods and Feeds: A Special Focus on Africa.in: Trends in Vital Food and Control Engineering. In Tech. 2012, Pp188-234.

[39] Shundo L. and Sabino M. Aflatoxin M_1 determination in milk by immunoaffinity column cleanup with TLC/HPLC. Brazilian Journal of Microbiology 2006; 37: 164-167.

[40] Abulu EO, Uriah N, Aigbefo HS, Oboh PA, Aggonlaho DE. Preliminary investigation on aflatoxin in cord blood of jaundiced neonates. West African Medicine , 1998; 17(3): 184-187.

[41] Sadeghi N, Oveisi MR, Jannat B, Hajimahmoodi M, Bonyani H, Jannat F. Incidence of Aflatoxin M1 in human breast milk in Tehran, Iran. Food Control 2009; 20: 75-78.

[42] Chen CP, Li, WJ and Peng KP. Determination of Aflatoxin M1 in Milk and Milk Powder Using High-Flow Solid-Phase Extraction and Liquid Chromatography-Tandem Mass Spectrometry. Journal of Agriculture Food Chemistry 2005; 53: 8474-8480.

[43] Sarmelnetoglu B, Kuplulu O and Celik HT, 2004. Detection of aflatoxin M_1 in cheese by ELISA. Food Chemistry 24: 981-984.

[44] Stark AA. Mycotoxins Molecular Mechanism of Detection of Aflatoxins and Other Mycotoxins . in M. Rai and A. Varma (eds.), Mycotoxins in Food, Feed and BioweaponsDOI: 10.1007/978-3-642-00725-5_2, # Springer-Verlag Berlin Heidelberg, 2010.

[45] Magliulo M, Mirasoli M, Simoni P, Lelli R, Portanti O and Roda A. Development and validation of an ultrasensitive chemiluminescent enzyme immunoassay for aflatoxinM1 in milk. Journal of Agriculture and Food Chemistry 2005; 53: 3300-3305.

[46] Kanungo L and Pal S, Sunil Bhand Miniaturised hybrid immunoassay for high sensitivity analysis of aflatoxin M1 in milk. Biosensors and Bioelectronics 2011; 26: 2601-2606.

[47] Krska R and Molinelli A. Rapid test strips for analysis of mycotoxins in food and feed. Analyt Bioanalytic Chem 2009; 393(1): 67-71.

[48] Kim HJ, Lee JE, Kwak BM, Ahn JH, Jeong SH. Occurrence Of Aflatoxin M1 In Raw Milk From South Korea Winter Seasons Using An Immunoaffinity Column And High Performance Liquid Chromatography. Journal of Food Safety 2009; 30(4): 804-813.

[49] Kim YM, Oh SW, Jeong SY, Pyo DJ, Choi EY. Development of an ultrarapid one-step fluorescence immunochromatographic assay system for the quantification of microcystins. Environmental Sciences and Technology 2003; 37: 2899–2904.

[50] Manetta AC; Di Giuseppe L; Giammarco, M.; Fusaro, I.; Simonella, A.; Gramenzi, A.; Formigoni, A. High performance liquid chromatography with post-column derivatisation and ultra violet detection for sensitive determination of aflatoxin M1 in milk and cheese. Journal of Chromatography A 2005; 1083: 219-222.

[51] Plattner RD, Bennett GA and Stubblefield RD, Identification of aflatoxins by quadrupole mass spectrometry/mass spectrometry. Journal of the Association of Official Analytical Chemistry 1984; 67: 734-738.

[52] Sorensen LK, Elbæk TH. Determination of mycotoxins in bovine milk by liquid chromatography tandem mass spectrometry. Journal of Chromatography B 2005; 820: 183-196.

[53] Kokkonen M, Jestoi M and Rizzo A. Determination of selected mycotoxins in mould cheeses with liquid chromatography coupled to tandem with mass spectrometry. Food Additives and Contaminants 2005; 22:449-456.

[54] Wilson TJ and Romer TRUse of the Mycosep multifunctional cleanup column for liquid-chromatographic determination of aflatoxins in agricultural products. Journal Association Official Analytical Chemistry 1991; 74: 951-956.

[55] Dragacci S, Grosso F and Gilbert J. Immunoaffinity column clean-up with liquid chromatography for determination of aflatoxin M1 in liquid milk: collaborative study. Journal Association Official Analytical Chemistry 2001; 84(2) 437-443

[56] Rodriguez valasco ML, Calogne Delso MM and OrdonezEscudero DELISA and HPLC determination of the occurence of aflatoxin M1 in raw cow's milk. Food Additives and Contaminants 2003; 20: 276-280.

[57] Dutton MF, Mwanza M, de Kock S and Khilosia LD. Mycotoxins in South African foods: a case study on aflatoxin M1 in milk. Mycotoxin Research 2012; 28: 17-23.

[58] Bhatnagar D, Cary JW, Ehrlich K, Yu J, Cleveland TE. Understanding the genetics of regulation of aflatoxin production and Aspergillus flavus development. Mycopathologia 2006; 262: 255–266.

[59] Shapira R, Paster N, Eyal O, Menasherov M, Mett A, Salomon R. Detection of aflatoxigenic moulds in grains by PCR. Applied Environmental Microbiology 1996; 62: 3270–3273.

[60] Chen RS, Tsay JG, Huang YF, Chiou RY. Polymerase chain reaction-mediated characterization of moulds belonging to the Aspergillus flavus group and detection of Aspergillus parasiticus in peanut kernels by a multiplex polymerase chain reaction. Journal of Food Proteins 2002; 65: 840–844

[61] Bothast RJ, Fennel DI. A medium for rapid identification and enumeration of Aspergillus flavus, and related organisms. Mycologia 1974; 66: 365–369

[62] Hara S, Fennell DI, Hesseltine CW. Aflatoxin-producing strains of Aspergillus flavus detected by fluorescence of agar medium under ultraviolet light. Applied Microbiology 1974; 27 2228–2223.

[63] Fente CA, Ordaz JJ, Va´zquez BI, Franco CM, Cepeda ANew additive for culture media for rapid identification of aflatoxin-producing Aspergillus strains. Applied Environmental Microbiology 2002; 67: 4858–4862

[64] Rojas-Dura´n TR, Fente CA, Va´zquez BI, Franco CM, Sanz-Medel A, Cepeda A Study of a room temperature phosphorescence phenomenon to allow the detection of aflatoxigenic strains in culture media. Internation Journal of Food Microbiology 2007; 225:249–258

[65] Stark AA. Molecular and biochemical mechanisms of action of acute toxicity and carcinogenicity induced by aflatoxin B2 and of the chemoprevention of liver cancer. In: Wilson CL (ed) Microbial food contamination. Boca-Raton, CRC, 2007; 227–246

[66] Stark AA, Essigmann JM, Demain AL, Skopek TR, Wogan GN. Aflatoxin B2 mutagenesis and adduct formation in Salmonella typhimurium. Proc Natl Acad Sci USA 76:2343–2347, 1979.

[67] Whitlow LW. Evaluation of Mycotoxin Binders Proceedings of the 4th Mid-Atlantic Nutrition Conference. Zimmermann, N.G., ed., University of Maryland, College Park, MD 20742, 2006.

[68] Munkvold G, Hurburgh C, Meyer J, Loy D, Robertson A. Aflatoxins in corn. Iowa State University extension, File: Pest Management 2–5, 2005.

[69] Degola F, Berni E, Dall'Asta C, Spotti E, Marchelli R, Ferrero I, Restivo FM. A multiplex RT-PCR approach to detect aflatoxigenic strains of Aspergillus flavus. Journal of Applied Microbiology 2007; 203:4 09–427.

[70] Yu JC, Hrdina A, Mancini C, Lai EP. Molecularly imprinted polypyrrole encapsulated carbon nanotubes in stainless steel frit for micro solid phase extraction of estrogenic compounds. Journal of Nanoscience Nanotechnology 2007; 7: 3095–3203

[71] Ngundi MM, Qadri SA, Wallace EV, Moore MH, Lassman ME, Shriver-Lake LC, Ligler FS, Taitt CR Detection of deoxynivalenol in foods and indoor air using an array biosensor. Environmental Science Technology 2006; 40: 2352–2356

[72] Olsson J, Bo¨rjesson T, Lundstedt T, Schnu¨rer J. Detection and quantification of ochratoxin A and deoxynivalenol in barley grains by GC-MS and electronic nose. International Journal Food Microbiology 2002; 72: 203–224

[73] Applebaum, R.S., Brackett, R.E., Wiseman, D.W. and Marth. EH. Reponses of dairy cows to dietary aflatoxin: Feed intake and yield, toxin content, and quality of milk of cows treated with pure and impure aflatoxin. Journal of Dairy Science 1982; 65: 1503-1508.

[74] Jackson PE and Groopman J. Aflatoxin and liver cancer Baillie Á Research Clinical Gastroenterology 1999; 13(4): 545-555.

[75] Motawee MM, Bauer J. and McMahon DJ. Survey of Aflatoxin M1 in Cow, Goat, Buffalo and Camel Milks in Ismailia-Egypt. Bull Environ Contam Toxicology 2009; 83: 766-769.

[76] Zinedine A, Brera C, Elakhdari S, Catano C, Debegnach F, Angelini S, De Santis B. Faid M, Benlemlih M, Minardi V and Miraglia M. Natural occurrence of mycotoxins in cereals and spices commercialized in Morocco. Food Control 2006; 17: 868–874.

[77] Atanda O, Oguntubo A, Adejumo O, Ikeorah J, Akpan I. Aflatoxin M1 contamination of milk and ice cream in Abeokuta and Odeda local governments of Ogun State, Nigeria. Chemosphere, 2007; 68: 1455-1458.

[78] Fallah AA. Assessment of aflatoxin M1 contamination in pasteurized and UHT milk marketed in central part of Iran. Food Chemistry and Toxicology 2010; 48 988–991.

[79] Dashti B, Al-Hamli S, Alomirah H, Al-Zenki S, Abbas AB, Sawaya WLevels of aflatoxin M1 in milk, cheese consumed in Kuwait and occurrence of total aflatoxin in local and imported animal feed. Food Control 2009; 20: 686-690.

[80] Ghanem I and Orfi M, 2009. Aflatoxin M1 in raw, pasteurized and powdered milk available in the Syrian market. Food Control 20: 603-605.

[81] Hussain I. and Anwar J, 2008. A study on contamination aflatoxin M1 in raw milk in the Punjab Province of Pakistan. Food. Contr. 19: 393-395.

[82] Sadia A, Jabbar MA, Deng Y, Hussain EA, Riffat S, Naveed S, Arif M, 2012. Survey of aflatoxin M1 in milk and sweets of Punjab, Pakistan Food Control 26: 235-240.

[83] Hussain I, Anwar J, Rafiq M, Munawa A, Munawar A and Kashif M, 2010. Aflatoxin M1 contamination in milk from five dairy species in Pakistan. Food Control 21: 122–124.

[84] Lopez CE, Ramos LL, Ramadan, SS and Bulacio LC, 2003. Presence of aflatoxin m1 in milk for human consumption in Argentina. Food Control, 14: 31-34.

[85] Garrido NS, Iha MH, Santos Ortolani MR and Duarte Fávaro RM. Occurrence of aflatoxinsM1 and M2 in milk commercialized in Ribeirão Preto-SP, Brazil, Food

Additives and Contaminants: Chemistry, Analysis, Control, Exposure and Risk Assessment 2003; 20: 70-73.

[86] Gurbay AS, Engin AB, Çaglayan A and Sahin G. Aflatoxin M1 levels in Commonly consumed cheese and yoghurt samples in Ankara, Turkey. Ecology of Food and Nutrition, 2006; 45: 449-459.

[87] Oliveira CAF and Ferraz JCO. Occurrence of aflatoxin M1 in pasteurised, UHT milk and milk powder from goat origin. Food Control 2007; 18: 375-378.

[88] Anfossi L, Baggiani C, Giovannoli C and Giraudi G. Occurence of Aflatoxin M1 in dairy products. Aflatoxins detection, measurement and control, 2011; ISBN: 978-953-307-711-6. ,

[89] Boudra H; Barnouin J; Dragacci S; Morgavi DP. Aflatoxin M1 and Ochratoxin A in raw bulk milk from French dairy herds. Journal of Dairy Science 2007; 90: 3197-3201.

[90] Decastelli D, Lai J, Gramaglia M, Monaco A, Nachtmann C, Oldano F, RuYer, Sezian A, Bandirola B. AXatoxins occurrence in milk and feed in Northern Italy during 2004–2005. Food Control 2007; 18 1263-1266.

[91] Martins HM and Guerra MM. Bernardo A six year survey (1999-2004) of the occurrence of aflatoxin M1 in dairy products produced in Portugal. Mycotoxin Research 2005; 21: 192-195.

[92] Asi MR, Iqbal SZ, Arino A and Hussain H. Effect of seasonal variations and lactation times on aflatoxin M1 contamination in milk of different species from Punjab, Pakistan Food Control 2012; 25: 34-38.

[93] Kamkar AA. study on the occurrence of aflatoxin M1 in raw milk produced in Sarab city of Iran. Food Control 2005; 16: 593-599.

[94] Ghiasian SA, Maghsood AH, Neyestani TR and Mirhendi SH. Occurrence of aflatoxin M1 in raw milk during the summer and winter seasons in Hamadan, Iran. Journal of Food Safety 2007; 27: 188-198.

[95] Heshmati A, and Milani J. Contamination of UHT milk by aflatoxin M1 in Iran. Food Control 2010; 21:19-22.

[96] Mwanza M. A comparative study of fungi and mycotoxin contamination in animal products from selected rural and urban areas of South Africa with particular reference to the impact of this on the health of rural black people. 2012, Thesis, University of Johannesburg Library

[97] Jensen AA and Slorach SA. Chemical contaminants in human milk. Florida, USA: CRC Press. 1991.

[98] Gong YY, Hounsa A, Egal S, Turner PC and Sutcliffe AE. Postweaning exposure to aflatoxin results to impaired child growth: a longitudinal study In Bennin, West Africa. Environmental Health Perspectives 2004; 112: 1033-5.

[99] Pier AC. Major biological consequences of aflatoxicosis in animal production. Journal of Animal Science 1992; 70: 8860-8867.

[100] Peraica M, Radic B, Lulic A and Pavlovic M. Toxic effects of mycotoxins in humans. Research Bulletin of the World Health Organisation 1999; 77: 754-766

[101] Weidenborner M. Mycotoxins and their metabolites in human and animals. Springer Science, Busness Media, LLC, 2011.

[102] Lee, Y. K., El-Nezami, H., Haskard, C. A., Gratz, S., Puong, K. Y., Salminen, S., et al. Kinetics of adsorption and desorption of aflatoxin B1 by viable and nonviable bacteria. Journal of Food Protection 2003, 66: 426-430.

[103] Peltonen, K., El-Nezami, H., Haskard, C., Ahokas, J., and Salminen, S. Aflatoxin B1 binding by dairy strains of lactic acid bacteria and bifidobacteria. Journal of Dairy Science 2001; 84: 1256-2152.

[104] Ayoub M. Sobeih AMK and. Raslan AA. Evaluation of aflatoxin M1 in raw, processed milk and some milk products in Cairo with special reference to its recovery. Researcher 2011; 3: 56-61. (ISSN: 1553-9865). http://www.sciencepub.net.

[105] Galvano F, Galofaro V, Ritieni A, Bognanno M, De Angelis A and Galvano GSurvey of the occurrence of aflatoxin M1 in dairy products marketed in Italy: second year of observation. Food Additives and Contaminants 2001; 18: 644-646.

[106] Bilandzic N, Varenina I and Solomun B. Aflatoxin M1 in raw milk in Croatia. Food Control 2010; 21: 1279-1281.

[107] Rastogi, S, Dwivedi, P.D, Pitt J.I. and Hocking A.DFungi and mycotoxins in foods. In Fungi of Australia, vol.1B, Introduction Fungi in the environment, ed. A.E. Orchard. Canberra, Autralia: Austrarian Biology Research Study, 1997; 315-342.

[108] Ruangwises N and Ruangwises S. Aflatoxin M1 Contamination in Raw Milk within the Central Region of Thailand. Bulletin of Environmenat Contaminants Toxicology 2010; 85: 195-198.

[109] Iha MH, Barbosa CB, Okada IA and Trucksess MW. Occurrence of aflatoxin M1 in dairy products in Brazil. Food Control 2011; 22: 1971-1974.

[110] Unusam N. Occurrence of aflatoxin M1 in UHT milk in Turkey. Food Chemistry and Toxicology 2006; 44: 1897-1900.

[111] Buldu HM, Koç AN and Uraz G. Aflatoxin M1 contamination in cow's milk in Kayseri (central Turkey). Turkish Journal of Veterinary Animal Science 2011; 35: 87-91

[112] Nuryono N, Agus A, Wedhastri S, Maryudani YB, Sigit Setyabudi FMC, Böhm J and Razzazi-Fazeli E. A limited survey of aflatoxin M1 in milk from Indonesia by ELISA Food Control 2009; 20: 721-724.

[113] Elzupir AO and Elhussein AM. Determination of aflatoxin M1 in dairy cattle milk in Khartoum State, Sudan. Food Control 2010; 21: 945-946.

[114] Elgerbi AM, Aidoo KE, Candlish AAG, Tester RF. Occurrence of aflatoxin M1 in randomly selected in North African milk and cheese samples. Food Additives and Contaminants 2004; 21: 592-597.

[115] ElKhoury A., Atoui A., Yaghi J. Analysis of aflatoxin M1 in milk and yoghurt and AFM1 reduction by lactic acid bacteria used in Lebanese industry. Food Control 2011; 22: 1695-1699.

[116] Torkar K.G and Vengus, T. The presence of yeasts, moulds and aflatoxin M1 in raw Milk and cheese in Slovenia. Food Control 2008; 19: 570-577

[117] Rahimi E, Bonyadian M, Rafei M and Kazemain HR. Occurrence of aflatoxin M1 in raw milk of five dairy species in Ahvaz, Iran. Food and Chemical Toxicology 2010; 48: 129–131.

[118] Abdulrazzaq YM,Osman N, Yousif ZM, Al-Falahi S. AflatoxinM1 in breast-milk of UAE women. Annals of Tropical Paediatric 2003; 23(3):173-9.

[119] Benedetti S, Iametti F, Bonomi S and Mannino A. Head space sensor array for the detection of aflatoxinM1 in raw ewe's milk. Journal of Food Protection 2005; 68: 1089-1092

[120] Dehkordi AJ and Pourradi N. Determination of Aflatoxin M1 in Breast Milk Samples in Isfahan, Iranian Journal of Isfahan Medical School 2012; 30:182

[121] Elzupir AO, Abas AA, Abueliz MH, Nima KM, Afaf MIA, Nuha Abd, FFJ, Smah AA, Nousiba,Y AA, Ahmed AM, Arwa Eltahir AAK and Khalil AG. Aflatoxin M1 in breast milk of nursing Sudanese mothers. Mycotoxin Research, 2012; 10.1007/s12550-012-0127-x.

[122] Keskin Y, Başkaya R, Karsli S, Yurdun T, Ozyaral O.Detection of aflatoxin M1 in human breast milk and raw cow's milk in Istanbul, Turkey. Journal of Food Proteins 2009; 2(4): 885-889.

[123] Yasar K, Ruhtan B, Karsli SK, Turkan Y, Oguz O. Detection of Aflatoxin M1 in Human Breast Milk and Raw Cow's Milk in Istanbul, Turkey. Journal Protection Science 2009; 72(4)885-889.

[124] Ghaisain SA and Maghsood AH. Infants exposure to aflatoxin M1 from mothers breast milk in iran. Iranian Journal of Public Health 2012; 41(3): 119-126.

[125] Mahdavi R. Nikniaz L. Arefhosseini SR, Vahed Jabbari M. Determination of aflatoxin M1 in breast mil samples in Tabriz-Iran. Matern Child Health Journal 2010; 14: 141-145.

[126] Polychronaki N, Turner PC, Mykkanen H, Gong Y, Amra H, Abdel-Wahhab M and E;l-Nezami H. Deterimation of Aflatoxin M1 in Breast milk in a selected group of Egyptian mothers. Food Additives and Contaminants 2006; 23 (23): 700-708.

[127] Tomarek RH, Shaban HH, Khalafallah OA, El SHazly MN. Assessment of exposure of Egyptian infant to aflatoxin M1 through breast milk. Journal of Egypt Public Health Association 2011; 86: 51-5.

[128] Goryacheva IY, DeSaeger S, Eremin SA, Van Peteghem C, Immunochemical methods for rapid mycotoxin detection: evolution from single to multiple analyte screening. A review. Food Additives and Contaminants 2007; 24: 1169-1183.

Section 2

Public Health Impact of Mycotoxins

Chapter 3

Mycotoxins-Induced Oxidative Stress and Disease

Hossam El-Din M. Omar

Additional information is available at the end of the chapter

http://dx.doi.org/10.5772/51806

1. Introduction

Mycotoxins are pharmacologically active mold metabolites produced in a strain-specific way that elicit some complicated toxicological activities [1]. More than 300 secondary metabolites have been identified while only around 30 have true toxic properties [2]. The chemical structures of mycotoxins vary significantly, but they are low molecular mass organic compounds [3]. Mycotoxins are small and quite stable molecules which are extremely difficult to remove and enter the food and feed chain while keeping their toxic properties [4]. So, the occurrence of mycotoxins is regulated by legal limits in all developed countries [5]. Mycotoxin contamination of the feed and food is a global problem because more than 25% of world grain production is contaminated by mycotoxins [6]. The synthesis of mycotoxins by moulds is genetically determined and closely related to primary metabolic pathways, such as amino acid and fatty acid metabolism. However, the actual toxin production is modulated by environmental factors such as substrate composition and quality, humidity and temperature. The occurrence of mycotoxins in animal feed exhibits a geographic pattern, for example *Aspergillus* species meet optimal conditions only in tropical and subtropical regions, whereas *Fusarium* and *Penicillium* species are adapted to the moderate climate. Worldwide trade with food and feed commodities results in a wide distribution of contaminated material [7].

Plant selections for mycotoxin resistance have not created any significant results in protection against grain mycotoxins. The major problem comes from the fact that there are no safe levels of mycotoxins, because of synergistic interactions of many mycotoxins [2]. There is sufficient evidence from animal models and human epidemiological data to conclude that mycotoxins cause an important hazard to human and animal health [1]. The toxic effect of mycotoxins on animal and human health depends on the type of mycotoxin; level and duration of the exposure; age, health, and sex of the exposed individual, genetics, dietary status, and interactions with other toxic insults. Thus, the severity of mycotoxin toxicity can be complicated by factors such as vitamin deficiency, caloric deprivation, alcohol abuse, and infectious disease **[1,3,8]**.

Mycotoxins according to their chemical structure exert a broad variety of biological effects. The nature and intensity of these effects depend on the actual concentration of an individual mycotoxin and the time of exposure **[7]**. Cell proliferation of all mycotoxin treated blood mononuclear cells was significantly decreased at the highest concentrations of mycotoxins, but this decrease was significantly stronger for different mixtures of mycotoxins **[9]**. In addition, feed commodities are often contaminated with more than one mycotoxin, as mould species produce different mycotoxins at the same time. These co-occurring mycotoxins can exert additive effects, as for example various trichothecenes, but may also act antagonistically, as for example, observed with feeds containing trichothecenes and zearalenone, and commodities, containing aflatoxins and cyclopiazonic acid **[7]**.

Mycotoxicoses are more common in underdeveloped countries and often remain unrecognized by medical professionals, except when huge numbers of people are involved **[3]**. In general, mycotoxin exposure is more likely to occur in parts of the world where poor methods of food handling and storage are common, where malnutrition is a problem, and where few regulations exist to protect exposed populations. The incidence of liver cancer varies widely from country to country, but it is one of the most common cancers in China, Philippines, Thailand, and many African countries. Worldwide, liver cancer incidence rates are 2 to 10 times higher in developing countries than in developed countries **[10]**. The occurrence of fumonisin B1 was correlated with the occurrence of a higher incidence of esophageal cancer in regions of Transkei (South Africa), China, and Northeast Italy **[3]**. In Africa and Asia where the occurrence of mycotoxins is common and a high percentage of the population is infected with hepatitis B or C mycotoxin reduction is obligatory **[8]**. One of the strategies for reducing the exposure to mycotoxins is to decrease their bioavailability by including various mycotoxins-adsorbing agents in the compound feed, which lead to reduction of mycotoxins uptake as well as distribution to the blood and target organs. Another strategy is the degradation of mycotoxins into non-toxic metabolites by using biotransforming agents such as bacteria/fungi or enzymes **[4]**.

Diagnosis of animal mycotoxicosis is based on experimental studies with specific toxins and specific animals, very often under well-defined toxicological laboratory conditions, so that the results of such studies can be far from real-life or natural situations. Furthermore, factors such as breeding, sex, environment, nutritional status, as well as other toxic entities can affect the symptoms of intoxication and may contribute to the significance of mycotoxin damage on economic output and animal health **[11]**. The economic costs of mycotoxins are impossible to determine accurately **[12]**, but the US Food and Drug Administration (FDA) estimated that in the US the mean economic annual cost of crop losses from the mycotoxins aflatoxins, fumonisins, and deoxynivalenol are $932million USD **[13]**. While mycotoxin associated losses in industrial countries are typically market losses as a result of rejected crops, developing countries suffer additionally from health impacts **[14]**. Diagnosis is very much dependent on receiving a sample of feed that was ingested prior to intoxication, but also on data from another representative group of animals of the facility and the results of a post-mortem examination **[11, 13]**.

In the following table, the mycotoxins of major concern as feed contaminants are aflatoxins, ochratoxin A, Fusarium toxins (trichothecenes like, deoxynivalenol, diacetoxyscipenol, nivalenol, T2-toxin/HT2-toxin, zearalenone and fumonisins) **[4]**. Moreover, the most predominant mycotoxigenic species in wheat grain were *A. flavus* with the ability to produce mycotoxins (aflatoxins B1, B2, G1 and G2 and sterigmatocystin) **[15]**.

Fungal species	Mycotoxin
Aspergillus flavus; A. parasiticus	Aflatoxins
A. flavus	Cyclopiazonic acid
A. ochraceus; Penicillium viridicatum; P. cyclopium;	Ochatoxin A
P. expansum	Patulin
Fusarium culmorum; F. graminearum; F. sporotrichioides	Deoxynivalenol
F. sporotrichioides; F. poae	T-2 toxin
F. sporotrichioides; F. graminearum; F. poae	Diacetoxyscirpenol
F. culmorum; F. graminearum; F. sporotrichioides	Zearalenone
F. moniliforme	Fumonisins
Acremonium coenophialum	Ergopeptine alkaloids

Table 1. The major toxigenic species of fungi and their mycotoxins [16]

2. Route of mycotoxins exposure

The most common route of exposure to mycotoxins is ingestion, but it may also involve dermal, respiratory, and parenteral routes, the last being associated with drug abuse **[17]**. In general, animals are directly exposed to mycotoxins through the consumption of mouldy feedstuffs, eating contaminated foods, skin contact with mould infected substrates and inhalation of spore-borne toxins **[1]**. Human exposure can be via one of two routes; direct exposure due to the consumption of mouldy plant products, or indirect exposure through the consumption of contaminated animal products containing residual amounts of the mycotoxin ingested by the food producing animals **[18]**. Human exposure to mycotoxins is further determined by environmental or biological monitoring. In environmental monitoring, mycotoxins are measured in food, air, or other samples; in biological monitoring, the presence of residues, adducts, and metabolites is assayed directly in tissues, fluids, and excretory products **[19]**. The risk of systemic toxicity resulting from dermal exposure increases in the presence of high toxin concentrations, occlusion, and vehicles which enhance penetration **[20]**. The main human and veterinary health load of mycotoxin exposure is related to chronic exposure **[2]**.

3. Mycotoxins metabolism and induction of oxidative stress

Biodegradation of mycotoxins with microorganisms or enzymes is considered as the best strategy for detoxification of feedstuffs. This approach is considered as environmental friendly approach in contrast to physicochemical techniques of detoxification. Ruminants are potential source of microbes or enzymes for mycotoxins biodegradation **[21]**. In vertebrate, mycotoxin is metabolized by cytochrome P450 enzymes to metabolite-guanine-N7 adduct **(Fig 1)**. The carcinogenic potency is highly correlated with the extent of total DNA adducts formed *in vivo* **[22]**.

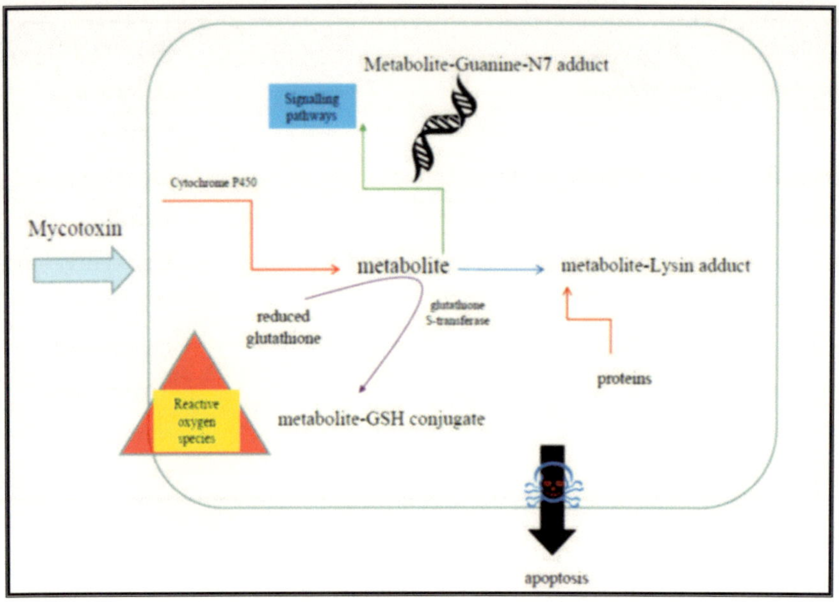

Figure 1. Mycotoxin metabolism in vertebrates **[23]**

Cytotoxicity and ROS generation are mechanisms of mycotoxins mediated toxicity. ROS are chemically reactive molecules containing oxygen. They are highly reactive due to the presence of unpaired electrons. ROS formed as a natural byproduct of the normal metabolism of oxygen have important roles in cell signaling and homeostasis. However, during times of environmental stress, ROS levels can increase dramatically as a result of oxidative stress **[24]**. Oxidative stress occurs when the concentration of ROS generated exceeds the antioxidant capability of the cell. In other words, oxidative stress describes various deleterious processes resulting from an imbalance between the excessive formation of ROS and limited antioxidant defenses **[25]**. Under normal conditions, ROS are cleared from the cell by the action of superoxide dismutase (SOD), catalase (CAT), or glutathione peroxidase (GPx). The main damage to cells results from the ROS-induced alteration of macromolecules such as polyunsaturated fatty acids in membrane lipids, proteins, and DNA. Additionally, oxidative stress and ROS can originate from xenobiotic bioactivation by prostaglandin H synthase (PHS) and lipoxygenases (LPOs) or microsomal P450s which can oxidize xenobiotics to free radical intermediates that react directly or indirectly with oxygen to produce ROS and oxidative stress **[26]** as in **Fig (2)**. Moreover, the cell can tolerate a small to moderate amount of oxidative stress by producing antioxidant molecules e.g vitamin A, C &E and GSH and activates enzymes e.g. CAT, SOD, GPx, glutathione reductase (GR) and glutathione S transferase (GST) to counteract the excess oxidants **[27]**. LPO may bring about protein damage and inactivation of membrane-bound enzyme either through direct attack by free radicals or through chemical modification by its end products **[28]**. Reduction of cellular viability by mycotoxins was correlated with increases of ROS generation and MDA formation in concentration and time dependent manner **[29]**. The importance of oxidative stress and LPO in mycotoxins toxicity was confirmed by the protective effects of natural antioxidants **[2]**. Sporidesmin, the mycotoxin responsible for 'facial eczema' in ruminants, contains a disulphide group which appears to be intimately involved in its toxic action. The dithiol form of sporidesmin has been shown readily to undergo autoxidation *in vitro* in a reaction which generates superoxide radical (O_2^-) **[30]**. GST found in the cytosol and microsomes catalyzes the conjugation of activated aflatoxins with GSH, leading to the excretion of aflatoxin **[31]**. Variations in the level of the GST as well as variations in the cytochrome P450 system are thought to contribute to the differences observed in interspecies aflatoxin susceptibility **[22, 32]**.

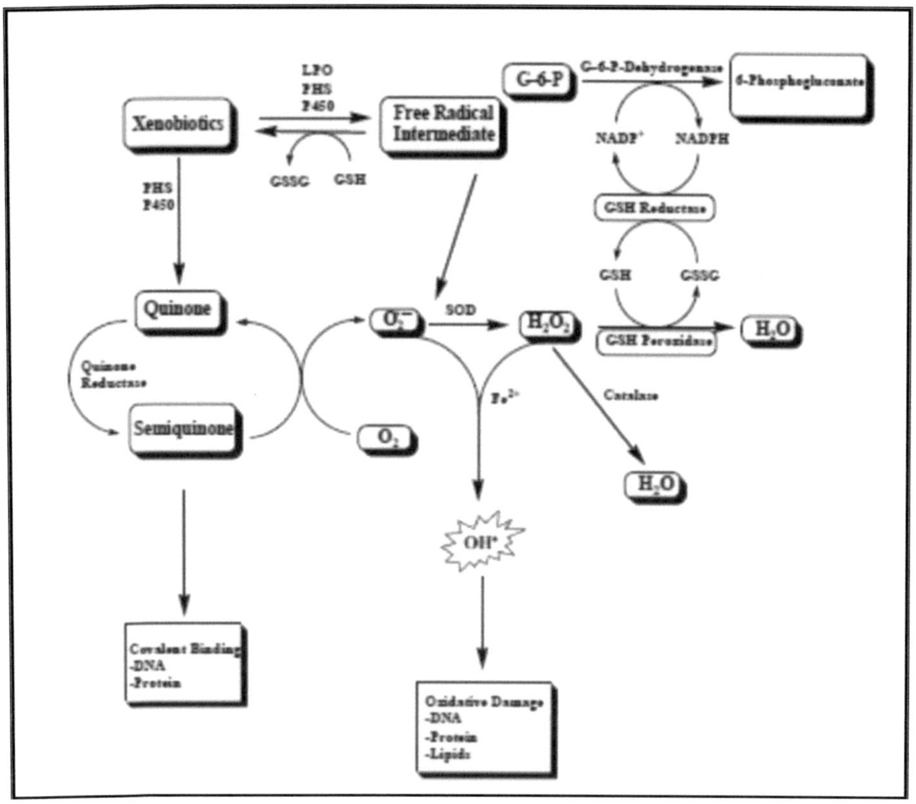

Figure 2. General pathways of ROS production and clearance **[26]**

4. Mycotoxin toxicity

The amount of mycotoxins needed to produce adverse health effects varies widely among toxins, as well as for each animal or person's immune system. Two concepts are needed to understand the negative effects of mycotoxins on human health: *Acute toxicity*, the rapid onset of an adverse effect from a single exposure. *Chronic toxicity*, the slow or delayed onset of an adverse effect, usually from multiple, long-term exposures. Mycotoxins can be acutely or chronically toxic, or both, depending on the kind of toxin and the dose. Membrane-active properties of various mycotoxins determine their toxicity. Incorporation of mycotoxins into membrane structures lead to alterations in membrane functions. In general, mycotoxins effects on DNA, RNA, protein synthesis and the pro-apoptotic action **(Fig. 3)** causing changes in physiological functions including growth, development and reproduction **[2]**. Clinicians often arrange mycotoxins by the organ they affect. Thus, mycotoxins can be classified as hepatotoxins, nephrotoxins, neurotoxins, immunotoxins, and so forth. Cell biologists put them into generic groups such as teratogens, mutagens, carcinogens, and allergens **[1]**.

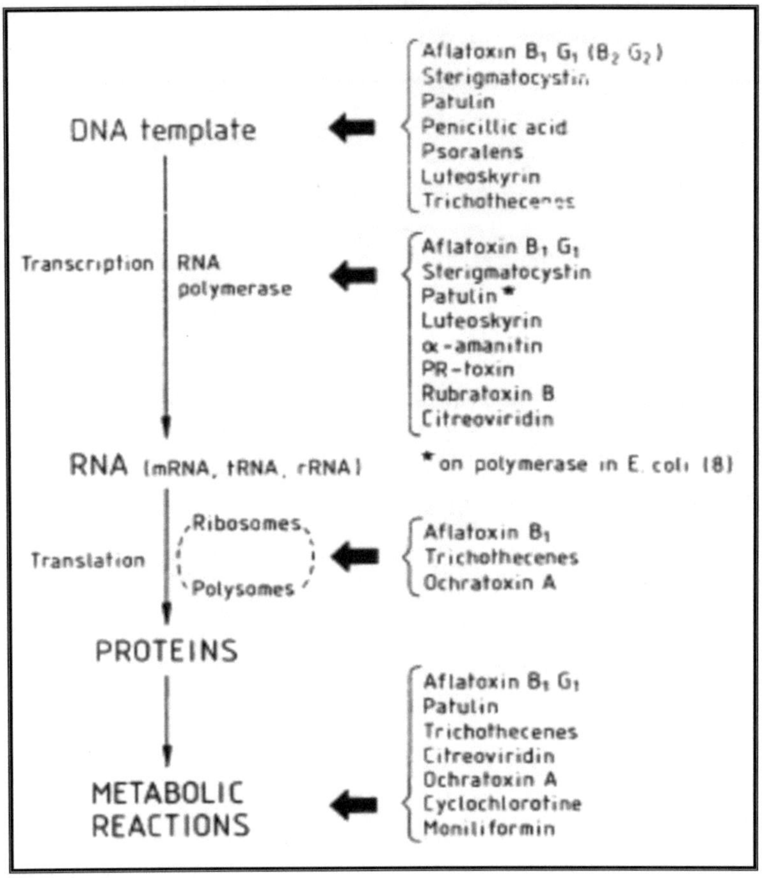

Figure 3. Mycotoxins affecting major sites in RNA and protein synthesis **[33]**

Aflatoxins

Aflatoxins occur in nuts, cereals and rice under conditions of high humidity and temperature. The two major *Aspergillus* species that produce aflatoxins are *A. flavus*, which produces only B aflatoxins, and *A. parasiticus*, which produces both B and G aflatoxins. Aflatoxins M1 and M2 are oxidative metabolic products of aflatoxins B1 and B2 produced by animals following ingestion, and so appear in milk, urine and faeces. Aflatoxicol is a reductive metabolite of aflatoxin B1. Aflatoxins are acutely toxic, immunosuppressive, mutagenic, teratogenic and carcinogenic compounds (classified as group 1 carcinogens according to the **International Agency for Research on Cancer (IARC) [34]**. Aflatoxins have been detected in the blood of pregnant women, in neonatal umbilical cord blood, and in breast milk in African countries, with significant seasonal variations **[35]**. The geographical and seasonal occurrence of aflatoxins in food and of kwashiorkor shows a remarkable similarity **[36]**. It has been hypothesized that kwashiorkor, a severe malnutrition disease, may be a form of pediatric aflatoxicosis **[37]**. Aflatoxins exposure accounts for about 40% of the load of disease in developing countries where a short lifespan is prevalent. Food systems and economics in developed country make the advance in aflatoxins management impossible **[38]**. The prevention of mycotoxins toxicity involves reduction of mycotoxin levels in foodstuffs and increasing the intake of diet components such as vitamins, antioxidants and substances known to prevent carcinogenesis **[39]**. The prevention of mycotoxin contamination of human foods could have a significant effect on public health in low-income countries due to enhanced food safety **[40]**. Chemoprotection against aflatoxins has been confirmed with the use of a number of compounds that either increase an animal's detoxification processes **[41]** or prevent the production of the epoxide that leads to cytotoxicity **[42]**. For the animal feed industries, a major focus has been on developing food additives that provide protection from the mycotoxins. One approach has been the use of esterified glucomanoses and other yeast extracts that provide chemoprotection by increasing the detoxification of aflatoxin **[41]**.

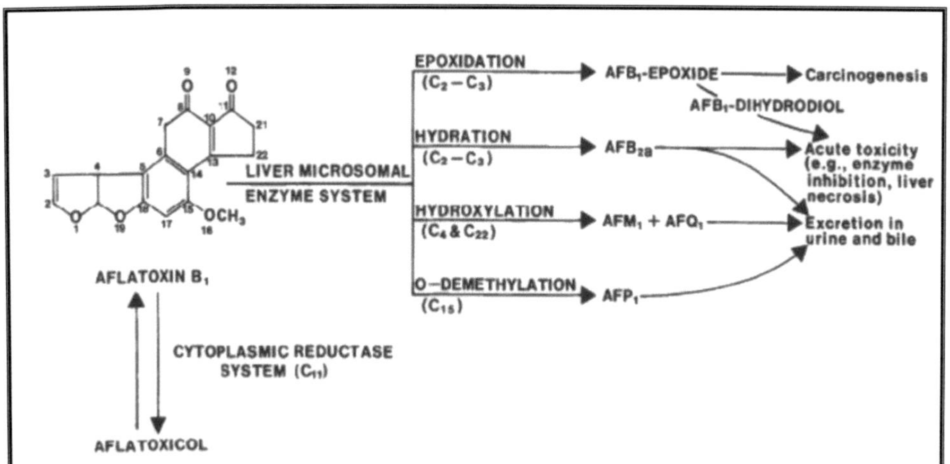

Figure 4. Metabolism of aflatoxin in liver **[46]**

After the absorption, highest concentration of the toxin is found in the liver **[43]**. Once in liver, aflatoxin B1 is metabolized by microsomal enzymes cytochrome P-450 3A4 to different metabolites through hydroxylation, hydration, demethylation and epoxidation. Variations in its catalytic activity of P-450 3A4 are important in issues of bioavailability and drug-drug interactions **[44]**. As in Fig (4) the hydroxylation of AFB1 at C4 or C22 produces, AFM1 and AFQ1, respectively. Hydration of the C2 – C3 double bond results in the formation of AFB2a which is rapidly formed in certain avian species **[45]**. AFP1 results from o-demethylation while the AFB1 – epoxide is formed by epoxidation at the 2,3 double bond Aflatoxicol is the only metabolite of AFB1 produced by a soluble cytoplasmic reductase enzyme system **[46]** .

The putative AFB1 epoxide is generally accepted as the active electrophilic form of AFB1 that may attack nucleophilic nitrogen, oxygen and sulphur heteroatoms in cellular constituents **[47]**. This highly reactive substance may combine with DNA bases such as guanine to produce alterations in DNA **[36]**. However, both humans and animals possess enzymes system, which are capable of reducing the damage to DNA and other cellular constituents caused by the 8,9-epoxide. For example GST mediates the conjugation reaction of the 8,9-epoxide to the endogenous compound GSH, this essentially neutralizes its toxic potential (**Fig. 5**). Animal species such as the mouse that are resistant to aflatoxin carcinogenesis have 3-5 times more GST activity than susceptible species such as the rat. Humans have less GST activity or 8,9-epoxide conjugation than rats or mice suggesting that humans are less capable of detoxifying this important metabolite **[48]**.

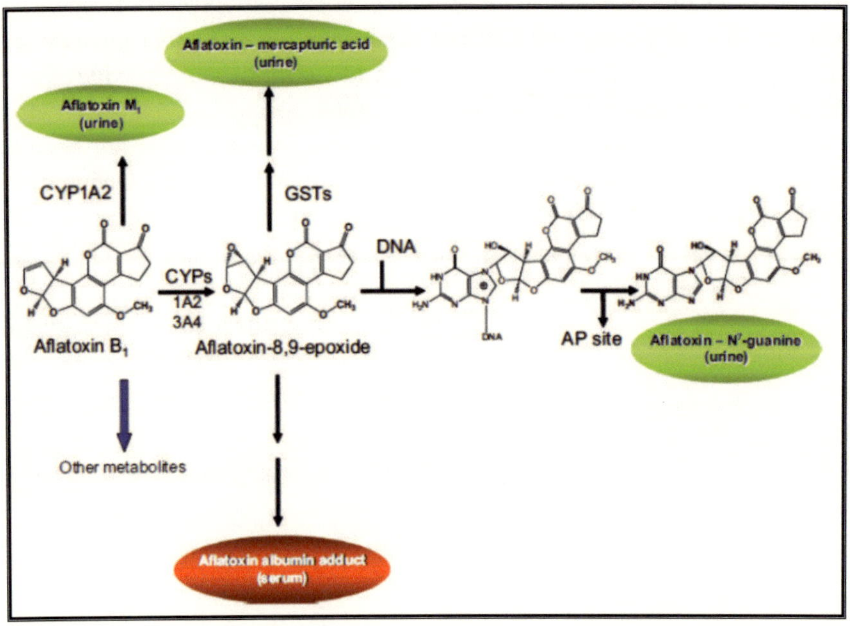

Figure 5. Biomarkers of aflatoxin exposure in an internal dose and a biologically effective dose. Biomarkers of exposure include aflatoxin M1, the internal dose includes the aflatoxin-mercapturic acid and aflatoxinalbumin adduct, and the biologically effective dose is reflected by the excretion of the aflatoxin-N7-guanine adduct formed by depurination leading to an apurinic (AP) site in DNA **[49]**.

The diseases caused by aflatoxin consumption are called aflatoxicosis. Acute aflatoxicosis results in death, however, chronic aflatoxicosis results in immune suppression and cancer **[19]**. Suppression of the cell-mediated immune response was mediated by altered cytokine expression **[50]**. Aflatoxins caused hepatotoxicity, nephrotoxicity and genotoxicity in somatic and germ cells, resulted in mitotic and meiotic delay in mice **[51]**. An increase in AFB1-8, 9-epoxide cause a significant increases in hepatic LPO level **[52]**. Peroxidation of membrane lipids initiated loss of membrane integrity; membrane bound enzyme activity and cell lysis **[53]**. LPO was significantly increased in the liver, kidney **[54]** and testis **[55]** of aflatoxin-treated mice as compared to controls. However, GSH levels declined significantly in the liver, kidney and testis after 45 days of aflatoxin treatment **[56]**. Moreover, AFB1 intake and expression of enzymes involved in AFB1 activation/detoxification may play an important role in hepatitis B virus-related hepatocarcinogenesis **[57]**. The results of a clinical trial suggest that chlorophyllin may have a role in preventing dietary exposure to aflatoxin B_1 by reducing its oral bioavailability **[58]**.

Srategies for reducing exposure and risk from aflatoxin in developing countries should be carefully tested and validated using clinical trial designs with biomarkers serving as objective endpoints. Clinical trials and other interventions are designed to translate findings from human and experimental investigations to public health prevention. Both primary (to reduce exposure) and secondary (to alter metabolism and deposition) interventions can use specific biomarkers as endpoints of efficacy. In a primary prevention trial, the goal is to reduce exposure to aflatoxins in the diet. A range of interventions includes planting pest-resistant varieties of staple crops, attempting to lower mould growth in harvested crops, improving storage methods following harvest, and using trapping agents that block the uptake of unavoidably ingested aflatoxins. In secondary prevention trials, one goal is to modulate the metabolism of ingested aflatoxin to enhance detoxification processes, thereby reducing internal dose and subsequent risk **[49] (Fig. 6)**.

Ochratoxin A (OTA)

Ochratoxins are the first major group of mycotoxins identified after the discovery of the aflatoxins **[59]**. OTA is found in a variety of plant food products such as cereals. Because of its long half life, it accumulates in the food chain **[60]**. OTA is absorbed passively throughout the gastrointestinal tract and actively in the kidneys. Highest amounts of OTA could be found in the blood and it is distributed in kidney, liver, muscle and adipose tissue in a decreasing order. The toxin is excreted primarily in the urine, and to a lesser degree in bile and also in milk. The half-life of experimentally orally ingested OTA is shorter than intravenously injected OTA **[61]**. According to IRAC **[34]** OTA is classified as group 1 carcinogens. Structure-activity studies suggested that the toxicity of OTA may be attributed to its isocoumarin moiety and lactone carbonyl group. OTA reduces the expression of several genes regulated by nuclear factor-erythroid 2 p45-related factor (Nrf2) and reduces the expression of antioxidant enzymes through inhibition of Nrf2 **[62, 63]**. OTA toxicity may be involved in the development of certain kidney diseases through generation of oxidative stress **[64]**. Chronic administration of low dose of OTA caused morphological and functional changes in proximal tubules and administration of date extract protects against OTA-induced tubule's tissue damage **[65]**. However, antioxidant treatment failed to prevent the development of OTA-induced tumors in animal models **[66]**. Indomethacin and aspirin were found to prevent OTA genotoxicity in the urinary bladder and kidney of mice **[67]**. OTA causes acute depletion of striatal dopamine and its metabolites, accompanying evidence of neural cell apoptosis in the substantia nigra, stratum and hippocampus **[68]**.

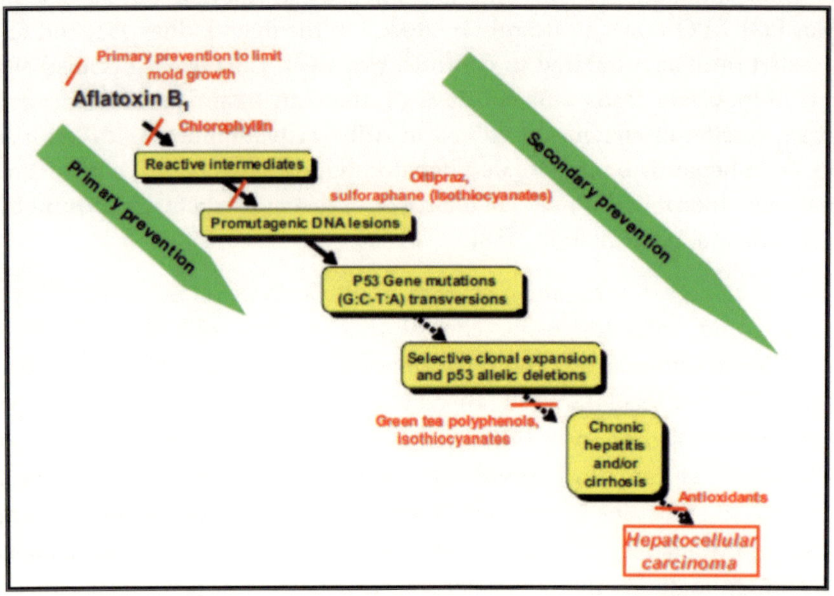

Figure 6. Strategies for reducing exposure and risk from aflatoxin in developing countries **[49]**

OTA has complex mechanisms of action that include oxidative stress, bio-energetic compromise, mitochondrial impairment, inhibition of protein synthesis, production of DNA single strand breaks and formation of OTA-DNA adducts **[69-71]**. OTA induced renal toxicity and carcinogenicity may be mediated by an Nrf2-dependent signal transduction pathway **[63]**. It is a mitochondrial poison causing mitochondrial damage, oxidative burst, LPO and interferes with oxidative phosphorylation **[72, 73]**. OTA was found to chelate ferric ions (Fe^3), facilitating their reduction to ferrous ions (Fe^2), which in the presence of oxygen, provided the active species initiating LPO **[74]**. OTA hydroquinone/ quinone couple was generated from the oxidation of OTA by electrochemical, photochemical and chemical processes resulting in redox cycling and in the generation of ROS **[75]**. OTA impairs the antioxidant defense of the cells making them more susceptible to oxidative damage **[62]** and a reduction in cellular antioxidant defense may contribute to the production of OTA-dependent oxidative damage **[76]**.

Studies carried out in several countries including Tunisia, Egypt and France, have indicated a link between dietary intake of OTA and the development of renal and urothelial tumours **[77- 81]**. OTA is known to affect the immune system in a number of mammalian species. The type of immune suppression experienced appears to be dependant on a number of factors, including the species involved, the route of administration, the doses tested, and the methods used to detect the effects **[82]**. OTA causes immunosuppression following prenatal, postnatal and adult-life exposures. These effects include reduced phagocytosis and lymphocyte markers **[83]** and increased susceptibility to bacterial infections and delayed response to immunization in piglets **[9]**. OTA induces apoptosis in a variety of cell types *in vivo* and *in vitro* that mediated through cellular processes involved in the degradation of DNA **[84]**. Moreover, the immunosuppressant activity of OTA is characterized by size reduction of vital immune organs, such as thymus, spleen, and lymph nodes, depression of antibody responses, alterations in the number and functions of immune cells, and modulation of cytokine production (TNF-α and Il-6). The immunotoxic activity of OTA probably results from degenerative changes and cell death following necrosis and apoptosis, in combination with slow replacement of affected immune cells, due to inhibition of protein synthesis **[85]**. Finally, it is proposed that a network of interacting epigenetic mechanisms, including protein synthesis inhibition, oxidative stress and the activation of specific cell signalling pathways is responsible for OTA carcinogenicity **[86] (Fig.7)**

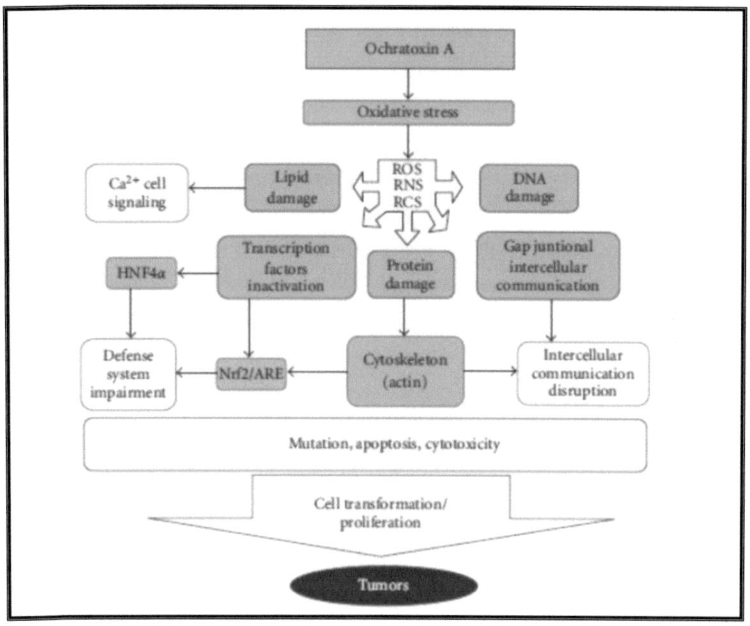

Figure 7. Scheme to illustrate the oxidative stress-mediated mode of action proposed for OTA. Increased production of ROS, RNS, and RCS is likely to originate either from direct redox reactions involving OTA or through the inhibition of cellular defenses such as through the inhibition of transcription factors as Nrf2 which regulates enzymes with antioxidant properties. The generation of radicals will induce macromolecular oxidative damage such as oxidized DNA bases which may be converted into mutation resulting into generation of transformed cells [66].

Trichothecenes

Trichothecenes (TCs) are mycotoxins produced mostly by members of the *Fusarium* genus and other genera (e.g. *Trichoderma, Trichothecium, Myrothecium* and *Stachybotrys*). By now, more than 180 different trichothecenes and trichothecene derivatives have been isolated and characterized **[87, 88]**. TCs were found in air samples collected during the drying and milling process on farms, in the ventilation systems of private houses and office buildings and on the walls of houses with high humidity **[89-90]**. They can be divided into four categories according to both their chemical properties and their producer fungi;

1. **Type A:** functional group other than a ketone at C8 position (e.g.; T-2, HT-2, DAS);
2. **Type B:** carbonyl functions at C8 position (e.g.; DON, NIV, FUS-X, 3-acetyl-deoxynivalenol, 15-acetyl-deoxynivalenol);
3. **Type C:** second epoxide group at C7, 8 or C9, 10; (e.g.; crotocin and baccharin);
4. **Type D:** macrocyclic ring system between C4 and C15 with two ester linkages (e.g.; satratoxin G, H, roridin A and verrucarin A) **[87, 91, 92]**.

TCs exposure leads to apoptosis both *in vitro* and *in vivo* in several organs such as lymphoid organs, hematopoietic tissues, liver, intestinal crypts, bone marrow and thymus **[91, 93]**. Acute high dose toxicity of TCs is characterized by diarrhea, vomiting, leukocytosis, haemorrhage, and circulatory shock and death, whereas chronic low dose toxicity is characterized by anorexia, reduced weight gain, neuroendocrine and immunologic changes **[91, 94]**. The myelotoxicity was considered highest for T-2 and HT-2 toxins and lowest for DON and NIV **[94]**. TCs are toxic to many animal species, but the sensitivity varies considerably between species and also between the different TCs **[93]**. Cellular effects on DNA and membrane integrity have been considered as secondary effects of the inhibited protein synthesis. The toxin binds to the peptidyl transferase, which is an integral part of the 60S ribosomal subunit of mammalian ribosome. TCs interfere with the metabolism of membrane phospholipids and increase liver LPO *in vivo*. Also, some TCs are shown to change the serotonin activity in the central nervous system, which is known to be related in the regulation of food intake **[88]**.

T-2 Toxin

T-2 toxin is a cytotoxic secondary fungal metabolite that belongs to TCs family produced by various species of *Fusarium* (*F. sporotichioides, F. poae, F. equiseti,* and *F. acuminatum*), which can infect corn, wheat, barley and rice crops in the field or during storage **[95]**. T-2 toxin is a well known inhibitor of protein synthesis through its high binding affinity to peptidyl transferase resulting in trigger of ribotoxic stress response that activate mitogen-activated protein kinases **[96]**. Moreover, T-2 toxin interferes with the metabolism of membrane phospholipids and increases liver LPO **[97]**. Also, T-2 toxin suppresses drug metabolizing enzymes such as GST **[98]**. T-2 toxin treated mice showed a time-dependent increase in ROS generation, depletion of GSH, increases in LPO and protein carbonyl content in the brain. Moreover, the gene expression profile of antioxidant enzymes showed a significant increase in SOD and CAT via the dermal route and GR and GPx via the subcutaneous route **[99]**. General signs of T-2 include nausea, emesis, dizziness, chills, abdominal pain, diarrhea, dermal necrosis, abortion, irreversible damage to the bone marrow, reduction in white blood cells and inhibition of protein synthesis **[100, 101]**. Moreover, the effects of T-2 toxins on the immune system include changes in leukocyte counts, delayed hypersensitivity, depletion of selective blood cell progenitors, depressed antibody formation and allograft rejection **[39]**. Also, T-2 toxin has a direct lytic effect on erythrocytes **[102]**. T-2 toxin can induce apoptosis in many types of cells bearing rapid rates of proliferation **[103]** and increased the expression of both oxidative stress and apoptosis related genes in hepatocytes of mice **[104]**. T-2 toxin induces neuronal cell apoptosis in the fetal and adult brain **[68]**. In this aspect, it suggested that dysfunction of the mitochondria and oxidative stress might be the main factor behind the T-2 toxin-induced apoptosis in the fetal brain **[105]**. ROS activate caspase-2 which play a crucial role in the control of apoptosis **[106, 107]**. Moreover, it was demonstrated that T-2 toxin induced cytotoxicity in HeLa cells is mediated by generation of ROS leading to DNA damage and trans activation of p53 protein expression which leads to shift in the ratio of Bax/Bcl-2 in favour of apoptosis and subsequent release of Cyt-c from mitochondria followed by caspase cascade **[99]**.

Fumonisins

Fumonisins produced by the fungus *Fusarium verticillioides*, a widespread fungal contaminants of various cereals, predominantly corn **[2, 108]**. Fumonisn B1 (FB1) and B2 are of toxicological significance, while the others (B3, B4, A1 and A2) occur in very low concentrations and are less toxic **[3]**. FB1 is poorly absorbed and rapidly eliminated in feces. Minor amounts are retained in liver and kidneys. FB1 does not cross the placenta and is not teratogenic *in vivo* in rats, mice, or rabbits, but is embryotoxic at high, maternally toxic doses **[109]**. FB1 has been linked to a number of diseases in humans and animals **[1, 40]**. FB1 increases oxidative DNA damage, as measured by increased DNA strand breaks and malondialdehyde adducts in rat liver and kidney *in vivo* **[111]**. As shown in Fig. (9) an alternative mechanism of action of FB1 involves the disruption of the de novo sphingolipid biosynthesis pathway by inhibition of the enzyme ceramide synthase **[68, 112]**. The inhibition of sphingolipid biosynthesis disrupts numerous cell functions and signaling pathways, including apoptosis and mitosis, thus potentially contributing to carcinogenesis through an altered balance of cell death and replication **[113]**. Disruption of sphingolipid metabolism leads to changes in the sphinganine to sphingosine ratio **[114]** as demonstrated in rat liver and mouse kidney at carcinogenic doses of FB1 **[115]**.

FB1-induced DNA damage and hepatocarcinogenesis in experimental models can be modulated by a variety of factors including nutrients, chemopreventive agents, and other factors such as food restriction and viral infection, as well as genetic polymorphisms **[118]**. In rat C6 glioma cells, FB1 inhibits protein synthesis, causes DNA fragmentation and cell death, increases 8-hydroxy-2'-deoxyguanosine, induces LPO, and cell cycle arrest **[119]**. Also, the signs of apoptosis were increased caspase-3 like protease activity and internucleosomal DNA fragmentation **[120]**. Furthermore, the disruption of membrane structure, the enhancement of membrane endocytosis, and the increase in membrane permeability caused by FB1 in macrophages provide additional insight into potential mechanisms by which the fumonisins might enhance oxidative stress and cellular damage **[121]**.

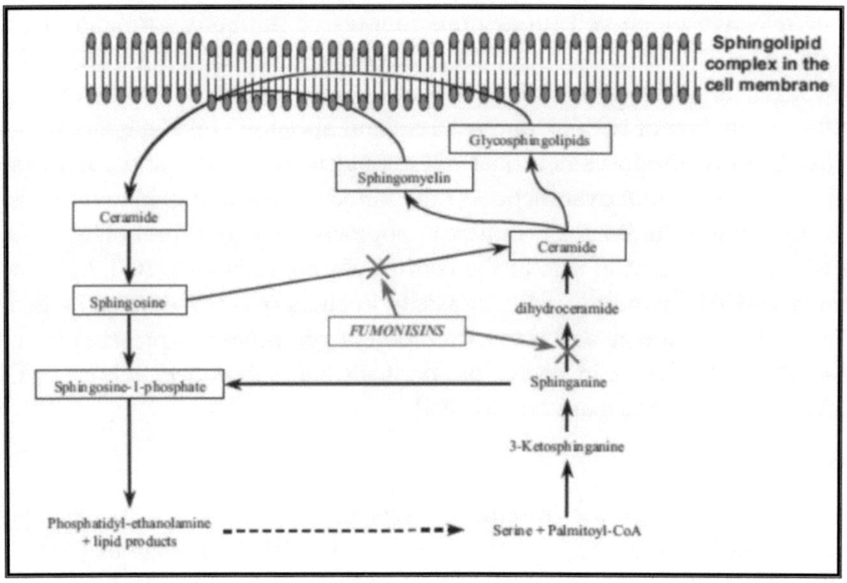

Figure 8. Pathway of de novo synthesis (not in boxes) and turnover of sphingolipids (boxed) in animal cells, and their inhibition by fumonisins. Fumonisns inhibit the synthesis of ceramides by specifically binding to sphingosine and sphinganine **[116, 117]**

Zearalenone

Zearalenone (ZEA) is produced mainly by *Fusarium graminearum* and related species, principally in wheat and maize. ZEA and its derivatives produce estrogenic effects in various animal species **[3].** The structure of the ZEA similar to steroids and binds to ER as an agonist. There are two major biotrasformation pathways for ZEA in animals (1) hydroxylation catalyzed by 3α- and 3β- hydroxysteroid dehydrogenase (HSDs) resulting in the formation of α- and β-ZOL; (2) conjugation of ZEA and its metabolites with glucuronic acid, catalyzed by uridine diphosphate glucuronyl transferase. Consequently, ZEA is a substrate for 3α-HSD and 3β-HSD present in many steroidogenic tissues, such as liver, kidney, testis, prostate, hypothalamus, pituitary, ovary, intestine **[122, 123]**. The adverse effects of ZEA are partly determined by the processes of elimination, because the biliary excretion and entero-hepatic cycling are important processes affecting the fate of ZEA and explaining a different sensitivity between animals **[124]**. α and β Zearalenol metabolites caused cytotoxicity by inhibiting cell viability, protein and DNA syntheses and inducing oxidative damage and over-expression of stress proteins. However, the ZEA metabolites exhibited lower toxicity than ZEA, with β zearalenol being the more active of the two metabolites **[125].** In addition, oxidative damage is likely to be evoked as one of the main pathways of ZEA toxicity which may initiate event at least in part contribute to the mechanism of ZEA induced genotoxic and cytotoxic effects **[126].** ZEA and its derivatives compete effectively with 17 β-E2 for the specific binding sites of the oestrogen receptors (ERs) occurring in different organs. Two subtypes of ER exist, ER-α and ERβ that are differently distributed in the body. Binding of ZEA and its derivatives initiate a sequence of events known to follow estrogen stimulation of target organs **[127, 128]**. So, the effect of ZEA and its metabolites depends upon the reproductive status (prepubertal, cycling or pregnant) of the affect animals **[123]**. ZEA do not induce apoptosis in porcine ovaries **[129]**, however, apoptosis is the principal mechanism contributing to germ cell depletion and testicular atrophy following ZEA exposure **[130]**. Moreover, ZEA has potent effects on the expression of chicken splenic lymphocytes cytokines at the mRNA level **[131]**.

Patulin

Patulin (PAT) is a toxic chemical contaminant produced by several species of mould, especially within *Aspergillus, Penicillium* and *Byssochlamys*. It is the most common mycotoxin found in apples and apple-derived products such as juice, cider, compotes and other food intended for young children. Exposure to this mycotoxin is associated with immunological, neurological and gastrointestinal outcomes **[132]**. PAT-induced nephropathy and gastrointestinal tract malfunction have been demonstrated in animal models **[133]**. The toxic effects of PAT on various cells related to its activity on SH groups **[134]**. Moreover, it suggested that PAT-induced apoptosis is mediated through the mitochondrial pathway without the involvement of p53 **[12]**. The interaction with sulfhydryl groups of macromolecules by PAT and the subsequent generation of ROS plays a primary role in the apoptotic process. The genotoxic effects might be related to its ability to react with sulfhydryl groups and to induce oxidative damage **[135]**. PAT was found to reduce the cytokine secretion of IFN-γ and IL-4 by human macrophages **[136]** and of IL-4, IL-13, IFN-γ, and IL-10 by human peripheral blood mononuclear cells and human T cells **[137]**. The clinical signs of PAT toxicosis are typical of the nervous syndrome. Animals present hyperaesthesia, lack of coordination of motor organs, problems with ingestion and digestion. At the molecular level, PAT alters ion permeability and/or intracellular communication, causing oxidative stress and cell death **(116)**.

Citrinin

Citrinin is a toxic metabolite produced by several filamentous fungi of the genera *Penicillium, Aspergillus* and *Monascus*, which has been encountered as a natural contaminant in grains, foods, feedstuffs, as well as biological fluids. Some analytical systems have been developed for its detection and quantification **[138]**. As one of mycotoxins, citrinin possesses antibiotic, bacteriostatic, antifungal and antiprotozoal properties. While it is also known as a hepato-nephrotoxin in a wide range of species **[139]**, *in vitro* studies have demonstrated that citrinin produced multiple effects on renal mitochondrial function and macromolecule biosynthesis that ultimately resulted in cell death **[140]**. Citrinin inhibited the oxygen consumption rate by about 45 % and inhibited the glucose utilization of BHK-21 cells by about 86 % due to alterations in mitochondrial function and in the glycolytic anaerobic pathway **[141]**. Citrinin occurred frequently together with another nephrotoxin–ochratoxin A in foodstuffs such as cereals, fruits, meat **[142]** and cheese **[143]**. Citrinin can act synergistically with ochratoxin A to depress RNA synthesis in murine kidneys **[144, 145]**. The simultaneous exposure of rabbits to citrinin with OTA even at sub-clinical dietary levels potentiated the OTA induced nephrotoxicity at ultrastructural level **[146]**. To avoid the direct/indirect intake of citrinin, it is important to develop detoxification methods for citrinin during food processing. So far, there have been several reports on the detoxification of citrinin. The investigation on thermal decomposition and detoxification showed that, in the presence of a small amount of water, heating citrinin at 130ºC caused a significant decrease in its toxicity to Hela cells **[147]**; whereas heating at 150ºC in water caused formation of highly toxic compounds **[148]**.

Ergot Alkaloids

The ergot alkaloids are among the most fascinating of fungal metabolites. They are classified as indole alkaloids and are derived from a tetracyclic ergoline ring system **[149]**. These compounds are produced as a toxic cocktail of alkaloids in the sclerotia of species of *Claviceps*, which are common pathogens of various grass species. Ergotism is still an important veterinarian problem. The principal animals at risk are cattle, sheep, pigs, and chickens. Clinical symptoms of ergotism in animals include gangrene, abortion, convulsions, suppression of lactation and hypersensitivity **[150]**. More recently, pure ergotamine has been used for the treatment of migraine headaches. Other ergot derivatives are used as prolactin inhibitors, in the treatment of Parkinsonism, and in cases of cerebrovascular insufficiency [**149]**. The therapeutic administration of ergot alkaloids may cause sporadic cases of human ergotism **[151]**. Ergotism is extremely rare today, primarily because the normal grain cleaning and milling processes remove most of the ergot so that only very low levels of alkaloids remain in the resultant flours. In addition, the alkaloids that are the causative agents of ergotism are relatively labile and are usually destroyed during baking and cooking **[3]**.

Satratoxin G

Satratoxin G is one of the most potent macrocylclic TCs produced by *Stachybotrys chartarum* **[152]**. Roridin A is a commercially available macrocyclic TC used as a stratoxin G substitute, and roridin L2 is a putative biosynthetic precursor of satratoxin **[153]**. Satratoxin G is potent inhibitors of eukaryotic translation that are potentially immunosuppressive. It rapidly binds small and large ribosomal subunits in a concentration- and time-dependent manner that was consistent with induction of apoptosis **[154]**. A signal transduction pathway in satratoxin-induced apoptosis in HL-60 cells involves, caspase-3 activation through activation of both caspase-8 and caspase-9 along with cytosolic release of cytochrome c and fragmentation of nucleosomal DNA by DFF-40/CAD **[155]**.

Roridin E

Roridin E is a well-known macrocyclic trichothecene mycotoxin possessing potent anti-proliferative activity against cancer cell lines **[156]**. Four new isolated from a marine-derived fungus, *Myrothecium roridum* strain 98F42 **[157]**. One of them, 12-deoxy derivative of roridin E, showed reduced cytotoxicity about 80-fold less than that of roridin E against human promyelocytic (HL-60) and murine leukemia (L1210) cell lines **[158]**. Treatment of rats with roridin E caused minimal toxicity on the hepatic and renal tissue, however, co administration of linoleic acid with roridin E resulted in increase toxicity due to increased incorporation to the cell membrane or inhibit its biotransformation **[159]**.

5. Mmycotoxins and apoptosis

Apoptosis is a process for maintenance of tissue homeostasis. Several processes, such as initiation of death signals at the plasma membrane, expression of pro-apoptotic oncoproteins, activation of death proteases and endonucleases combine to cause cell termination. ROS may play a major role in apoptosis. GSH depletion increases the % of apoptotic cells **[160]**. In general, apoptosis is considered as a common mechanism of toxicity of various mycotoxins **[68]**. TCs induce apoptosis response via mitochondrial and non-mitochondrial mechanisms **[161]**. The amphophilic nature of TCs facilitates their cytotoxic effect on cell membranes and inside the cell interact with ribosome and mitochondria causing inhibition of protein synthesis **[162]**. FB_1 and OTA are able to induce apoptosis and necrosis in porcine kidney PK15 cells **[163]**. This is because the structure of FB_1 resembles sphingoid bases which regulate cell growth, differentiation, transformation and apoptosis, and so it is not surprising that FB_1 can alter growth of certain mammalian cells. The involvement of the TNF signal transduction pathway in FB1 induced apoptosis in African green monkey kidney fibroblasts has been shown **[164]**. Moreover, TNF-α production is responsible for FB1 induced apoptosis in mice primary hepatocytes **[165]**. Over expression of cytochrome P450-sensitized hepatocyte to TNFα-mediated cell death was associated with increased LPO and GSH depletion **[166]**. FB1 was reported to increase induction of cytochrome P450 isoforms and caused peroxidation of membrane lipids in isolated rat liver nuclei as well as GSH depletion of in pig kidney cells **[167-169]**. GSH depletion is known to activate c-Jun N-terminal kinase through redox inhibition of GST, which normally binds to and inhibits stress kinases **[170]**. Stimulation of apoptosis and necrosis in porcine granulosa cells by ZEA is dose-dependent manner via a caspase-3- and caspase-9-dependent mitochondrial pathway **[171]**. At the molecular level, fumonisins inhibit ceramide synthase and disrupt sphingolipid metabolism therefore influence apoptosis and mitosis **[109]**. The immunotoxic activity of OTA probably results from degenerative changes and cell death following necrosis and apoptosis in combination with slow replacement of affected immune cells due to inhibition of protein synthesis **[85]**. Moreover, PAT induce DNA damage and cell cycle arrest along with intrinsic pathway mediated apoptosis which may have dermal toxicological implications **[172]**.

Satratoxin H is thought to induce apoptosis of PC12 cells through the activation of p38 mitogen activated protein kinase and c-Jun N-terminal kinase in GSH-sensitive manner **[173]**. Chemoprotective effects of flavonoid compounds against aflatoxins were confirmed in hens **[174]**. Moreover, cysteine and GSH has protective effect against PAT in the incident of rumen microbial ecosystem, however vitamin C and ferulic acid did not demonstrate an effect **[175]**. Metallothioneins (MTs) are four major isoforms found in cytoplasm, lysosomes, mitochondria and nuclei of mammalian cells **[176]**. MT-1 and 2 have ubiquitous tissue distribution particularly in liver, pancreas, intestine, and kidney, whereas MT-3 is found in brain and MT-4 in skin **[177]**. MT can play important role in the process of mycotoxins detoxification probably by redistribution of significant ions to transcriptional factors and interactions with oxygen radicals that may be generated by mycotoxins **[23]**. Nivalenol, a trichothecene mycotoxin induces apoptosis in HL60 cells and that intracellular calcium ion plays a role in the nivalenol-induced secretion of IL-8 from this cell line **[178]**.

6. Mycotoxins as therapeutics compound

Cumulative knowledge about toxins structure and mechanism of action, as well as recent progress in the fields of cell biology, immunology, molecular biology and nanotechnology, enabled the development of different targeting strategies that are vital for converting a lethal toxin into a therapeutic agent. **Fig. 9** showed three targeting strategies in toxin based therapy. i- Ligand targeted toxins upon administration to patients are internalized and intoxicate diseased cells, sparing healthy cells that do not display the target on their surface. ii- protease activated toxins: the toxin is engineered to be cleaved and activated by a disease-related intracellular or extracellular protease. Toxin cleavage may enhance cell-binding and/or translocation, stabilization or catalytic activity of the toxic moiety specifically in protease expressing cells, leading to their suppression. iii- toxin based suicide gene therapy: a DNA construct, encoding for a toxic polypeptide whose expression is regulated by a specific transcription regulation element, is delivered to a heterogeneous cell population **[179]**.

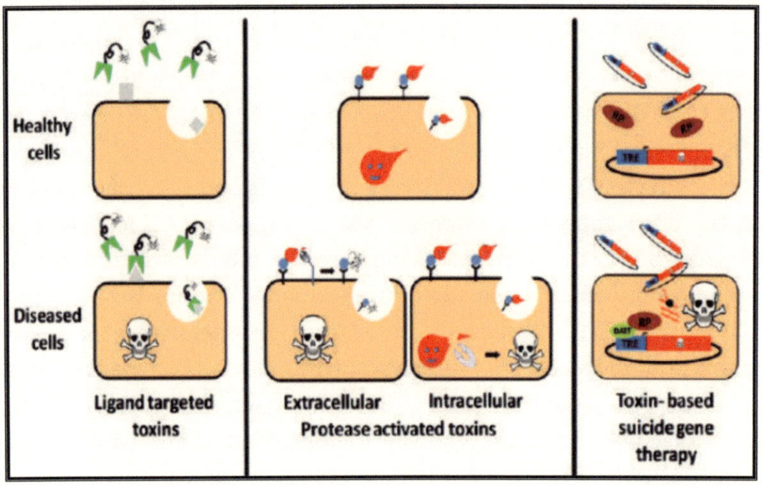

Figure 9. Three targeting strategies in toxin based therapy **[179]**.

Because of their pharmacological activity, some mycotoxins or mycotoxin derivatives have found use as antibiotics, growth promoters, and other kinds of drugs. Ergocryptine is an ergot alkaloid that affects dopaminergic activity principally by interacting with D2-type receptors **[180]**. The bromation derivative has increased dopamine agonist activity, and is used against Parkinsonism and to reduce growth hormone secretion and milk production **[181]**. Ergotamine was among the most effective available agents for relieving migraine attacks **[182]**. Ergometrine and the semi-synthetic methylergometrine have been widely used for the prevention and treatment of excessive uterine bleeding following birth and also to initiate delivery **[183]**. Lysergic acid diethylamide is a serotonin receptor agonist **[184]** and can also interact with dopamine receptors to make it a useful tool for probing the biochemical basis for behaviour **[185]**. Methysergide a semi-synthetic ergot alkaloid is a serotonin antagonist used in the treatment of migraine and is used for daily preventive therapy rather than in acute cases **[184]**. The TCs have been associated with various biological properties, such as antiviral especially as inhibitors of the replication of Herpes, antibiotic, antimalarial, antileukemic and immunotoxic **[59,186]**. Mycoestrogenic zearalenone is suspected to be a triggering factor for central precocious puberty development in girls. Due to its chemical resemblance to some anabolic agents used in animal breeding, ZEA may also represent a growth promoter in exposed patients **[187]**. Development of cyclosporine A as immunosuppressive drug has been traced back to the stimulus derived from the first highly-active cyclopeptides from *Amantia mushrooms* **[188]**.

7. Conclusion

Mycotoxins are produced in a strain-specific way, and elicit some complicated and overlapping toxigenic activities in sensitive species that include carcinogenicity, inhibition of protein synthesis, immunosuppression, dermal irritation, and other metabolic perturbations. Mycotoxins usually enter the body via ingestion of contaminated foods, but inhalation of toxigenic spores and direct dermal contact are also important routes. There is sufficient evidence from animal models and human epidemiological data to conclude that mycotoxins pose an important danger to human and animal health. Trichothecenes cause protein synthesis inhibition via binding to the 18s rRNA of the ribosomal large subunit as a major mechanism underlying induction of cell apoptosis. T-2 toxin triggers a ribotoxic response through its high binding affinity to peptidyl transferase which is an integral part of the 60 s ribosomal subunit and interferes with the metabolism of membrane phospholipids and increases liver lipid peroxides. SH is thought to induce caspase-3 activation and apoptosis through the activation of MAPK and JNK in a GSH-sensitive manner. FB_1-induced inhibition of ceramide synthesis can result in a wide spectrum of changes in lipid metabolism and associated lipid-dependent pathways. OTA has complex mechanisms of action that include mitochondrial impairment, formation of OTA-DNA adducts and induction of oxidative stress and apoptosis through caspase activation. Accordingly, the strict control of food quality, in both industrialized and developing countries, is therefore necessary to avoid mycotoxicosis.

Author details

Hossam El-Din M. Omar
Zoology Department, Faculty of Science, Assiut University, Egypt

8. References

[1] Bennett JW, Klich M. Mycotoxins. Clinical Microbiology Reviews 2003; 16 (3): 497–516.
[2] Surai PF, Mezes M, Melnichuk SD, Fotina TI. Mycotoxins and animal health: From oxidative stress to gene expression. *Krmiva 2008; 50*: 35–43.
[3] Peraica M, Radic B, Lucic A, Pavlovic M. Toxic effects of mycotoxins in humans. Bull. WHO 1999; 77:754–766.

[4] EFSA (2009): Annual Report of European Food Safety Authority, ISBN: 978-92-9199-211-9 doi:10.2805/3682.

[5] Reverberi M, Ricelli A, Zjalic S, Fabbri AA, Fanelli C. Natural functions of mycotoxins and control of their biosynthesis in fungi. Appl Microbiol Biotechnol 2010; 87:899–911.

[6] Fink-Grenmels J, Georgiou NA. Risk assesment of mycotoxins for the consumer. In: Ennen G, Kuiper HA, Valentin A, eds. Residues of Veterinary Drugs and Mycotoxins in Animal Products. NL-Wageningen Press 1996 p 159-74.

[7] Fink-Grenmels, J . Mycotoxins: Their implications for human and animal health. Veterinary Quarterly 1999; 21(4):115-120.

[8] Bryden WL.Mycotoxins in the food chain: human health implications. Asia Pac J Clin Nutr 2007; 16(1):95-101.

[9] Stoev S, Denev S, Dutton M, Nkosi B. Cytotoxic effect of some mycotoxins and their combinations on human peripheral blood mononuclear cells as measured by the MTT assay. The Open Toxinology Journal 209; 2: 1-8.

[10] Henry SH, Bosch FX, Troxell TC, Bolger PM. Reducing liver cancer-global control of aflatoxin. Science 1999; 286:2453–2454.

[11] Binder EM, Tan LM, Chin LJ, Handl J, Richard J. Worldwide occurrence of mycotoxins in commodities, feeds and feed ingredients. Animal Feed Science and Technology,2007; 137: 265–282.

[12] Wu TS, Liao YC, Yub FY, Chang CH, Liu BH. Mechanism of patulin-induced apoptosis in human leukemia cells (HL-60). Toxicology Letters 2008; 183:105–111.

[13] CAST Report. Mycotoxins: risks in plant, animal, and human systems. In: J.L. Richard, G.A. Payne (Eds.), Council for Agricultural Science and Technology Task Force Report 2003; No. 139, Ames, Iowa, USA. ISBN 1-887383-22-0.

[14] Wu F. Mycotoxins risk assessment for the purpose of setting International Regulatory Standards. Environ. Sci. Technol. 2004; 38 (15): 4049–4055.

[15] Afifi MM, Abdel-Mallek AY, El-Shanawany AA, Khattab SMR .Fangal populations and myctotoxins of wheat grains imported to Egypt. Ass.Univ. Bull.Envir. Res.2012; 15(1):31-52.

[16] D'mello, JPE, Macdonald AMC. Mycotoxins. Animal Food Sci. Technol. 1997; 69, 155-166.

[17] Peraica M, Domijan AM. Contamination of food with mycotoxins and human health. Arh. Hig. Rada. Toksikol. 2001; 52: 23–35.

[18] Boutrif E, Bessy C. Global significance of mycotoxins and phycotoxins. In: *Mycotoxins and phycotoxins in perspective at the turn of the millennium*. Koe, W.J., Samson, R.A., van Egmond, H.P., Gilbert, J. and Sabino, M. (eds.). Ponsen and Looyen, Wageningen, The Netherlands 2001,p. 3-16.

[19] Hsieh D . Potential human health hazards of mycotoxins. In: Natori S, Hashimoto K, Ueno Y (Eds.). Mycotoxins and Phytotoxins. Third Joint Food and Agriculture Organization/ W.H.O./United Nations Environment Program International Conference of Mycotoxins. Elsevier, Amsterdam, The Netherlands 1988; p. 69-80.

[20] Kemppainen RJ, Thompson FN, Lorenz MD, Munnell JF, Chakraborty PK. Effects of prednisone on thyroidal and gonadal endocrine function in dogs. *Journal of Endocrinology,* 1983; 96:293-302.

[21] Upadhaya SD, Park MA, Ha JK. Mycotoxins and Their Biotransformation in the Rumen. A review. Asian-Aust. J. Anim. Sci.2010; 23 (9): 1250-1260.

[22] Eaton DL, Groopman DJ, ed.; 1994). The toxicology of aflatoxins: human health, veterinary, and agricultural significance. Academic Press, San Diego, Calif.

[23] Vasatkova A, Krizova S, Adam V, Zeman L, Kizek R. Changes in metallothionein level in rat hepatic tissue after administration of natural mouldy wheat. Int. J. Mol. Sci., 2009; 10: 1138-1160.

[24] Devasagayam TPA, Tilak JC, Boloor KK, Sane Ketaki S, Ghaskadbi Saroj S, Lele RD ."Free Radicals and Antioxidants in Human Health: Current Status and Future Prospects". *Journal of Association of Physicians of India 2004;* 52: 796.

[25] Sies H. Oxidative stress: from basic research to clinical application. *Am. J. Med.*, 1991; *91*: 31S–38S.

[26] Tafazoli, S. Mechanisms of drug-induced oxidative stress in the hepatocyte inflammation model, Doctor of Philosophy, Department of Pharmaceutical Sciences, University of Toronto, 2008.

[27] Halliwell B, Gutteridge JMC. Free Radicals in Biology and Medicine. Fourth Edition, Oxford University Press, Oxford, UK, 2007.

[28] Halliwell B, Gutteridge JMC. *Free Radicals in Biology and Medicine*, 3rd ed.; Oxford University Press: New York, NY, USA, 1999.

[29] Ferrer E, Juan-Garcia A, Font G, Ruiz MG. Reactive oxygen species induced by beauvericin, patulin and zearalenone in CHO-K1 cells. Toxicology *in Vitro;* 2009, 23: 1504–1509

[30] Munday R. Studies on the mechanism of toxicity of the mycotoxin, sporidesmin. I. Generation of superoxide radical by sporidesmin.Chemico-Biological Interactions; 1982, 41(3): 361-374.

[31] Raj HG, Prasanna HR, Mage PN, Lotlikar PD. Effect of purified rat and hamster hepatic glutathione S-transferases on the microsome mediated binding of aflatoxin B1 to DNA. Cancer Lett.; 1986, 33:1–9.

[32] Eaton DL, Ramsdel HS. Species and diet related differences in aflatoxin biotransformation, p. 157–182. *In* D. Bhatnagar, E. B. Lillehoj, and D.K. Arora (ed.), Handbook of applied mycology, vol. 5, mycotoxins in ecological systems. Marcel Dekker, Inc., New York, N.Y.;1992.

[33] Kiessling KH. Biochemical mechanism of action of mycotoxins. Pure & Appl. Chem.;1986, 58(2): 327-338.

[34] IARC. Overall evaluations of carcinogenicity: an updating of IARC Monographs volumes 1 to 42. Report of an IARC Expert Committee. Lyon, International Agency for Research on Cancer, 1987 (IARC Monographs on the Evaluation of Carcinogenic Risks to Humans, Supplement 7).

[35] Maxwell SM, Apeagyei F, de Vries HR, Mwanmut DD, Hendrickse RG. Aflatoxins in breast milk, neonatal cord blood and sera of pregnant women. J. Toxicol. Toxin. Rev.; 1989, 8: 19-29.

[36] Hendrickse RG. Kwashiorkor: the hypothesis that incriminates aflatoxins. Pediatrics; 1991, 88: 376-379.

[37] Hendrickse RG. Of sick turkeys, kwashiorkor, malaria, perinatal mortality, heroin addicts and food poisoning: research on the influence of aflatoxins on child health in the tropics. Ann. Trop. Med. Parasitol.; 1997, 91:787– 793.

[38] Williams JH, Phillips TD, Jolly PE, Stiles JK, Jolly CM, Aggarwal D. Human aflatoxicosis in developing countries: a review of toxicology, exposure, potential health consequences, and interventions. Am.J.Clin.Nutr.; 2004, 80:1106-1122.

[39] Creppy EE. Update of survey, regulation and toxic effects of mycotoxins in Europe. Toxicology Letters; 2002, 127: 9–28.

[40] Murphy PA, Hendrich S, Landgren C, Bryant CM. Food mycotoxins: an update. Journal of Food Science; 2005, 71: 52-R65.

[41] Kensler TW, Davis EF, Bolton MG. Strategies for chemoprotection against aflatoxin-induced liver cancer. In: Eaton D, Groopman JD, eds. The toxicology of aflatoxins:humanhealth, veterinary, and agricultural significance. London: Academic Press; 1993, p. 281–306.

[42] Hayes JD, Pulford DJ, Ellis EM, McLeod R, James RF, Seidegard J. Regulation of rat glutathione S-transferase A5 by cancer chemopreventive agents: mechanisms of inducible resistance to aflatoxin B1. Chem Biol Interact; 1998, 112:51–67.

[43] Mintzlaff HJ, Lotzsch R, Tauchmann F, Meyer W, Leistner L. Aflatoxin residues in the liver of broiler chicken given aflatoxin-containing feed. Fleischwirtschaft; 1974, 54: 774-778.

[44] Guengerich FP. Cytochrome P450s and other enzymes in drug metabolism and toxicity. *The AAPS Journal* ; 2006, 8 (1) Article 12 (http://www.aapsj.org).*pp.E101-E110.*

[45] Patterson DSP, Allcroft R. Metabolism of aflatoxins in susceptible and resistant animal species. Fd. Cosmet. Toxicol 1970, 8: 43.

[46] Dhanasekaran D, Shanmugapriya S, Thajuddin N Panneerselvam A. Aflatoxins and aflatoxicosis in human and animals. In aflatoxins - biochemistry and molecular biology, Guevara-Gonzalez, R.G. (editor), ISBN 978-953-307-395-8, InTech, Published, 2011, PP.221-254.

[47] Guengerich FP, Johnsen WW, Ueng YF, Yamazaki H, Shimada T. Involvement of cytochrome P450, glutathione S-transferase and epoxide hydrolase in the metabolism of aflatoxin B1 and relevance to risk of human liver cancer. Environ Health Persp, 1996, 104: 557-562.

[48] Verma RJ. Aflatoxin Cause DNA Damage. Int J Hum Genet; 2004, 4(4): 231-236.

[49] Groopman JD, Thomas W, Kensler TW, Wild CP. Protective interventions to prevent aflatoxin-induced carcinogenesis in developing countries. Annu. Rev. Public Health; 2008, 29:187–203.

[50] Meissonnier GM, Pinton P, Laffitte J, Cossalter AM, Gong YY, Wild CP, Bertin G, Galtier P, Oswald I. Immunotoxicity of aflatoxin B1: impairment of the cell-mediated response to vaccine antigen and modulation of cytokine expression. Toxicol. Appl. Pharmacol.; 2008, 231, 142–149.

[51] Deabes MM, Darwish HR, Abdel-Aziz KB, Farag IM, Nada SA, Tawfek N S. Protective effects of *Lactobacillus rhamnosus GG* on aflatoxins-induced toxicities in male albino mice. J Environment Analytic Toxicol.; 2012, 2:132. doi:10.4172/2161-0525.1000132.

[52] Toskulkao C, Taycharpipranai S, Glinsukon T. Enhanced hepatotoxicity of aflatoxin B1 by pretreatment of rats with ethanol. Res Comm Chem Pathol Pharmacol; 1982, 36: 477-482.

[53] Toskulkao C, Glinsukon T. Hepatic lipid peroxidation and intracellular calcium accumulation in ethanol potentiated aflatoxin B1 toxicity. J Pharmacobio Dyn, 1988, 11:191-197.

[54] Verma RJ, Nair A. Vitamin E prevents aflatoxin induced lipid peroxidation in liver and kidney. Med Sci Res; 1999, 27: 223.

[55] Verma RJ, Nair A. Ameliorative effect of vitamin E on aflatoxin-induced lipid peroxidation in the testis of mice. Asian J Androl; 2001, 3: 217.

[56] Patel JW. Stimulation of cyclophosphamide induced pulmonary microsomal lipid peroxidation by oxygen. Toxicology; 1987, 45: 71.

[57] Yu MW, Lien JP, Chiu YH, Santella RM, Liaw YF, Cher CJ. Effect of aflatoxin metabolism and DNA adduct formation on hepatocellular carcinoma among chronic hepatitis B carriers in Taiwan. Journal of Hepatology; 1991, 27: 320-330.

[58] Sudakin DL. Dietary Aflatoxin Exposure and Chemoprevention of Cancer: A Clinical Review. Clinical Toxicology; 2003, 41(2):195-204.

[59] Bra¨se S, Encinas A, Keck J, Nising CF. Chemistry and Biology of Mycotoxins and Related Fungal Metabolites. Chem. Rev. 2009, *109*, 3903–3990.

[60] Pfohl-Leszkowicz A, Manderville RA. Ochratoxin A: An overview on toxicity and carcinogenicity in animals and humans. Mol. Nutr. Food Res. 2007, *51*, 61–99.

[61] Marquardt RR, Frohlich AA. A review of recent advances in understanding ochratoxicosis. Journal of Animal Science, 1992, 70, 3968-3988.

[62] Cavin C, Delatour T, Marin-Kuan M, Holzhauser D, Higgins L, Bezencon C, Guignard G, Junod S, Piguet D, Richoz-Payot J, Gremaux E, Hayes JD, Nestler S, Mantle P, Schilter B. Reduction in antioxidant defences may contribute to ochratoxin A toxicity and carcinogenicity. Toxicol. Sci.; 2007, 96 (1), 30–39.

[63] Boesch-Saadatmandi C, Wagner AE, Graeser AC, Hundhausen C, Wollram S, Rimbach G. Ochratoxin A impairs Nrf2-dependent gene expression in porcine kidney tubulus cells. J. Anim. Phys. Anim. Nutr;.2009, *93*: 547–555.

[64] Krogh P. Role of ochratoxin in disease causation. Fd Chem Toxic; 1992, 30: 213–224.

[65] Ali A, Abdu S.Antioxidant protection against pathological mycotoxins alterations on proximal tubules in rat kidney. Functional Foods in Heals and Disease; 2011, 4:118-134.

[66] Marin-Kuan M, Ehrlich V, Delatour T, Cavin C, Schilter B. Evidence for a role of oxidative stress in the carcinogenicity of ochratoxin A. Journal of Toxicolog, 2011: 1-15.

[67] Obrecht-Pumio S, Grosse Y, Pfohi-Leszkowicz A, Dirheimer G. Protection by indomethacin and aspirin against genotoxicity of ochraoxin A, particularly in the urinary bladder and kidney. Arch Toxicol. 1996; 70:244-248

[68] Doi K, Uetsuka K. Mechanisms of mycotoxin-induced neurotoxicity through oxidative stress-associated pathways. Int. J. Mol. Sci.;2011, *12*: 5213-5237

[69] Dirheimer G, Creppy EE. Mechanism of action of ochratoxin A, IARC Sci. Publ., 1991, 115: 171-175.

[70] Gautier JC, Holzhaeuser D, Markovic J, Gremaud E, Schilter B, Turesky RJ. Oxidative damage and stress response from ochratoxin exposure in rats. Free Radic. Biol. Med.,2001, *30*: 1089–1098.

[71] Bryan NS, Rassaf T, Maloney RE, Rodriguez CM, Saijo F, Rodriguez JR, Feelisch M. Cellular targets and mechanisms of nitros(yl)ation: An insight into their nature and kinetics *in vivo.* Proc. Natl. Acad. Sci. USA; 2004, *101*: 4308–4313.

[72] Mantle PG. Risk assessment and the importance of ochratoxins. International Biodeterioration and Biodegradation, 2000, 50: 143-146.

[73] Petzinger E, Ziegler K. Ochratoxin A from a toxicological perspective. Journal of Veterinary Pharmacolocy Therapeutics, 2000, 23, 91-98.

[74] Omar RF, Hasinoff BB, Mejilla F, Rahimtula AD. Mechanism of ochratoxin A stimulated lipid peroxidation. Biochemical Pharmacology, 1990, 40: 1183-1191.

[75] Dai J, Park G, Wright MW, Adams M, Akman SA, Manderville RA. Detection and characterization of a glutathione conjugate of ochratoxin A. Chem. Res. Toxicol., 2002, 15 (12), 1581–1588.

[76] Stemmer K, Ellinger-Ziegelbauer H, Ahr HJ, Dietrich DR. Carcinogen- specific gene expression profiles in short-term treated Eker and wild-type rats indicative of pathways involved in renal tumorigenesis. Cancer Res., 2007, 67: 4052–4068.

[77] Abdelhamid AM. Occurrence of some mycotoxins (aflatoxin, ochratoxin, citrinin, zearalenon and vomitoxin) in various Egyptian feeds. Archive in Animal Nutrition, 1990, 40, 647.

[78] Maaroufi K, Achour A, Hammami M, el May M, Betheder AM, Ellouz F, Creppy EE Bacha H. Ochratoxin A in human blood in relation to nephropathy in Tunisia. Human and Experimental Toxicology, 1995, 14, 609-614.

[79] Fillastre JP. Néphrotoxicité expérimentale et humaine des ochratoxines. Bulletin Académie Nationale de Médecine, 1997, 181, 1447.

[80] Godin M, Fillastre JP, Le Gallicier B, Pauti MD. Ochratoxin-induced nephrotoxicity in animals and humans, Semaine des Hopitaux, 1998, 74, 800-806.

[81] Wafa EW, Yahya RS, Sobh MA, Eraky I, El Baz H, El Gayar HAM, Betbeder AM, Creppy, EE. Human ochratoxicosis and nehropathy in Egypt: a preliminary study. Human and Experimental Toxicology, *1998,* 17, 124-129.

[82] [82]- O'Brien E, Dietrich DR. Ochratoxin A: The continuing enigma. Critical Reviews in Toxicology, 2005, 35:33–60.

[83] Müller G, Kielstein P, Rosner H, Berndt A, Heller M, Köhler H. Studies on the influence of combined administration of ochratoxin A, fumonisin B1, deoxynivalenol and T-2 toxin on immune and defence reactions in weaner pigs. Mycoses, 1999, 42, 485–493.

[84] Seegers JC, Boehmer LH, Kruger MC, Lottering ML, De Kock M. A comparative study of ochratoxin A induced apoptosis in hamster kidney and HELA cells. Toxicol. Appl. Pharmacol., 1994, 129:1–11.

[85] Alanati, L., Petzinger, E. Immunotoxic activity of ochratoxin A. J. Vet. Pharmacol. Therap., 2006, 29: 79–90.

[86] Marin-Kuan M, Cavin C, Delatour T, Schilt B. Ochratoxin A carcinogenicity involves a complex network of epigenetic mechanisms. Toxicon, 2008, 52:195–202 .

[87] Sudakin DL. Trichothecenes in the environment: Relevance to human health. *Toxicol. Lett.,*2003, *143*: 97-107.

[88] Eriksen GS, Pettersson H. Toxicological evaluation of trichothecenes in animal feed. Anim. Feed Sci. Technol., 2004, *114*: 205-239.

[89] Croft WA, Jarvis BB, Yatawara CS. Airborne outbreak of trichothecene toxicosis. Atmospheric Environment, 1986, 20, 549-552.

[90] Nikulin M, Pasanen AL, Berg S, Hintikka EL. Stachybotrys atra growth and toxin production in some building materials and fodder under di!erent relative humidities. Applied and Environmental Microbiology, 1994, 60: 3421-3424.

[91] Pestka JJ. Deoxynivalenol:toxicity, mechanisms and animal health risks. Anim. Feed Sci.Technol., 2007, *137*, 283-298.

[92] Yazar S, Omurtag GZ. Fumonisins, Trichothecenes and Zearalenone in Cereals. Int. J. Mol. Sci.,2008, *9*, 2062-2090.

[93] Eriksen GS. *Metabolism and Toxicity of Trichothecenes*, Doctoral thesis, Uppsala, Sweden, 2003.

[94] Larsen JC, Hunt J, Perin I, Ruckenbauer P. Workshop on trichothecenes with a focus on DON: Summary report. Toxicol. Lett., 2004, 153: 1-22.

[95] Desjardins AE, Hohn TM, McComic SP. Trichothecene biosynthesis in *Fusarium* species: chemistry, genetics, and significance. Microbiol. Mol. Biol. Rev., 1993, *57*: 595–604.

[96] Shifrin VI, Anderson P. Trichothecene mycotoxins trigger a ribotoxic stress response that activates c-jun N-terminal kinase and p38 mitogen-activated protein kinase and induces apoptosis. J. Biol. Chem., 1999, *274*: 13985–13992.

[97] Chang IM, Mar WC. Effect of T-2 toxin on lipid peroxidation in rats: Elevation of conjugated diene formation. Toxicol. Lett., 1988, *40*: 275–280.

[98] Guerre P, Eeckhoutte C, Burgat V, Galtier P. The effects of T-2 toxin exposure on liver drug metabolizing enzymes in rabbit. Food Addit. Contam., 2002, *17, 1019-1026.*

[99] Chaudhary M, Rao PV. Brain oxidative stress after dermal and subcutaneous exposure of T-2 toxin in mice. Food Chem. Toxicol., 2010, *48*: 3436–3442.

[100] Pacin A, Reale C, Mirengui H, Orellana L, Boente G. Subclinic effect of the administration of T-2 toxin and nivalenol in mice. Mycotoxin Research, 1994, *10*: 34-46.

[101] Moss MO. Mycotoxin review-2. *Fusarium*. Mycologist, 2002, *16*, 158-161.

[102] Gyongyossy-Issa MIC, Khanna V, Khachatourians GC. Characterisation of hemolysis induced by T-2 toxin. Biochim. Biophys. Acta.,1985, 838: 252-256.

[103] Shinozuka J, Suzuki M, Noguchi N, Sugimoto T, Uetsuka K, Nakayama H, Doi K. T-2 toxin-induced apoptosis in hematopoietic tissues of mice. Toxicol. Pathol.,1998, *26*: 674–681.

[104] Shinozuka J, Miwa S, Fujimura H, Toriumi W, Doi K. Hepatotoxicity of T-2 Toxin, Trichothecene Mycotoxin. In *New Strategies for Mycotoxin Research in Asia (Proceedings of ISMYCO Bangkok '06)*; Kumagai, S., Ed.; Japanese Association of Mycotoxicology: Tokyo, 2007, pp. 62–66

[105] Sehata S, Kiyosawa N, Makino T, Atsumi F, Ito K, Yamoto T, Teranishi M, Baba Y, Uetauka K, Nakayama H, Doi K. Morphological and microarray analysis of T-2 toxin-induced rat fetal brain lesion. Food Chem. Toxicol., 2004, *42*: 1727–1736.

[106] Annunziato L, Amoroso S, Pannaccione A, Cataldi M, Pignataro G, D'Alessio S, Sirabella R, Second A, Sibaud L, DiRenzo GF. Apoptosis induced in neuronal cells by oxidative stress: role played by caspases and intracellular calcium ions. Toxicol. Lett.,2003, *139*: 125–133.

[107] Huang P, Akagawa K, Yokoyama Y, Nohara K, Kano K, Morimoto K. T-2 toxin initially activates caspase-2 and induces apoptosis in U937 cells. Toxicol. Lett., 2007, *170*: 1–10.

[108] Wild CP, Gong YY. Mycotoxins and human disease: a largely ignored global health issue. Carcinogenesis, 2010, 31(1):71–82.

[109] Voss KA, Riley RT, Norred WP, Bacon CW, Meredith FI, Howard PC, Plattner RD, Collins TF, Hansen DK, Porter JK. An overview of rodent toxicities: liver and kidney effects of fumonisins and *Fusarium moniliforme*. Environ Health Perspect.,2001,109 (2):259–266.

[110] Howard PC, Eppley RM, Stack ME, Warbritton A, Voss KA, Lorentzen RJ, Kovach RM, Bucci TJ. Fumonisin B1 carcinogenicity in a 2-year feeding study using F344rats and B6C3 F1 mice. Environ. Health Perspect., 2001,109: 277–282.

[111] Abel S, Gelderblom WCA. Oxidative damage and fumonisin B1-induced toxicity in primary rat hepatocytes and liver *in vivo*. Toxicology, 1998,131, 121 - 131

[112] Merrill AH, Sullards MC, Wang E, Voss KA, Riley RT. Sphingolipid metabolism: roles in signal transduction and disruption by fumonisins. Environ. Health Perspect., 2001, 109(2):283–289.

[113] Stockmann-Juvala H, Savolainen A. A review of the toxic effects and mechanisms of action of fumonisin B1. Hum. Exp. Toxicol., 2008, 27: 799–809.

[114] Riley RT, Enongene E, Voss KA, Norred WP, Meredith FI, Sharma RP, Spitsbergen J, Williams DE, Carlson DB, Merrill AH, Jr. Sphingolipid perturbations as mechanisms for fumonisin carcinogenesis. Environ. Health Perspect., 2001, 109: 301–308.

[115] Voss KA, Howard PC, Riley RT, Sharma RP, Bucci TJ, Lorentzen RJ. Carcinogenicity and mechanism of action of fumonisin B1: a mycotoxin produced by *Fusarium moniliforme* (=*F. verticillioides*). Cancer Detect. Prevent., 2002, 26: 1-9.

[116] Riley RT. Mechanistic interactions of mycotoxins: theoretical consideration. In: Sinha KK, Bhatanagar D (Eds.), Mycotoxins in Agriculture and Food Safety. Marcel Dekker, Inc, Basel, New York, 1998, pp. 227–254.

[117] Yiannikouris A, Jouany JB. Mycotoxins in feeds and their fate in animals: a review. Anim. Res., 2002, 51: 81–99.

[118] Wang JS, Groopman DJ. DNA damage by mycotoxins. Mutation Research,1999, 424: 167–181.

[119] Mobio TA, Anane R, Baudrimont I, Carratū MR, Shier TW, Dano SD, Ueno Y, Creppy EE. Epigenetic properties of fumonisin B1: cell cycle arrest and DNA base modification in C6 glioma cells. *Toxicol. Appl. Pharmacol.* 2000, *164*, 91–96.

[120] Stockmann-Juvala H, Mikkola J, Naarala J, Loikkanen J, Elovaara E, Savolainen K. Fuminisin B1-induced toxicity and oxidative damage in U-118MG glioblastoma cells. Toxicology, 2004, *202*: 173–183.

[121] Ferrante MC, Meli R, Raso GM, Esposito E, Severino L, Carlo GD, Lucisano A. Effect of fumonisin B1 on structure and function of macrophage plasma membrane. Toxicology Letters, 2002, 129: 181–187.

[122] Olsen M. Metabolism of zearalenone in farm animals. In *Fusarium mycotoxins, taxonomy and pathogenicity,* 1st Ed.; Chelkowsi, J., Ed.; Elsevier: Amsterdam-Oxford-New York, 1989, pp. 167–177.

[123] Minervini F, Dell'Aquila MD. Zearalenone and reproductive function in farm animals. Int. J. Mol. Sci, 2008, *9*: 2570-2584.

[124] D'Mello JPF, Placinta CM, MacDonald AMC. *Fusarium* mycotoxins: A review of global implications for animal health, welfare and productivity. Anim. Feed Sci. Technol., 1999, *80*: 183-205.

[125] Ben Othmen ZO, El Golli E, Abid-Essefi S, Bacha H. Cytotoxicity effects induced by zearalenone metabolites, α zearalenol and β zearalenol, on cultured vero cells. Toxicology, 2008, 252: 72–77.

[126] Hassen W, Ayed-Boussema I, Oscoz AA, Lopez AD, Bacha H. The role of oxidative stress in zearalenone-mediated toxicity in Hep G2 cells: Oxidative DNA damage, gluthatione depletion and stress proteins induction. Toxicology, 2007, 232: 294-302.

[127] Kuiper-Goodman T, Scott PM, Watanabe H. Risk assessment of the mycotoxin zearalenone. Reg. Toxicol. Pharmacol., 1987, *7*: 253–306.

[128] Kuiper-Goodman T, Hilts C, Billiard SM, Kiparissis Y, Richard ID, Hayward S. Health risk assessment of ochratoxin A for all age-sex strata in a market economy. Food Addit. Contam. Part A Chem. Anal. Control Expo. Risk Assess., 2010, *27*: 212–240.

[129] Wasowiczi K, Gajecja M, Calka J, Jakimiuk E, Gajecki M. Influence of chronic administration of zearalenone on the processes of apoptosis in the porcine ovary. Vet. Med. Czech, 2005, *50 (12): 531–536.*

[130] Kim II-H, Son HY, Cho SW, Chang-Su Ha, CS, Kang BH. Zearalenone induces male germ cell apoptosis in rats. Toxicology Letters, 2003, 138: 185-192.

[131] Wang YC, Deng JL, Xu SW, Peng X, Zuo ZC, Cui HM, Wang Y, Ren ZH. Effects of zearalenone on IL-2, IL-6, and IFN-γ mRNA levels in the splenic lymphocytes of chickens. The Scientific World Journal, 2012: 1-5.

[132] Puel O, Galtier P, Oswald IP. Biosynthesis and toxicological effects of patulin. Toxins, 2010, *2*: 613-631.

[133] Mahfoud R, Maresca M, Garmy N, Fantini J. The mycotoxin patulin alters the barrier function of the intestinal epithelium: mechanism of action of the toxin and protective effects of glutathione. Toxicol. Appl. Pharmacol., 2002, 181: 209–218.

[134] Liu F, Ooi V, Chang S. Free radical scavenging activities of mushroom polysaccharides extracts. Life Sci., 1996, 60(10): 763- 771.

[135] [135]- Liu BH, Wu TS, Yu FY, Su CC. Induction of oxidative stress response by the mycotoxin patulin in mammalian cells. Toxicol. Sci., 2007, 95(2):340-347.

[136] Wichmann G, Herbarth O, Lehmann I.: The mycotoxins citrinin, gliotoxin, and patulin affect interferon-gamma rather than interleukin-4 production in human blood cells. Environ. Toxicol., 2002, *17*: 211–218.

[137] Luft P, Oostingh GJ, Gruijthuijsen Y, Horejs-Hoeck J, Lehmann I, Duschl A. Patulin Influences the Expression of Th1/Th2 Cytokines by Activated Peripheral Blood Mononuclear Cells and T Cells Through Depletion of Intracellular Glutathione. Environ. Toxicol., 2008, *23*: 84–95.

[138] Yu FY, Liao YC, Chang CH and Liu BH. Citrinin induces apoptosis in HL-60 cells via activation of the mitochondrial pathway. Toxicology Letters, 2006,161: 143-151

[139] Berndt WO. Ochratoxin–citrinin as nephrotoxins. In Llewellyn GC, Rear PCO (Eds.), Biodeterioration Research 3 New York, USA: Plenum Press, 1999, PP.55-56.

[140] Chagas GM, Oliveira MBM, Campello AP, Kluppel MLW. Mechanism of citrinin-induced dysfunction of mitochondria. III. Effects on renal cortical and liver mitochondria swelling. Journal of Applied Toxicology, 1995, 15: 91–95.

[141] Chagas GM, Kluppel MLW, Oliveira MBM. Citrinin affects the oxidative metabolism of BHK-21 cells. Cell Biochem and Function, 1995, 13(4):257-271.

[142] Nishijima, M. In Kurata H & Ueno Y (Eds.), Toxigenic fungi. Amsterdam, Netherlands, 1984, PP.172-181.

[143] Vazquez BI, Fente C, Franco C, Cepeda A, Prognon P, Mahuzier G. Simultaneous high-performance liquid chromatographic determination of ochratoxin A and citrinin in cheese by time-resolved luminescence using terbium. Journal of Chromatography A, 1996, 727: 185–193.

[144] Sansing GA, Lillehoj EB, Detroy RW. Synergistic toxic effect of citrinin, ochratoxin A and penicillic acid in mice. Toxicon, 1976, 14:213-220.

[145] Glahn RP, Shapiro RS, Vena VE, Wideman RF, Huff WE. Effects of chronic ochratoxin A and citrinin toxins on kidney function of single comb white leghorn pullets. Poultry Science, 1989, 68(9): 1205–1211.

[146] Kumar M, Dwivedi P, Sharma AK, Singh ND, Patil RD. Ochratoxin A and citrinin nephrotoxicity in New Zealand White rabbits: an ultrastructural assessment. Mycopathologia, 2007, 163: 21–30.

[147] Kitabatake N, Trivedi AB, Doi E. Thermal decomposition and detoxification of citrinin under various moisture conditions. Journal of Agricultural and Food Chemistry, 1991, 39(12): 2240–2244.

[148] Trivedi AB, Doi E, Kitabatake N. Toxic compounds formed on prolonged heating of citrinin under watery conditions. Journal of Food science, 1993, 58(1): 229–231.

[149] Bennett JW, Bentley R. Pride and prejudice: the story of ergot. Perspect. Biol. Med., 1999, 42:333-355.

[150] Lorenz K. Ergot on cereal grains. Crit. Rev. Food Sci. Nutr., 1979, 11:311-354.

[151] Cabellero-Granado FJ, Viciana P, Cordero E, Gomez-Vera M.J, del Nozal M, Opez-Cortes LF. Ergotism related to concurrent administration of ergotamine tartrate and ritonavir in an AIDS patient. Antimicrob. Agents Chemother., 1997, 41:1297.

[152] Yang GH, Jarvis BB, Chung YJ, Pestka JJ. Apoptosis induction by satratoxins and other trichothecene mycotoxins: Relationship to ERK, p38 MAPK, and SAPK/JNK activation. Toxicol. Appl. Pharmacol., 2000, 164: 149–160.

[153] Nielsen KF. Mycotoxin production by indoor molds. Fungal Genetics Biology, 2003, 39: 103-117.

[154] Bae HK, Shinozuka J, Islam Z, Pestka JJ. Satratoxin G Interaction with 40S and 60S Ribosomal Subunits Precedes Apoptosis in the Macrophage. Toxicol Appl Pharmacol., 2009, 237(2): 137–145.

[155] Nagase M, Shiota T, Tsushima A, Murshedul M, Fukuoka S, Yoshizawa T, Sakato N. Molecular mechanism of satratoxin-induced apoptosis in HL-60 cells: activation of caspase-8 and caspase-9 is involved in activation of caspase-3. Immunology Letters, 2002, 84: 23-27.

[156] Oda T, Xu JKU, Nakazawa T, Namikoshi M. 12- -Hydroxyl group remarkably reduces Roridin E cytotoxicity. Mycoscience, 2010, 51:317–320.

[157] Xu J, Takasaki A, Kobayashi H, Oda T, Yamada J, Mangindaan REP, Ukai K, Nagai H, Namikoshi M. Four new macrocyclic trichothecenes from two strains of marine-derived fungi of the genus Myrothecium. J Antibiot, 2006, 59:451–455.

[158] Namikoshi M, Akano K, Meguro S, Kasuga I, Mine Y, Takahashi T, Kobayashi H. A new macrocyclic trichothecene, 12,13-deoxyroridin E, produced by the marine-derived fungus Myrothecium roridum collected in Palau. J Nat Prod. 2001, 64:396–398.

[159] Omar HM, El-Sawi NM, Meki ARMA. Acute toxicity of the mycotoxin roridin E on liver and kidney of rats. J. Appl. Anim. Res., 1997, 12:145-152.

[160] Kam PCA , Ferch NI. Apoptosis: mechanisms and clinical implicat. Anaesthesia, 2000, 55: 1081-1093.

[161] Rocha O, Ansari K, Doohan FM. Effects of trichothecene mycotoxins on eukaryotic cells: A review. Food Additives and Contaminants, 2005, 22(4): 369–378.

[162] Pace JG, Watts MR, Canterbury WJ. T-2 mycotoxin inhibits mitochondrial protein synthesis. Toxicon, 1988, 26:77–85.

[163] Klaric MK, Rumora L, Ljubanvic D, Pepeljnjak S. Cytotoxicity and apoptosis induced by fumonisin B1, beauvericin and ochratoxin A in porcine kidney PK15 cells: effects of individual and combined treatment. Arch Toxicol., 2008, 82:247–255.

[164] Jones C, Ciacci-Zanella JR, Zhang Y, Henderson G, Dickman M. Analysis of fumonisin B1-induced apoptosis.Environ Health Perspect., 2001, 109 (2): 315–320.

[165] Sharma N, Suzuki H, He Q, Sharma RP. Tumor necrosis factor α -mediated activation of c-Jun NH2-terminal kinase as a mechanism for fumonisin B1 induced apoptosis in murine primary hepatocytes. J Biochem. Molecular Toxicology, 2005, 19 (6):359-367.

[166] Liu H, Jones BE, Bradham C, Czaja MJ. Increased cytochrome P-450 2E1 expression sensitizes hepatocytes to c-Jun-mediated cell death from TNF-α. Am J Physiol Gastrointest Liver Physiol, 2002, 282:G257–G266.

[167] Martinez-Larranaga MR, Anadon A, Diaz MJ, Fernandez R, Sevil B, Fernandez-Cruz ML, Fernandez MC, Martinez MA, Anton R. Induction of cytochrome P4501A1 and P4504A1 activities and peroxisomal proliferation by fumonisin B1. Toxicol Appl Pharmacol., 1996, 141:185–194.

[168] Kang YJ, Alexander JM. Alterations of the glutathione redox cycle status in fumonisin B1-treated pig kidney cells. J Biochem Toxicol, 1996, 11:121–16.

[169] Sahu SC, Eppley RM, Page SW, Gray GC, Barton CN, O'Donnel Lmw. Peroxidation of membrane lipids and oxidative DNA damage by fumonisin B1 in isolated rat liver nuclei. Cancer Lett, 1998, 125:117–121.

[170] Adler V, Yin Z, Fuchs SY, Benezra M, Rosario L, Tew KD, Pincus MR, Sardana M, Henderson CJ,Wolf CR, Davis RJ, Ronai Z. Regulation of JNK signaling by GSTp. EMBO J; 1999, 18:1321–1334

[171] Zhu L, Yuan H, Guo C, Lu Y, Deng S, Yang Y, Wei Q, Wen L, He Z. Zearalenone induces apoptosis and necrosis in porcine granulosa cells via a caspase-3- and caspase-9-dependent mitochondrial signaling pathway. Journal of Cellular Physiology, 2012, 227(6):1814-1820.

[172] Saxena N, Ansari KM, Kumar R, Dhawan A, Dwivedi PD, Das M. Patulin causes DNA damage leading to cell cycle arrest and apoptosis through modulation of Bax, P53 and P21/waf1 proteins in skin of mice. Toxicology and Applied Pharmacology, 2009, 234:192-201.

[173] Nusuetrong P, Pengsuparp T, Meksuriyen D, Tanitsu M, Kikuchi H, Mizugaki M, Shimazu KI, Oshima Y, Nakahata N, Yoshida M. Satratoxin H generates reactive oxygen species and lipid peroxides in PC12 cells. Biol. Pharm. Bull., 2008, 31: 1115-1120.

[174] Coulombe RA, Guarisco JA, Klein PJ, Hall JO. Chemoprevention of aflatoxicosis in poultry by dietary butylated hydroxytoluene. Anim. Feed Sci. Technol., 2005,*121*: 217-225.

[175] Morgavi DP, Boudra H, Jouany JP, Graviou D. Prevention of patulin toxicity on rumen microbial fermentation by SH-containing reducing agents. J. Agric. Food Chem., 2003, *51*: 6906-6910.

[176] Eckschlager T, Adam V, Hrabeta J, Figova K, Kizek R. Metallothioneins and Cancer. Curr Protein Pept Sci, 2009, 10: 360–375.

[177] Davis SR, Cousins RJ. Metallothionein expression in animals: A physiological perspective on function. J. Nutr., 2000, 130: 1085-1088.

[178] Nagashima H, Nakagawa H, Iwashita K. Mycotoxin nivalenol induces apoptosis and intracellular calcium ion-dependent interleukin-8 secretion but does not exert mutagenicity. In Ikura K et al. (eds.), Animal Cell Technology: Basic & Applied Aspects, 2009, pp.301-306.

[179] Shapira A, Benhar I. Toxin-based therapeutic approaches. Toxins, 2010 *2*: 2519-2583.

[180] Rowell PP, Larson BT. Ergocryptine and other ergot alkaloids stimulate the release of [3H] dopamine from rat striatal synaptosomes. Journal of Animal Science, 1999, 77(7): 1800-6.

[181] Samuelsson G. Drugs of natural origin. 4th ed. Apotekar societeten. Stockholm, 1999.

[182] Eadie MJ. Ergot of rye-the first specific for migraine. Journal of Clinical Neuroscience, 20, 11 (1): 4-7.

[183] De Costa C. St Anthony's Fire and living ligatures: a short history of ergometrine. The Lancet, 2002, 359: 1768-70.

[184] Nichols CD, Garcia EE, Sanders-Bush E. Dynamic changes in prefrontal cortex gene xpression following lysergic acid diethylamide administration. Molecular Brain Research, 2003, 111 (1-2): 182-188.

[185] Nichols CD, Sanders-Bush EA. Single dose of lysergic acid diethylamide influences gene expression patterns within the mammalian brain. Neuropsychopharmacology, 2002, 26 (5): 634-642.

[186] Hart C. Forged in St. Anthony's Fire: drugs for migraine. Modern drug discovery, 1999, 2 (2): 20- 31.

[187] Kupchan SM, Streelman DR, Jarvis BB, Dailey RG, Jr, Sneden ATJ. Isolation of potent new antileukemic trichothecenes from Baccharis megapotamica. J Org Chem., 1977, 42(26):4221-4225

[188] Hughes BJ, Hsieh GC, Jarvis BB, Sharma RP. Effects of macrocyclic trichothecene mycotoxins on the murine immune system. Arh. Environ. Contam. Toxicol, 1989, 18: 388-395.

[189] Massaer F, Meucci V, Saggese G, Soldani G. High growth rate of girls with precocious puberty exposed to estrogenic mycotoxins. J Pediatr; 2008, 152: 690-695.

[190] Kapoor VK. Natural toxins and their therapeutic potential. Indian Journal of Experimental Biology., 2010, 8: 228-237.

Chapter 4

Avian Mycotoxicosis in Developing Countries

Adeniran Lateef Ariyo, Ajagbonna Olatunde Peter, Sani Nuhu Abdulazeez and Olabode Hamza Olatunde

Additional information is available at the end of the chapter

http://dx.doi.org/10.5772/56050

1. Introduction

Avian mycotoxicosis refers to all the diseases caused by the effect of mycotoxin in birds. These diseases may not be pathognomonic and sometimes subclinical and difficult to diagnose. The problem is worldwide but effort will be made to localise the effect of these diseases in developing countries. Developing countries have more than 50% of total meat and egg production in global poultry market: [1]. The global poultry meat market is 86.8 million tonnes, consisting of chicken: 85.6%, turkey: 6.8%; duck: 4.6%; goose and guinea fowl: 2.6%.

Years	world	Developed countries	Developing countries	Share (%) of developing countries
1970	15	11	4	26
1975	19	13	5	31
1980	26	18	8	31
1985	31	21	10	33
1990	41	26	15	37
1995	55	28	26	48
2000	69	33	36	53
2005	81	37	44	55
(Increase %)	437	227	1,043	-

Table 1. Development of poultry meat production in developed and developing countries (million tonnes).

Years	world	Developed countries	Developing countries	Share (%) of developing countries
1970	20	15	5	24
1975	22	16	6	27
1980	26	18	8	32
1985	31	19	12	39
1990	35	19	16	46
1995	43	17	25	59
2000	51	18	33	64
2005	59	19	40	68
(Increase %)	195	29	758	-

Source: [1]

Table 2. Development of poultry hen egg production in developed and developing countries (million tonnes)

The world market poultry meat and egg market is been influenced by the production and managemental style from the developing countries. Avian mycotoxicosis is a great constraint in poultry industry, because the disease is characterized by immunosuppresion, hepatotoxicity, nephrotoxicity, loss of egg production, mutagenicity and tetratogenicity.

Mycotoxin are antinutritive factor present in feed ingredients and in concentrated feed, they are a group of secondary fungal metabolites of low molecular weight, diverse and ambiguous in nature, which are specifically implicated in causing toxic effect in animals and man [2,3]. Mycotoxicosis has been a major but unrecognized food safety issue for several centuries. They are naturally occurring contaminants that causes health related problems when it gets into the body through natural route of ingestion, inhalation or may be absorbed through the skin [4]. They are endogenously generated in foods as a result of secondary metabolism [5]. These metabolites are synthesized in or on food surfaces and transported through the food chain[6]. Mycotoxin production takes place in the mycelium after active fungal growth, but may accumulate in specialized structures such as sclerotia, conidia or in surrounding area [7]. Animal studies have shown that, besides acute effects, mycotoxins can cause carcinogenic, mutagenic and teratogenic effects. Mycotoxins-contaminated poultry feed can lead to the transfer of toxins through meat and egg to human beings.

The Food and Agriculture Organization [8] estimating that as much as 25% of the world's Agricultural commodities are contaminated with mycotoxins, leading to significant economic losses. Mycotoxigenic fungi genera include; *Aspergillus, Penicillium* and *Fusarium.* The important mycotoxin in the developing countries include aflatoxins, ochratoxins, citrinin, T-2 toxin, deoxynivalenol (DON), fumonisins and zearalenone.

Fungi genera	Associated mycotoxin
Aspergillus	Aflatoxin, Ochratoxins, cyclopiazonic acid, patulin, sterigmatocystin, gliotoxin, citrinin.
Peniccillium	Ochratoxin, citrinin, patulin, penicillic acid, cyclopiazonic acid, penitrem A, griseofulvin.
Fusarium	Fumonisins, moniliformin, zearalenone, zearalenol, deoxynivalenol, nivalenol, 15- acetyldeoxynivalenol, 3-acetydeoxynivalenol, T-2 toxin, iso T-2 toxin, acetyl T-2 toxin, t-2 triol, T-2 tetraol, fusarenon- X, diacetoxyscripentriol, neosalaniol, fusaric acid.
Claviceps	Ergot alkaloids.

[9]

Table 3. Showing fungi genera and the associated mycotoxin.

2. Avian aflatoxicosis

2.1. Aetiology

Avian aflatoxicosis is a disease of poultry caused by aflatoxin. Aflatoxins (AF) are widely distributed toxins produced by *Aspergillus*. Of the over 180 species of Aspergillus, only a few are aflatoxigenic. After the discovery of AF in the 1960s, A. flavus and *A. parasiticus* of the section *Flavi* were the only known AF producers producing the B and B/G types of AF, respectively [10]. Other aflatoxigenic species that subsequently emerged are *A. nomius* (B and G types), *A. bombycis* (B and G AF), *A. ochraceoroseus*, and *A. pseudotamarii* (B type), but they occur less frequently [11,12]. *A. tamarii, A. parvisclerotigenus* (B types*), A. rambellii* and certain members of *Aspergillus subgenus Nidulantes* namely: *Emericella venezualensis* [13] and *E. astellata* [14] have now been included in the growing list of aflatoxigenic species. *A. arachidicola* sp. Nov. and *A. minisclerotigenes sp.* Nov that produce both forms of the toxin, are the latest emerging aflatoxigenic species. The unexpected new comer is *A. niger*, an ochratoxin (OT) producer which was discovered over four decades ago but was never associated with AF synthesis. However, in a search for aflatoxigenic fungi in Romanian medicinal herbs, [15] showed the capacity of some strains of *A. niger* to produce AFB1 [16].

AFBI is a member of aflatoxin group is one of the most carcinogenic natural product formed in nature [17]. AF has been detected in most countries of the world. Four toxins soon identified: Aflatoxin B1, B2, G1, G2-blue or green florescence under UV-light.• AflatoxinB1most important -highly carcinogenic and widespread occurrence in foods •(B1> M1> G1> B2> M2~ G2). Aflatoxin M1: hydroxylated product of B1appears in milk, urine, and feces as metabolic product

2.2. Factor enhancing AF prevalence in feed ingredients and poultry feed

There are several factors enhancing the prevalence of aflatoxigenic fungi and aflatoxin production in developing countries. The factor include the following:

The food materials must be infected by aflatoxigenic fungi which deposit the toxins on feed ingredients and concentrated feeds.

The substrate which may be feed ingredients and concentrated feeds posseses a source of energy in the form of carbohydrates and organic and inorganic source of nitrogen, trace elememts and moisture for growth of mould and toxin production [8].

Among cereal, the size and integrity of the seed coat also affects the susceptibility of fungal infection and mycotoxin formation [18]

The environmental condition favouring mould growth and AF production are hot and humid conditions, the optimal temperature varies between 24^{0}Cand 28^{0}C [19] and seed moisture content of at least 17.5% [20]. These conditions that favours mould growth are present in most developing countries.

Soil type also affect the level of AF contamination of crops for example, light sandy soil support rapid growth of fungi [21]

Presence of other microorganism either bacteria for example presence of *Streptococcus lactis* and *Lactobacillius casei* causes reduction in AF production by *A. parasiticus* [20]. Meanwhile fungal metabolites like rubratoxin and cerulenin enhances AF production [16].

Agricultural practices also affect AF contamination of feed ingredient. Off season harvesting and harvesting system that enhances seed breakage would also increase the degree of AF production [22].

A well aerated storage condition used in most developing country to store feed ingredients increases metabolism and subsequent AF production [23].

2.3. Occurrence of AF

AF has been found as contaminants in animal feed ingredient worldwide. The occurrence in developing countries is more because there is no strict food and feed quality control programmes to reduce the burden of AF. Also their environmental condition presented as hot and humid climate makes most developing country vulnerable to AF in poultry feed. Among the four AF that are of significance in poultry include; AFB1, B2, G1and G2. AFB1 was detected mostly from animal and feed ingredients from developing countries. Among the feeds ingredients, sorghum, wheat, maize were the most investigated, data on groundnut cake, cotton seed meal and fish meal showed high level of AF contamination. The highest level of AFB1 contamination of feed ingredient were reported in corn from Pakistan 25µg/kg [24], Nigeria wheat was found to be contaminated with 17.10-20.53 µg /kg [25].

Higher level of contamination of AF were found in the animal feed than the feed ingredient possibly because of the storage condition which allowed growth and proliferation of mycotoxigenic fungi. In Nigeria AF was detected in poultry feed at 0.0-67.9 µg/kg [26], wheat 17.10-20.53 µg/kg [25], millet 1370-3475 µg/kg [23].

AF contamination of feed and feed ingredients has been a major concern in many developing country like Pakistan where concentration ranging from 24-37.62 µg/kg were found in poultry feed and poultry feed ingredient [24].

Commodity	Country	Type of AF	Incidence	Range (µg/kg)	Mean level ±SD (µg/kg)	References
Poultry/livestock	Nigeria	AFB1	6/13	0.0-67.9	15.5	[26]
Animal feed	Kenya	AFB1	703/830	0.9-595	8.9-46.0	[27]
Animal feed	South Africa	AF	17/23	0.8-156	39.8	[28]
Poultry feed	Morocco	AFB1	14/21	0.3-58	8.4	[29]
Sorghum	Malawi	AFB1	2/15	1.7-3.0	2.35 ±0.65	[30]
Wheat	Kenya	AFB1	23/50	0-7	1.93	[31]
Wheat	Tunisia	AFs	15/51	4.0-12.9	6.7±2.4	[32]
Wheat	Nigeria	AFB1	-	17.10-20.53	19.00±1.67	[25]
Wheat	Algeria	AFB1	30/53	0.13-37.42	>5	[33]
Wheat	South Africa	AFB1	13/238	0.5-2.0	>2	[34]
Maize	Ghana	AF	30/30	6.20-29.50	13-596	[35]
Maize	Uganda	AF	22/49	1.00-1000	-	[22]
Millet	Nigeria	AFB1	12/49	1370.28-3495	2587.47±78.23	[23]
Mouldy Sorghum	Nigeria	AFB1	93/168		199.51±26	[36]
Poultry feed	Pakistan	AFB1	60%		37.62	[24]
Corn	Pakistan	AFB1	8/13		25	[24]
Rice broken	Pakistan	AFB1	3/5		21	[24]
Wheat	Pakistan	AFB1	3/5		19	[24]
Cotton seed meal	Pakistan	AFB1	5/5		22	[24]
Fish meal	Pakistan	AFB1	3/5		24	[24]
Broiler starter (Crumbs)	Pakistan	AFB1	6/11		20	[24]
Broiler starter (Mash)	Pakistan	AFB1	8/14		21	[24]
Layer Starter (Crumbs)	Pakistan	AFB1	16/30		26	[24]
Layer Grower (Crumbs)	Pakistan	AFB1	3/7		23	[24]
Layer Grower (Mash)	Pakistan	AFB1	3/5		32.5	[24]
Layers (Crumbs)	Pakistan	AFB1	23/60		21	[24]
Layers (Mash)	Pakistan	AFB1	25/58		23.5	[24]
Poultry Feed	China	AFB1	38.2		29.7	[37]
Poultry Feed	South Africa	Aflatoxin	22/62		0.7±0.7	[38]
Maize	Morroco	AFB1	16/20		1.57±0.78	[29]

[16]

Table 4. Showing occurrence of AF in animal feed and feed ingredients in developing countries

An unacceptably high level of concentration of AF that ranges from 1-1000 μg/kg was found in maize from Uganda[22] About 70% of wheat samples investigated in Algeria were contamination at a range of 0.13-3742mg/kg [33]

Animal species	Clinical signs Performance effect	Gross pathology	Histopathology	References
Duckling	inappetance, reduced growth. abnormal vacuolation, feather. picking, discoloration of leg/feet. lameness, ataxia, convulsion.	Liver enlarged, pale and shrunken. Kidney enlarged and pale Hydropericardium, ascitis.		[40]
Turkey	inappetance, unsteady gait, Recumbency, anaemia.	body in good condition, generalized and edema. Liver and kidney Congested enlarged and firm. Gallbladder was full.		[41, 42]
Chicken	Same in turkey and duckling Increase mortality Loss of production Increased susceptibility to infectious disease and vaccination failure.	Same in turkey and duckling	Fatty vacuolation of the liver. Karyomegaly and prominent nucleoli in hepatocytes, Bile duct proliferation.	[40-44]
Chicken (broiler)	impared performance lower testis weight and Semen volume, Spermatocrit and Testosterone value.		Abnormal spermatozoa, cessation of spermatogenesis in seminiferous tubules.	[45-46]

Table 5. Main clinical signs, performance and pathological features in food producing animals exposed to AF in selected studies.

2.4. Pharmacological interaction

Aflatoxicosis has effect on plasma half-life, thus it affects drug effect in the body. [47] observed that chlortetracycline plasma concentrations were lowered due to decreased drug binding to plasma protein [48]. Though opinion differed considerably on sparing or aggravating effect caused by the addition of chlortetracycline to feed contaminated with aflatoxin [49,50].

2.5. Metabolism and residues

In broilers, metabolites of aflatoxins BI and B2 concentrated in kidney and liver but cleared within 4 days. Then metabolism of Aflatoxin B1 into conjugated aflatoxins B2a and Ml occurred in the liver, which will be metabolized to aflatoxicol [51-54]. Aflatoxin BI was excreted in the bile, urine, and feces as 6 major metabolites [55]. The half-life of aflatoxin BI in laying hens is about 67 hours [56], though feed: egg transmission is about 5000:1 [57]. Most aflatoxin excreted through the bile and intestine, but aflatoxin BI and aflatoxicol were detected in ova and eggs for 7 days or longer [58-59]. Aflatoxin BI accumulated in reproductive organs and its subsequent transmission to eggs and hatched progeny (yolk sac and liver) in poultry[60]. It is well established that AFB_1 is both carcinogenic and cytotoxic. For example, synthesis of both RNA and DNA was inhibited when AF (5mg/kg of feed) was given to rats over a 6-week-period. The activated AFB_1 metabolite (i.e. AFB_1-8, 9-epoxide) forms a covalent bond with the N_7 of guanine [61] and forms AFB_1-N_7-guanine adducts in the target cells. The results are G_T transversions, DNA repair, lesions, mutations and subsequently tumor formation [57]. The reactive epoxide can also be hydrolyzed to AFB_1-8, 9-dihydrodiol which ionizes to form a Schiff's base with primary amine groups in the proteins [58]. The short-lived epoxide AFB_1 has also been associated with coagulopathy due to reduced synthesis of vitamin K and other clotting factors as a result of sub-lethal intoxication of animals [62]. With regard to the cytotoxic effects, AFB_1 has been shown to induce lipid peroxidation in rat livers leading to oxidative damage to hepatocytes [63]. A more recent study [64], has demonstrated that AFB_1 can inhibit cyclic nucleotide phosphodiesterase activity in the brain, liver, heart, and kidney tissues.

3. Avian ochratoxicosis

3.1. Aetiology

This is a disease of bird caused by Ochratoxins. Ochratoxins are among the most toxic mycotoxins to poultry. They are nephrotoxins found in grains and feeds worldwide [65- 66]. Ochratoxins are isocoumarin compounds linked to L-b-phenylalanine and are designated A, B, C, and D, because of their methyl and ethyl esters. Ochratoxin A (OTA) is the most common and most toxic, and is relatively stable. OTA production is dependent on different factors such as temperature, water activity (*a*w) and medium composition, which affect the physiology of fungal producers. In cool and temperate regions, OTA is mainly produced by *Penicillium verrucosum* [67, 68] or *P. Nordicum* [69, 70]. *P. verrucosum* mainly contaminates plants such as cereal crops, whereas *P. nordicum* has been mainly detected in meat products and cheese [69]. In tropical and semitropical regions, OTA is mainly produced by *Aspergillus ochraceus* [71-73]. *A. ochraceus* is also referred to as *A. allutaceus* var *allutaceus* [71]. *A. ochraceus* have been reported in a large variety of matters like nuts, dried peanuts, beans, spices green coffee beans and dried fruits, but also in processed meat and smoked and salted fish [71]. Two other species of *Aspergillus section nigri, A. niger* var *niger* [74-75] and *A. carbonarius*[76,77] have been reported as OTA producers. The OTA contamination of substrate such as cereals, oilseeds and mixed feeds in warm zones is thought to be due to *A.niger* var *niger* in addition to *A. ochraceus* species [78], whereas *A. carbonarius* seems to be more common in grapes, raisins and coffee [79-80].

Recently, [81] isolated two new OTA producing *Aspergillus* species from coffee beans. These species, *A. lacticoffeatus* and *A. sclerotioniger*, need further investigations and are provisionally accepted in section *Nigri*. In addition, another *Aspergillus* species, *A. alliaceus* also named *Petromyces alliaceus* isolated from onions [82] has been previously reported as OTA producer under laboratory conditions [83]. This species has been suspected to be responsible for the occasional OTA contamination in Californian figs [84, 85] an Argentinean medicinal herbs [67]. The biosynthetic pathway for OTA has not yet been completely established. However, labeling experiments using both 14C- and 13C-labelled precursors showed that the phenylalanine moiety originates from the schikimate pathway and the dihydroisocoumarin moiety from the pentaketide pathway. The first step in the synthesis of the isocoumarin polyketide consists in the condensation of one acetate unit (acetyl-CoA) to four malonate units. Recent data showed that this step requires the activity of a polyketide synthase [86]. Moreover, the gene encoding polyketide synthase appears to be very different between *Penicillium* and *Aspergillus* species [86]. In *A. ochraceus,* the gene of polyketide synthase is expressed only under OTA permissive conditions and only during the early stages of the mycotoxin synthesis [86]. No such data are presently available on *penicillium*. In *Penicillium* species, ' [86]' observed that *P.nordicum* and *P. verrucosum* use two different polyketide synthases for OTA synthesis. This difference is probably related to the *P. verrucosum* ability to produce citrinin, also a polyketide-based mycotoxin, in addition to OTA.

Destined Specie	Country	Type of samples	Type of Grain composition	LOD (LOQ)	Incidence (%)	Average	Range	References
Poultry	Kuwait	Raw ingredients	Wheat bran	5	10/14(71.4%)	4.6	n.d. -12.1	[87]
			soybean meal		18/21(85.8%)	7.9	n.d – 40	
			Yellow maize		31/32 (96.8%)	6.38	n.d.–14.5	
		Feed	Layer mash	-	20/20 (100%)	9.6	5-16.7	
			broiler starter		13/14 (93%)	8.0	nd-9.1	
			Broiler finisher	-	17/19 (90%)	6.1	nd-14.3	
Poultry	Venezuela	Concentrated feed	-	-	47 /50 (94%)	-	2.56 -31.98	[88]
Poultry	Argentina	Feed	Corn (60%)	10	38%	27		[89]
Poultry	China	Feed			61.5%	7.0		[37]
Poultry	India	Raw ingredients	Wheat		4/12 (33.3%)	60.75	n.d. -98	[90]
			Maize		5/12 (41.7%)	104.4	n.d. -140	
			Rice		3/12 (25%)	20	n.d. -25	
			Sorghum		2/12 (16.7%)	34	n.d. -38	
			Barley		3/12 (25%)	26	n.d. -38	
			Grams		2/12 (16.7%)	12.5	n.d - 15	
			Ground nut		2/12 (16.7%)	39	n.d.48	
			Millet		3/12 (25%)	2.5	n.d. -3	
			Cotton seed meal		2/10 (20%)	31	n.d. -42	
			Soybean meal		2/10 (20%)	31	n.d. -42	
			Rapeseed meal		2/10 (20%)	19	n.d. -28	
			Sunflower meal		3/10 (30%)	49	n.d. -68	
			Guar meal		2/10 (20%)	21	n.d. -22	
			Corn gluten meal		2/10 (20%)	21	n.d. -22	

Source: [91]

Table 6. Showing the occurrence of Ochratoxin in developing countries in a selected surveys.

3.2. Occurrence of ochratoxin

OTA was reported by [90] in raw ingredient for making poultry feed were found to be contaminated at range of 00-140 μg/kg in maize 00-98mg/kg in wheat followed by sunflower meal at 00-68 μg/kg. The incidence in India ranges from 16-41% [90]. Also high level of contamination was reported in soya meal from Kuwait n-d-40 μg/kg [87]. [88] reported a contamination level of 2.56-31.98 μg/kg in Venezuela concentrated poultry feed investigated.

Animal specie	Production Phase (age)	Experimental (dosage)	Clinical signs and (duration)performance effects	Gross pathology	References
Laying hens) (*Isa brown*	Laying (28 week-old)	Artificially contaminated feed (100-2000) ug/kg (30 days)	Decrease of egg mean weight Decrease of number of eggs placed Shell decalcification/thinning Egg altered conformation	Kidney Congestion and hemorrhages Increased size Liver - Yellowish	[92]
Broiler chickens	Fattening (6 day-old)	Artificially contaminated feed (100-2000) μg/kg (28 days)	Decreased growth rate Reduced feed consumption Decreased feed conversion Reduced serum protein and albumin.	Not evaluated	[93]
Laying hen (*Isa brown)*	Laying (11month old)	Naturally contaminated diet (160-332) ug/kg	Debility Reduced egg production	Kidneys Congestion Hemorrhage Renomegalia Liver yellowish color Diffuse Hepatomegalia Scattered necrotic foci Congestion Hemorrhage	[94]
Broiler chickens	Fattening (1 day-old)	Artificially contaminated Feed (0-800) ug/kg (5 weeks)	Significantly decreased of -Body weight -Feed consumption - Feed conversion ratio - Increased mortality	Not assessed	[95]

Source: [91]

Table 7. Showing the main clinical signs, performance and pathological features in poultry exposed to OTA in selected studies

4. Funmonism

4.1. Aetiology

The fumonism, are food borne carcinogenic mycotoxin that affect animals and man. They are evaluated as group 2B component carcinogen [96]. It has various analog. Twenty eight fumonisin analogs separated into four main groups, as fumonisin A, B, C, and P series has been identified. The fumonisin B (FB) analogs, comprising toxicologically important FB_1, FB_2, and FB_3, are the most abundant naturally occurring fumonisins, with FB_1 predominating and usually being found at the highest levels [96] in feed ingredients and poultry feed in world wide. FB_1 accounts for about 80% of the total fumonisins produced inthis substrates, while FB_2 usually makes around 20% and FB_3 usually makes up from about 5% when cultured on corn or rice or in liquid medium [97-100].

Different *Fusarium* species have been reported to produce fumonisins

4.2. Occurrence of fumonisin

FB1 a potent carcinogen was found in maize investigated from developing countries like Argentina, Benin, Egypt, Nepal, Honduras, Malawi, Zambia Botswana, and Tanzania at a range between 35- 65,000 μg/kg. [101-109]. Poultry feed investigated in china was contaminated with 1854.3mg/kg(37).

No doubt the climatic condition to the agricultural practices in these country allow the growth of fungi and subsequent elaboration of toxin in their substrate.

Country	Nature of samples	Number of samples Positive/total	Highest level (μg/kg)	References
Argentina	maize	16/17	2000	[101]
Benin	maize	20/21	2310	[102]
Egypt	maize	2/2	2380	[103]
Nepal	maize	12/24	4600	[104]
Honduras	Maize	24/24	6555	[105]
Zambia	maize	20/20	1710	[102]
China	Poultry Feed	82%	1854.3	[37]
Botswana	Maize		35-255	[106]
Mozambique	Maize		240-296	[106]
Malawi	Maize		ND-115	[106]
Tanzania	Maize		ND-160	[106]
Honduras	Maize		68-6555	[107]
Uruguay	Maize		ND-3688	[108]
Coastarica	Maize		1700-4780	[109]

Table 8. Occurrence of FB1 In Feed Ingredient In Developing Countries

Animal Species	Type of toxin	Clinical signs	Gross pathology	Histopathology	References
Laying hen	FB1	Black sticky diarrhea Reduction in food intake, egg production and body weight. Lameness, increased mortality and impaired immunity.	Kidney, pancreas and liver enlargement. Enlargement of proventiculus. Atrophy of lymphoid Organ. Rickets.	Liver has multifocal necrosis of hepatocytes hyperplasia of hepatocytes and bile ductules. Intestine had villous atrophy Globlet cell hyperplasia lymphoid cell depletion from thymus.	[110] [111]
	FB1+ FB2 + moliniformin.			Decrease in blood cell counts Haemoglobin, PCV and white Blood cell count. Abnormal erythrocyte Formation	[112]
Chicken Embryo	FB1	100% mortality	pathological changes in liver, heart, lung, Musculoskeletal system, Intestine, testis and brain		[113]
Duckling	FBs		slightly swollen and Reddened liver, low body fat And loss of weight		[113, 114]
Turkey And poult	FB1	loss of weight	cerebral encephalomalasia	increased sphingamine to Sphingosine ratio in the Serum by distrupting Biosynthesis of ceramide and sphingolipid metabolism Hepatocellular and biliary hyperplasia	[115, 116]

Table 9. Showing the main clinical signs, performance and pathological features in poultry exposed to fumonism in selected studies

5. Fusariotoxin poisoning

Synonyms Fusariomycotoxicosis, trichothecene mycotoxicosis, T-2 toxicosis, vomitoxicosis, zearalenone toxicosis. They are responsible for various diseases of birds in developing countries.

5.1. Aetiology

The trichothecenes include deoxynivalenol (DON), 3, monoacetyldeoxynivalenol (3-AcDON), 15, mono-acetyldeoxynivalenol (15-AcDON), nivalenol (NIV), HT-2 toxin (HT-2), neosolaniol (NEO), T-2 toxin (T-2), T-2 tetraol and T-2 triol, diacetoxyscirpenol (DAS), MAS-monoacetoxyscirpenol (MAS) and fusarenone-X.

Different fungi species of the general *Fusarium* are responsible for the production of this group of mycotoxins. Major producers of trichothecenes are F. *graminearum, F. culmorum, F. cerealis, F. poae*.

5.2. Occurrence of trichothecenes

Occurrence of trichothecenes in feed ingredients and poultry feed in developing countries is as a result of ubiquitous nature of the fungi which are generally found when certain cereal crops like maize, wheat, corn, millet where grown under stressful condition such as drought. These mould occur in soil, hay and especially grains undergoing microbial and possibly enzymatic degradation [20]. Direct contamination or indirect contamination of feed may occur. Direct contamination occur when the poultry feed were infected with mycotoxigenic fungi.

Indirect contamination may be as a result of fungi elaborating its toxin into the substrate, the incriminating fungi may be removed but the toxin remained in the poultry feed made from such feed ingredients.

Since moulded feed are part of the diet of animal in developing counties, thus all poultry feed are suspect and may contain different level of Trichotheceus toxin.

DON has been reported in maize from Nigeria, South Africa, Argentina, Brazil Pakistan at different concentration that ranges from 0.05-2650 mg/kg [116-120].

6. Diagnosis

Diagnosis is made through observing the appropriate field signs, finding gross as well as microscopic tissue lesions, and detecting the suspected toxin in grains, forages, or the ingesta of affected animals. However, the tests required to detect these toxins are complex and few diagnostic laboratories offer tests for multiple trichothecenes in developing countries. The samples of choice include both refrigerated and frozen carcasses for necropsy examination and a representative sample of the suspected contaminated grain source. Because the toxin is produced under cold conditions, the grain sample should be frozen rather than refrigerated for shipment to the diagnostic laboratory.

Country	Feed samples	Type of toxin	Range (µg/kg)	References
Nigeria	Maize	DON	9.5-745.1	[116]
	Maize	3-acDON	0.7-72.4	
	Maize	DAS	1.0-51.0	
Poland	Wheat	DON	2-40	[121]
	Wheat	NIV	0.01	
	Wheat	ZEN	0.01-2	
Bulgaria	Wheat	DON	up to 1.8	[122]
	Wheat	ZEN	up to 0.12	
Finland	Feed and grains	DON	0.007-0.3	[123]
	Feed and grain	ZEN	0.022-0.095	
Norway	Wheat	DON	0.45-4.3	[124]
Netherland	Wheat	DON	0.020-0.231	[125]
	Wheat	NIV	0.007-0.203	
	Wheat	ZEN	0.002-0.174	
South Africa	Maize	DON	up to 1.83	[126]
	Maize	NIV	up to 0.37	
South Africa	Cereals and Animal feed	ZEN	0.05-8.0	[117]
Philippine	Maize	NIV	0.018-0.102	[127]
	Maize	ZEN	0.059-0.505	
Thailand	Maize	ZEN	0.923	[127]
Korea	Maize	DON	Mean-0.145	[128]
	Maize	NIV	Mean-168	
Vietnam	Maize powder	DON	1.53-6.51	[129]
	Maize powder	NIV	0.78-1.95	
China	Maize	DON	0.49-3.10	[129]
	Maize	NIV	0.6	
Japan	Wheat	DON	0.029-11.7	[130]
	Wheat	NIV	0.01-4.4	
	Wheat	ZEN	0.053-0.51	
New Zealand	Maize	DON	Max 3.4-8.5	[131]
	Maize	NIV	Max 4.4-7.0	
	Maize	ZEN	Max 2.7-10.5	
U.S.A	Wheat	DON	up to 9.3	[132]
Canada	Wheat and barley	DON	up to 0.5	[133]
	Wheat and barley	ZEN	up to 0.3	
	Maize	DON	0.02-4.09	[134]
Argentina	Wheat	DON	0.10-9.25	[118]
Brazil	Wheat	DON	0.47-0.59	[119]
	Wheat	NIV	0.16-0.40	
	Wheat	ZEN	0.04-0.21	
Pakistan	Maize	Nivalenol	500-2650	[120]
	Maize	DON	136-2656	
	Maize	3-ac DON	100-850	
	Maize	ZON	1250	
	Maize	15ac DON	100	
	Maize	DAS	364-750	
	Maize	HT-2	100-500	
	Maize	T-2	143-1125	

Table 10. Occurrence of Trichothecenes in Feed Ingredients In Developing Countries

Domestic Animal	Type of toxin	clinical signs	Gross lesions	Histopathology	References
Domestic poultry		Gastrointestinal bleeding Neurological abnormality Flaccid paralysis, weakness Of the neck and wing muscles Characteristic drooping head And wings. Immune suppression which May predispose bird to Secondary bacteria infection	Skin and mucosal surface inflammation which affected subcutaneous fluid over head and neck. Multiple haemorrhage and pale area in skeletal muscle.		[136]
Chicken	DAS T-2 toxin	necrotic lesion on the tongue reduces growth rate and efficiency	Lesion in palatine, sublingual, internal angle of the tongue.		[137]
	DAS	feed refusal Haemorrhagic disorder Prolong clothing time Mild diarrhea, fatigue, ataxia Poor feathering, poor feather Quality and soft bones, Subcutaneous edema, Degeneration of neck muscle.	Enlargement of liver, and gallbladder. perivascular edema of brain, depletion of lymphocyte in thymus and bursa of fabriciuos	it affects Coagulation factors VII, prothrombin fibrinogen	[138]
	T-2 And Aflatoxin	Decrease egg production increase egg shell breakage			[139]
Duck	DON	100% mortality and high Concentration	dehydration and heamorrhage along the intestinal epithelium		[140]
	T-2 toxin	reduced body weight		altered serum And plasma Level	[141]
	DON	reduced egg production			[142]
Goose And turkey	T-2 toxin	decrease egg production	degenerative changes in ovaries Interruption of maturation of Follicle. Peritonitis, bleeding, Wrapped oviducts, necrosis and Spleen amilodiosis. Catarrhal Enteritis.		

Table 11. Showing the main clinical signs, gross and histopathological changes in some poultry species.

7. Management of avian mycotoxicosis

This involves various practises that reduces fungal contamination of feedstuff and possible use of mycotoxin binders in feed. The clinical signs seen in avian mycotoxicosis are not pathognomonic so the presence of toxin in feed with the associated clinical signs may help clinician to make effective diagnosis and withdrawal of contaminated feed can help to ameliorated the disease condition. Preventive and control of mould in feed is key to achieving control of avian mycotoxicosis.

Following good agricultural practices during both pre-harvest and post-harvest conditions would, minimize the problem of contamination by mycotoxins such as aflatoxins, ochratoxin and trichothecene mycotoxins. These include appropriate drying techniques, maintaining proper storage facilities and taking care not to expose grains.

7.1. Prevention and control of mycotoxins in stored grains and seeds

7.1.1. Dry the feed ingredients

Fungi cannot grow or mycotoxins be produced in properly dried foods, so efficient drying of commodities and maintenance of the dry state is an effective control measure against fungal growth and mycotoxin production.

To reduce or prevent production of most mycotoxins, drying should take place as soon after harvest and as rapidly as feasible. The critical water content for safe storage corresponds to a water activity (a_w) of about 0.7. Maintenance of feeds below 0.7 a_w is an effective technique used throughout the world for controlling fungal spoilage and mycotoxin production in foods.

Problems in maintaining an adequately low a_w often occur in the tropics, where high ambient humidity make control of commodity moisture difficult. Where grain is held in bags, systems that employ careful drying and subsequent storage in moisture-proof plastic sheeting may overcome this problem.

While it is possible to control fungal growth in stored commodities by controlled atmospheres or use of preservatives or natural inhibitors, such techniques are almost always more expensive than effective drying, and are thus rarely feasible in developing countries.

7.1.2. Avoid grain damage

Damaged grain is more prone to fungal invasion and therefore mycotoxin contamination. It is thus important to avoid damage before and during drying, and in storage. Drying of maize on the cob, before shelling, is a very good practice.

Insects are a major cause of damage. Field insect pests and some storage species damage grain on the head and promote fungal growth in the moist environment of the ripening grain. In storage, many insect species attack grain, and the moisture that can accumulate from their activities provides ideal conditions for the fungi. To avoid moisture and mould problems, it is essential that numbers of insects in stored grain be kept to a minimum. Such problems are compounded if the grain lacks adequate ventilation, particularly if metal containers are used.

7.1.3. Ensure proper storage conditions

While keeping commodities dry during storage in tropical areas can be difficult, the importance of dry storage cannot be overemphasized. On a small scale, polyethylene bags are effective; on a large scale, safe storage requires well-designed structures with floors and walls impermeable to moisture. Maintenance of the water activity of the stored commodity below 0.7 is crucial.

In tropical areas, outdoor humidities usually fall well below 70% on sunny days. Appropriately timed ventilation, fan-forced if necessary, will greatly assist the maintenance of the commodity at below 0.7 aw. Ideally, all large-scale storage areas should be equipped with instruments for measuring humidity, so that air appropriate for ventilation can be selected.

Sealed storage under modified atmospheres for insect control is also very effective for controlling fungal growth, provided the grain is adequately dried before storage, and provided diurnal temperature fluctuations within the storage are minimised.

If commodities must be stored before adequate drying this should be for only short periods of no more than, say, three days. Use of sealed storage or modified atmospheres will prolong this safe period, but such procedures are relatively expensive and gaslight conditions are essential.

A proven system of storage management is needed, with mycotoxin considerations an integral part of it. A range of decision-support systems is becoming available covering the varying levels of sophistication and scale involved.

7.2. Control

Control of mycotoxin in poultry feed is important and it should be hinged on eliminating mycotoxin from the food chain. Mycotoxygenic fungi are naturally found in soil and air, which makes it difficult to prevent their contamination of agriculture commodities. Nevertheless attempts should be made to control factors that affects the growth of mycotoxigenic fungi and the subsequent toxin production. Factors which include warm temperature between (20°c to 30°c), high moisture content (20-25%), water activity (a_w) of about 0.7aw and relative humidity of 70% and above. These factors enhance fungi growth and mycotoxin production (143,145).

Before harvesting of crops damage to grains as a result of field insect pest and some storage species damage grains and promote fungal growth in the environment of ripening grain. Strategies used in various preventive measure in poultry feed involves good agronomic practices, detoxification of mycotoxin in grains use of mould inhibitors, genetic approach through improved breeds of plants.

7.2.1. Physical decontamination

Decontamination of mycotoxin from cereal crops used in the production of poultry feed can be classified as physical decontamination, biological decontamination and chemical decontamination [146]. [145] suggest the following method of elimination of mycotoxin in grains which include, Density segregation and floatation, cleaning and washing, seiving, dehulling, hand picking, irradiation, milling, thermal degeneration.

[147] observed that washing using distill water resulted in 65%-95% reduction of DON (16-24mg/kg) and 2% to 61% of ZEN (0.9-1.6mg/kg) in contaminated barley and corn.

Density segregation in certain liquid or fractionation by specific gravity help to segregate fungi infected and mycotoxin contamination grains used in the production of poultry feed.[148]. It was also observed that fumonisms present in broken corn kernels is about 10 fold higher than that in intact corn therefore the separation based on the size has been suggested. [147, 146]

Irradiation is also a useful tool in inactivation of some mycotoxin reported ultrasonication been used in contaminated corn without affecting the grain composition. Several workers reported the use of Gamma irradiation to reduce Zearelenone DON and T-2 toxin in corn, wheat. [148-150]

7.2.2. Biological decontamination

This involved systemic degradation of toxins leading to a less toxin product. [151] reports a fungus yeast *Expoliata spinnifera* was able to grow on fumonisin B1as a sole of carbon source. The hydrolysis of fumonisin B1 yields free Tricarboxylic acid and aminopental, the intermediate aminopentol undergo oxidative deamination. *Sacchromyces cerevisiae* ferment zearalenone converting it into beta-zearelenol, which has less activity compared to the parent compound.[152]

Feed additive like mycotoxin inactivates trichothecenes by enzymatic decontamination of the 12-13 epoxy ring, and zealenone by the enzymatic opening of the lactone ring [148-152]

7.2.3. Detoxification of mycotoxin feed

Moist ozone and dry ozone were able to reduce DON concentration in contaminated corn up to 90% and 70% respectively [153]. [154] reports 79% reduction in fumonism level in corn.

Author details

Adeniran Lateef Ariyo and Ajagbonna Olatunde Peter

Department of Physiology and Biochemistry, Faculty of Veterinary Medicine, University of Abuja, Nigeria

Sani Nuhu Abdulazeez

Department of Veterinary Pathology, Faculty of Veterinary Medicine, University of Abuja, Nigeria

Olabode Hamza Olatunde
Department of Veterinary Microbiology, Faculty of Veterinary Medicine, University of Abuja, Nigeria

8. References

[1] Simons P. Global production, Consumption and International market of Poultry meat and eggs. World's Poultry Science Association (WPSA) Poultry Seminar, Lonovala, In September 12 2009
[2] Moss M O. Mycotoxic fungi. In: Microbial Food Poisoning. Elley, A. R. (Ed) Chapman and Hall. London, Glassgow, New York, Tokyo, Melbourne, Madras. 1992 ; Pp 73-106.
[3] D'Mello JPF. Mycotoxins in cereal grains, nuts and other plant products. In: Food Safety Contaminants and Toxins. D'Mello, J P. F.(Ed).Cromwell Press, Trowbridge, UK; 2003. 65-90.
[4] Pitt J I. What are mycotoxins? Mycotoxin News 7:1.1996
[5] Scimeca J A. Naturally occurring orally active dietary carcinogens. In: Handbook of humantoxicology. Massaro, E. J. (Ed), Boka Raton, New York, U.S.A.; 1997. Pp 409-466.
[6] van Egmond HP, Speijers GJA. Survey of data on the incidence and levels of ochratoxin A in food and animal feed worldwide. Natural Toxins 1994; 3: 125-144.
[7] Bhatnagar D, Yu J. Ehrlich K. C. Toxins of filamentous fungi. Chemical Immunology 2002; 81: 167-206.
[8] FA O 1983. Post harvest losses in quality of food grains. Food and Agriculture Organisation (Food and Nutrition Paper No 29; 1983. p. 103.
[9] DeVries JW., Trucksess MW., Jackson LS. Mycotoxins and Food Safety. Kluwer Academic/Plenum Publishers, New York, NY, USA. 2002.
[10] Blount WP. Turkey X disease Turkeys. Journal of the British Turkey Association 1961; *9, 55-58.*
[11] Peterson SW, Ito Y, Horn BW, Goto T. *Aspergillus bombycis*, a new aflatoxigenic species and genetic variation in its sibling species, A. nomius. Mycologia 2001; 93, 689–703.
[12] Ito Y, Peterson SW, Wicklow DT, Goto T. *Aspergillus pseudotamarii,* a new Aflatoxin producing species in *Aspergillus* section *Flavi*. Mycological Research 2001; 105, 233–239.
[13] Frisvad JC, Skouboe P, Samson RA. Taxonomic comparison of three different groups of aflatoxin producers and a new efficient producer of aflatoxin B1, sterigmatocystin and 3-O-methylsterigmatocystin, *Aspergillus rambellii sp.* nov Systematic Applied Microbiology 2005; 28, 442–453.
[14] Frivad JC, Samson RA, Smedsgaard J. Emericella astellata, a new producer of aflatoxin B1, B2 and sterigmatocystin. Letters in Applied Microbiology 2004; 38, 440–445.
[15] Mircea C, Poiata A, Tuchilus C, Agoroae L, Butnaru E, Stanescu U. Aflatoxigenic fungi isolated from medicinal herbs Toxicology Letters 2008; 180: 32-246.
[16] Makun HA, Dutton MF, Njobeh PB, Gbodi TA, Ogbadu GH. Aflatoxin Contamination in Foods and Feeds: A Special Focus on Africa .Intech; 2012.

[17] D'Mello JPF. Mycotoxins in cereal grains, nuts and other plant products. In: Food Safety Contaminants and Toxins. D'Mello, J P. F.(Ed).Cromwell Press, Trowbridge, UK; 2003. 65-90.

[18] Stössel P. Aflatoxin contamination in soybeans: role of proteinase inhibitors, zinc availability, and seed coat integrity. Applied and Environmental Microbiology 1986; 52, 68–72.

[19] Schindler AF. Temperature limits for production of aflatoxin by twenty-five isolates of *Aspergillus flavus* and *Aspergillus parasiticus*. Journal of Food Protection. 1977; 40:39–40.

[20] Ominski KH., Marquardi RR., Sinha RN., Abramson D . Ecological aspects of growth and mycotoxin production by storage fungi. In: Miller, J.D and Trenholm, HL. Mycotoxins in grains: Compounds other than aflatoxins. Eagan Press, St. Paul Minnesota, USA.1994; 287-314.

[21] Codex Alimentarius Commission. Code of Practice for the Prevention and Reduction of Aflatoxin Contamination in Peanuts. 2004. Retrieved August, 2012 from http://www.codexalimentarius.net/download/standards/10084/CXC_055_2004e. pdf.

[22] Kaaya NA., Warren HL. A review of past and present research on aflatoxin in Uganda African Journal of Food Agriculture Nutrition and Development 2005, 18 pages (On Line Free Access)

[23] Agboola S.D 1992. Post harvest technologies to reduce mycotoxin contamination of food crops. In Z.S.C Okoye (ed) Book of proceedings of the first National Workshop on Mycotoxins held at University Jos, on the 29th November, 1990, 73-88.

[24] Anjum MA., Khan SH., Sahota AW, Sardar R. Assessment of Aflatoxin B1 in commercial poultry feed and feed ingredients. The journal of animal and plant sciences 2012; 22, 268-272.

[25] Odoemelam SA., Osu CI. Aflatoxin B1 contamination of some edible grains marketed in Nigeria. E-Journal of Chemistry 2009; 6 (2):308-314.

[26] Adebayo-Tayo BC, Ettah AE. Microbiological quality and aflatoxin B1 level in poultry and livestock feeds. Nigerian Journal of Microbiology, 2010; 24(1): 2145 – 2152.

[27] Kang'ethe EK., Lang.a KA. Aflatoxin B1 and M1 contamination of animal feeds and milk from urban centers in Kenya. African Health Sciences 2009; 9 (4): 218-226

[28] Mngadi PT, Govinden R, Odhav B. Co-occurring mycotoxins in animal feeds. African Journal of Biotechnology 2008; 7 (13): 2239-2243.

[29] Zinedine, A Juan, C Soriano, JM Moltó, JC Idrissi, L and Mañes. J. Limited survey for the occurrence of aflatoxins in cereals and poultry feeds from Rabat, Morocco International Journal of Food Microbiology 2007; 115, 124–127.

[30] Matumba L, Monjerezi M, Khonga EB, Lakudzala DD. Aflatoxins in sorghum, sorghum malt and traditional opaque beer in southern Malawi. Food Control 2011; 22, 266-268

[31] Muthomi JW, Ndung'u JK, Gathumbi JK, Mutitu EW, Wagacha JM. The occurrence of *Fusarium species* and mycotoxins in Kenyan wheat. Crop Protection 2008; 27, 1215– 1219.

[32] Ghali R, Khlifa KH, Ghorbel H, Maaroufi K, Hedilli A. Incidence of aflatoxins, ochratoxin A and zearalenone in Tunisian foods. Food Control 2008; 19, 921–924.

[33] Riba A., Bouras N., Mokrane S., Mathieu F., Lebrihi A., Sabaou N. *Aspergillus section Flavi* and aflatoxins in Algerian wheat and derived products. Food and Chemical Toxicology 2010; 48, 2772–2777

[34] Mashinini K, Dutton MF. The incidence of fungi and mycotoxins in South Africa wheat and wheat-based products Journal of Environmental Science and Health Part B, 2006; 41:285-296

[35] Akrobortu DE. Aflatoxin contamination of maize from different storage locations in Ghana. An M.Sc. Thesis submitted to the Department of Agricultural Engineering, Kwame Nkrumah University of Science and Technology, Ghana. 2008; 27-32.

[36] Makun HA, Gbodi TA, Akanya HO, Sakalo AE, Ogbadu HG. Fungi and some mycotoxins contaminating rice (Oryza sativa) in Niger state, Nigeria. African Journal of Biotechnology 2007; 6(2):99–108

[37] Njobeh PB., Dutton MF., Aberg AT., Haggblom P. Estimation of multi-mycotoxin contamination in South African compound feeds. Toxins 2012; 4, 836-848.

[38] Binder EM. managing the risk of mycotoxins in modern feed production Animal Science and Technology. 2007; 133:149-166.

[39] Anjum AD. Outbreak of infectious bursar disease in vaccinated chickens due to aflatoxicosis. Indian Veterinary Journal 1994; 71:322-324.

[40] Asplin FD, Carnaghan RBA. The toxicity of certain groundnut meals for poultry with special reference to their effect on ducklings and chickens. Veterinary Record 1961; 73:1215-1219.

[41] Siller WG, Ostler DC. The histopathology of an entero- hepatic syndrome of turkey poults. Veterinary Record 1961; 73:134-138.

[42] Wannop CC. The bistopathology of turkey "x" disease in Great Britain. Avian Disease 1961; 5:371-381.

[43] Archibald RM, Smith HJ, Smith JD. Brazilian groundnut toxicosis in Canadian broiler chickens. Canadian Veterinary Journal 1962; 3:322-325.

[44] Batra PA, Pruthi K, Sandana IR. Effect of aflatoxin B1 on the efficacy of turkey herpesvirus vaccine against Marek's disease. Reseach in Veterinary Science 1991 ;51:115-119.

[45] Sharlin 1S, Howarth B, Jr. Wyatt RD. Effect of dietary aflatoxin on reproductive performance of mature White Leghorn males. Poultry Science 1980; 59:1311-1315.

[46] Ortalatli M, Ciftci MK, Tuzcu M, Kaya A. The effects of aflatoxin on the reproductive system of roosters. Research in Veterinary Science 2002; 72:29-36.

[47] Larsen C, Acha M, Ehrich M. Research note: Chlortetracycline and aflatoxin interaction in two lines of chicks. Poultry Science 1988; 67: 1229-1232.

[48] Smith IW, Hill CH, Hamilton PB. The effect of dietary modifications on aflatoxicosis in the broiler chicken. Poultry Science 1971; 50:768-774.

[49] Basic Food Safety for Health Workers.WHO. 1999

[50] Chipley IR, Mabee MS, Applegate KL, Dreyt"us.i MS. Further characterization of tissue distribution and metabolism of (I4C) aflatoxin BI in chickens. Applied Microbiology 1974; 28:1027-1029.

[51] Patterson OSP, Roberts BA. The in vitro reduction of allatoxins Bland 82 by soluble avian liver enzymes. Food Additive and Contaminant 1971; 9:821-831.

[52] Dutton ME. Fumonisins, Mycotoxins of Increasing Importance:Their Nature and Their Effects. Pharmacology and Therapeutics. 1996; 70(2) 137-161

[53] Harland EC, Cardeilhac PT. Excretion of carbon14-labeled aflatoxin BI via bile, urine. and intestinal contents of the chicken. American Journal of Veterinary Research 1975; 36:909-912.

[54] Sawhney DS, Vadehra DV, Baker RC. The metabolism of [14C] aflatoxins in laying hens. Poultry Science 1973; 52:1302-1309.

[55] Oliveira CA, Kobashigawa E, Reis TA, Mestieri L, Albuquerque R, Correa B. Aflatoxin B I residues in eggs of laying hens fed a diet comaining different levels of the mycotoxin. Food Additive and Contaminant 2000; 17:459-462.

[56] Jacobson WC, Wiseman HG. The transmission of aflatoxin BI into eggs. Poultry Sciience 1974; 53:1743-1745.

[57] Trucksess MW, Stoloff L, Young K, Wyatt RD, Miller BL. Aflatoxicol and aflatoxins B I and MI in eggs and tissues of laying hens consuming aflatoxin-contaminated feed. Poultry Science 1983; 62:2176--2182.

[58] Sova Z, Fukal L, Trefuy D, Prosek I, Slamova A. Bl aflatoxin (AFBI) transfer from reproductive organs of farm birds into their eggs and hatched young. Conference of European Agriculture 1986;7:602-603.

[59] Lillehoj EB, Aalund O, Hald B. Bioproduction of 14C Ochratoxin A in submerged culture, Applied Environmental Microbiology. 1978; 36 : 720–723..

[60] Foster PL, Eisenstadt E, Miller JH. Base substitution mutations induced by metabolically activated aflatoxin B1. Proceeding of National Academic of Science 1983; 80 : 2695–2698.

[61] Raney KD, Meyer DJ, Ketterer B, Harris TM, Guengerich FP. Glutathione conjugation of aflatoxin B-1 exo- and endo-epoxides by rat and human glutathione-S-transferases. Chemical Research Toxicology 1992; 5 :470–478.

[62] Bababunmi EA, Thabrew I, Bassir O. Aflatoxin induced coagulopathy in different nutritionally classified animal species. World Review of Nutrition and Diet 1997; 34 : 161–181.

[63] Shen M, Ong CN, Shi CY. Involvement of reactive oxygen species in aflatoxin B1-induced cell injury in cultured rat hepatocytes. Toxicology 1997; 99 :115–123

[64] Bonsi GP, Agusti-Tocco M, Palmery M, Giorgi M. Aflatoxin B_1 is an inhibitor of cyclic nucleotide phosphodiesterase activity. General Pharmacoogy 1991; 32: 615–619.

[65] Dwivedi P, Burns RB. The natural occurrence of ochratoxin A and its effects in poultry. A review. Part I. Epidemiology and toxicity. World Poultry Science Journal 1986; 42:32-47.

[66] Rosa C A R, Ribeiro J M M, Fraga M J, Gatti M, Cavaglieri L R, Magnoli C E, Dalcero A M, Lopez C WG. Mycoflora ofpoultry feeds and ochratoxin-producing ability of isolated *Aspergillus* and *Penicillium species.* Veterinary Microbiology 2006; 113:89-96.

[67] Rizzo I, Vedoya G, Maurotto S, Haidukowski M, Varkavsky E. Assessment of oxinogenic fungi on Argentinean medicinal herbs, Microbiology Research 2004; 159:113–120.

[68] Sawhney DS, Vadehra DV, Baker RC. The metabolism of [14C] aflatoxins in laying hens. Poultry Science 1973; 52:1302-1309.

[69] Larsen TO, Svendsen A, Smedsgaard J. Biochemical characterization of ochratoxin A-roducing strains of the genus Penicillium, Applied Environmental Microbiology 2001; 67: 3630–3635.

[70] Castella G, Larsen TO, Cabanes J, Schmidt H, Alboresi A, Niessen L, Geisen R. Molecular characterization of ochratoxin A producing strains of the genum Penicillium, Systemic and Applied Microbiology 2002; 25 : 74–83

[71] Kozakiewicz Z. Aspergillus species on stored products, Mycological paper no. 161, CAB International Mycological Institute, Kew, UK, 1989, p. 1.

[72] Pardo E, Mar´ın S, Ramos AJ, Sanchis V. Effect of water activity and temperature on mycelial growth and ochratoxin A production by isolates of Aspergillus ochraceus onirradiated green coffee beans, Journal of Food Protection 2005; 68 : 133–138.

[73] Basic Food Safety for Health Workers.WHO. 1999

[74] Abarca M, Bragualt M R, Castella G, Cabanes F J. Ochratoxin A production by strains of Aspergillus niger var niger, Applied Environmental Microbiology 1994; 60: 2650–2652.

[75] Belli N, Marin S, Sanchis V, Ramos AJ. Influence of water activity and temperature on growth of isolates of *Aspergillus section nigri* obtained from grapes, International Journal Food Microbiology 2004; 96 : 19–27.

[76] Teren J, Varga J, Hamari Z. Immunochemical detection of Ochratoxin A in black Aspergillus strain, Mycopathologia 1996;134 :171–176.

[77] Mitchell D, Parra R, Aldred D, Magan N. Water and temperature relations of growth and ochratoxin A production by Aspergillus carbonarius strains from grapes in Europe and Israel, Journal Applied Microbiology 2004; 97: 439–445.

[78] Rosa C A R, Ribeiro J M M, Fraga M J, Gatti M, Cavaglieri L R, Magnoli C E, Dalcero A M, Lopez C WG. Mycoflora Of poultry feeds and ochratoxin-producing ability of isolated *Aspergillus* and *Penicillium species.* Veterinary Microbiology 2006; 113:89-96.

[79] Accensi F, Abarca M.L, Cabanes FJ. Occurrence of Aspergillus species in Mixed feeds and component raw materials and their ability to produce ochratoxin A, Food Microbiology 2004; 21 : 623–627.

[80] Beg MU, Al-Mutairi M, Beg KR, Al-Mazeedi HM, Ali LN, Saeed T, 2006. Mycotoxins in poultry feed in Kuwait. Archive of Environmental Contaminant. Toxicology 2006; 50, 594–602.

[81] Cabanes FJ, Accensi F, Bragualt MR, Abarca ML, Minguez G, Pons S. What is the source of ochratoxin A in wine? International Journal Food Microbiology 2002;79 : 213–215.

[82] Samson RA, Houbraken JAMP, Kujipers AFA, Frank JM, Frisvard, JC. New ochratoxin A or sclerotium producing species in *Aspergillus section Nigri,* Study.Mycology 2004;50 : 45–61.

[83] Moss MO. Mode of formation of ochratoxin A, Food Additive and Contaminant. 1996;13 : 5–9.

[84] ayman P, Baker JL, Doster MA, Michailidis TJ, Mahoney NE. (2002).Ochratoxin production by the *Aspergillus ochraceus* group and *Aspergillus alliaceus*, Applied Environmental Microbiology 2002; 68 : 2326–2329.

[85] Varga J, Rigo K, Toth B, Teren J, Kozakiewicz Z. Evolutionary relationships among Aspergillus species producing economically important mycotoxins, Food Technology and Biotechnology 2003; 41 : 29–36.

[86] Callaghan JO, Caddick MX, Dobson AD. A polyketide synthase gene required for ochratoxin A biosynthesis in *Aspergillus ochraceus*, Microbiology 2003;149 : 3485–3491.

[87] Beg MU., Al-Mutairi M., Beg KR., Al-Mazeedi HM., Ali LN., Saeed T. Mycotoxins in poultry feed in Kuwait. Archive of Environmental Contaminant & Toxicology. 2006;50, 594–602

[88] Figueroa S, Centeno, S, Calvo MA, Rengel A, Adelantado C. Mycobiodata and concentration of ochratoxin A in concentrated poultry feed from Venezuela. Pakistan Journal of Biological Science 2009; 12: 589–594

[89] Dalcero A, Magnoli C, Hallak C, Chiacchiera SM, Palacio G, Rosa CAR. Detection of ochratoxin A in animal feeds and capacity to produce this mycotoxin for *Aspergillus section Nigri* in Argentina. Food Additives and Contaminants. 2002; 19 (11), 1065–1072.

[90] Zafar, F., Yasmin, N., Hassan, R., Naim, T., Qureshi, A.A. A study on the analysis of ochratoxin A in different poultry feed ingredients. Pakistan Journal of Pharmaceutical Sciences 2001;14, 5–7.

[91] Duarte SC, Lino CL, Pena A. Ochratoxin A in feed of food-producing animals: An undesirable mycotoxin with health and performance effects. Veterinary Microbiology 2011; 154, 1–13.

[92] Bozzo G., Bonerba E, Ceci E, Colao V, Tantillo G. Determination of ochratoxin A in eggs and target tissues of experimentally drugged hens using HPLC–FLD. Food Chemistry 2011; 126, 1278–1282.

[93] Sakthivelan SM, Rao GVS. Effect of ochratoxin A on body weight, feed intake and feed conversion in broiler chicken. Veterinary Medical Int. 2010; 1–4.

[94] Bozzo G, Ceci E, Bonerba E, Desantis S, Tantillo G. Ochratoxin A in laying hens: high-performance liquid chromatography detection and cytological and histological analysis of target tissues. Journal of Applied Poultry Research 2008; 17, 151–156.

[95] Elaroussi MA, Mohamed FR, Barkouky EME, Atta AM, Abdou AM, Hatab MH. Experimental ochratoxicosis in broiler chickens. Avian Pathology 2006; 35, 263–269.

[96] International Agency for Research on Cancer. 1993. Toxins derived from *Fusarium moniliforme*: fumonisins B_1 and B_2 and *Fusarium* C, p. 445-466. *In* IARC Monographs on the evaluation of the carcinogenic risks to humans: some naturally occurring substances: food items and constituents, heterocyclic aromatic amines and mycotoxins, vol. 56. International Agency for Research on Cancer, Lyon, France.

[97] Marasas WFO. Fumonisins: history, worldwide occurrence and impact, p. 1-17. *In* L. S. Jackson, J. W. DeVries, and L. B. Bullerman (ed.), Fumonisins in food. Plenum Press, New York, N.Y; 1996.

[98] Branham, B. E., and R. D. Plattner. 1993. Alanine is a precursor in the biosynthesis of fumonisin B_1 by *Fusarium moniliforme*. Mycopathologia 124:99-1

[99] Marín S, Sanchis V, Magan N. Water activity, temperature, and pH effects on growth of *Fusarium moniliforme* and *Fusarium proliferatum* isolates from maize. Canadian Journal of Microbiology 1995a; 41:1063-1070.

[100] Marín S, Sanchis, V, Vinas I, Canela R, Magan N. Effect of water activity and temperature on growth and fumonisin B_1 and B_2 production by *Fusarium proliferatum* and *F. moniliforme* in grain. Letter of Applied Microbiology 1995b; 21:298-301.

[101] Sydenham EW, Shephard G S, Thiel P G, Marasas, W E, Rheeder J I, Peralta C E, Gonzalez H L, Resnik S L. Fumonisins in Argentinian field trial corn. Journal of Agriculture and Food Chemistry 1993; 41: 891-895.

[102] Doko M B, Rapior S, Visconti A, Schjoth J E. Incidence and levels of fumonisin contamination in maize enotypes grown in Europe and Africa. Journal of Agriculture and Food Chemistry 1995. 43: 429-434.

[103] Sydenham E W, Shephard G S, Thiel PG, Marasas W F 0, Stockenstrom S. Fumonisin contamination of ommercial corn-based human foodstuffs. Journal of Agriculture and Food Chemistry 1991; 39: 2014-2018.

[104] Ueno Y, Aoyama S, Suglaru Y, Wang D S, Lee U S, Hirooka EY, Ham S, Karki T, Chcn G, Yu S Z. A limited survey of fumonisins in corn and corn-based products in Asia countries. Mycotoxin. Research 1993; 9: 27- 34

[105] Julian A M, Wareing IW, Phillips SI, Medlock V F, MacDonald M V, del Rio L E. Fungal contamination and selected mycotoxins in pre and postharvest maize in Honduras. Mycopathologia 1995; 129: 5-16.

[106] Doko MB., Canet C., Brown N., Sydenham EW., Mpuchane S., Siame B A. Natural co-occurrence of fumonisins and zearalenone in cereals and cereal-based foods from eastern and southern Africa. Journal of Agriculture and Food Chemistry.1996; 44, 3240-3243.

[107] Julian A M, Wareing IW, Phillips SI, Medlock V F, MacDonald M V, del Rio L E. Fungal contamination and selected mycotoxins in pre and postharvest maize in Honduras. Mycopathologia 1995; 129: 5-16.

[108] Pineiro MS., Silva GE., Scott PM., Lawrence GA., Stack ME. Fumonisin level in Uruguayan corn products. Journal of AOAC International 1997; 80, 825-828.

[109] Viquez OM., Castell-Pere M.E., Shelby RA. Occurrence of fumonisin B1 in maize grown in Costa Rica. Journal of Agriculture and Food Chemistry. 1996; 44, 2789-2791.

[110] Prathapkumar S H, RaoVS, Paramkishanand UR, Bha RV. Disease outbreak in laying hens arising from the consumption of fumonisin-oontaminated food. Br Poultry Science 1997; 38:475-479.

[111] Chatterjee D S, MukheJjee K, Dey A. Nuclear disintegration in chicken peritoneal macrophages exposed to fumonisin BI from Indian maize. Applied Microbiology 1995; 20:184-185.

[112] Dombrink-Kurtzman MA, Javed T, Bennett G A, Richard J L, Cow L, Buck W B. Lymphocyte cytotoxicity and erythrocytic abnormalities induced in broiler chicks by fumonisins B, and B1 and moniliformin from *Fusarium proliferatum.* Mycopathologia 1993; 124: 47-54.

[113] Javed I, Bennett G A, Richard J L, Dombrink Kurtzman MA, Cote L M, Buck W B. Mortality in broiler chicks on feed amended with *Fusarium proliferatum* culture materials or with purified fumonisin B and moniliformin. Mycopathologia; 1993; 123: 171-184.

[114] Marasas,VI E. Mycotoxicological investigations on corn produced in esophageal cancer areas in Transkei. In: Cancer of the Esophagus, 1982 Vol. 1, pp. 29-40, Pfeiffer, C J (ed.) CRC Press Inc, Boca Raton.

[115] Vesonder R, Halihurton J, Golinski P. Toxicity of field samples and *Fusarium moniliforme* from feed associated with equine- leucoencephalomalacia Archive of Environmental Contaminant 1989; 18: 439-442.

[116] Adejumo TO, Hettwer U, Karlovsky P. Occurrence of Fusarium species and trichothecenes in Nigerian maize. International Journal of Food Microbiology. 2007; 116: 350–357

[117] Dutton MF., Kinsey A. A note on the occurrence of mycotoxins in cereals and animal feedstuffs in Kwazulu Natal, South Africa 1984-1993. South Africa Journal of Animal Science. 1996; 26, 53-57.

[118] Pacin AM., Resnik SL., Neira MS., Molto G., Martinez E. Natural occurrence of deoxynivalenol in wheat, wheat flour and bakery products in Argentina. Food Additive and Contaminant. 1997; 14, 327-331.

[119] Furlong EB., Soares LMV., Lasca CC., Kohara EY., 1995. Mycotoxins and fungi in wheat harvested during in test plots in the state of Sao Paulo Brazil. Mycopathologia 1990; 131, 185-190.

[120] Salma K, Nafeesa Q H, Tahira I, Sultana N, Sultana K, and Ayub N. Natural occurrence of aflatoxins, zearalenone and Trichothecenes in maize grown in Pakistan, Pakistan Journal of Botanical 2012; 44(1): 231-236

[121] Perkowski J., Plattner RD., Golinski P., Vesonder RF. Natural occurrence of deoxynivalenol, 3-acetyldeoxynivalenol, 15-acetyl-deoxynivalenol, nivalenol, 4,7-dideoxynivalenol and zearalenone in Polish wheat. Mycotoxin Research. 1990; 6, 7-12.

[122] Vrabcheva T., Gebler R., Usleber E., Martlbauer E. First survey on the natural occurrence of Fusarium mycotoxins in Bulgarian wheat. Mycopathologia. 1996; 136, 47-52.

[123] Hietaniemi V., Kumpulainen J. Contents of Fusarium toxins in Finnish and imported grains and feeds. Food Additive and Contaminants. 1991; 8, 171-182.

[124] Langseth W., Elen O. Differences between barley, oats and wheat in the occurrence of deoxynivalenol and other trichothecenes in Norwegian grain. J. Phytopathology. 1996; 144, 113-118.

[125] Tanaka T., Yamamoto S., Hasegawa A., Aoki N., Besling JR., Sugiura, Y., Ueno Y. A survey of the natural occurrence of Fusarium mycotoxins, deoxynivalenol, nivalenol and zearalenone, in cereals harvested in The Netherlands. Mycopathologia. 1990; 110, 19-22.

[126] Rheeder JP., Sydenham EW., Marasas WFO., Thiel PG., Shephard GS., Schlechter M., Stockenstrom S. .. Viljoen JH. Fungal infestation and mycotoxin contamination of South African commercial maize harvested in 1989 and 1990. South Africa Journal of Science.1995; 91, 127-131.

[127] Yamashita A., Yoshizawa T., Aiura Y., Sanchez PC., Dizon EI., Arim, RH., Sardjono, , 1995. Fusarium mycotoxins (fumonisins, nivalenol and zearalenone) and aflatoxins in corn from southeast Asia. Biological science.Biotechnology. Biochemistry. 1995; 59, 1804-1807.

[128] Ryu JC., Yang JS., Song YS., Kwon OS., Park J., Chang IM. 1996. Survey of natural occurrence of trichothecene mycotoxins and zearalenone in Korean cereals harvested in 1992 using gas chromatography/ mass spectrometry. Food Additive and Contamination. 1996; 13, 333-341.

[129] Wang DS., Liang YX., Iijima K., Sugiura Y., Tanaka T., Chen G., Yu SZ., Ueno Y. Cocontamination of mycotoxins in corn harvested in Haimen, a high risk area of primary liver cancer in China. Mycotoxins 1995b; 41, 67-70.

[130] Yoshizawa T. Geographic difference in trichothecene occurrence in Japanese wheat and barley. Bull. Institute of. Comprehensive Agricultural Science. Kinki University 1997; 5, 23-30.

[131] Lauren DR., Jensen DJ., Smith WA., Dow BW., Sayer ST. Mycotoxins in New Zealand maize: a study of some factors influencing contamination levels in grain New Zealand. Journal of Crop and Horticultural Science. 1996; 24, 13-20.

[132] Fernandez C., Stack ME., Musser SM. Determination of deoxynivalenol in 1991 U.S. winter and spring wheat by high-performance thin-layer chromatography. Journal of AOAC Institute.1994; 77, 628-630.

[133] Stratton GW., Robinson AR., Smith HC., Kittilsen L., Barbour M. Levels of five mycotoxins in grains harvested in Atlantic Canada as measured by high performance liquid chromatography. Architecture of Environmental Contamination and Toxicology.1993; 24, 399-409.

[134] Scott PM. Multi-year monitoring of Canadian grains and grain-based foods for treichothecenes and zearalenone. Food Additive and Contaminant. 14, 333-339.

[135]

[136] Diaz G.J., Squires E. J., Julian R. J. And Boermans H.J. Individual and combined effects of T-2 toxin and DAS in laying hens and Broiler Poultry Science 1994; 35; 393 - 405

[137] Brake J, Hamilton PB, Kittrell R S. Effects of the Trichothecene Mycotoxin Diacetoxyscirpenol on Feed Consumption, Body Weight, and Oral Lesions of Broiler Breeders. Poultry Science, 2000; 79:856–863

[138] Ademoyero A. A, Hamilton PB. Influence of degree of acetylation of scirpenol mycotoxins on feed refusal by chickens. Poultry Science 1989; 68:854–856.

[139] Jakić-Dimić D, Nešić K, Šefer D. Mycotoxicoses of poultry caused by Trichothecenes. Biotechnology in Animal Husbandry 2011; 27 (3), p 713-719. DOI: 10.2298/BAH1103713J

[140] Rafai P, Pettersson H, Bata A, Papa Z, Glavits S, Tubolys S,Vanyi A, Sooss P. Effect of dietary T-2 fusariotoxin concentrations on the health and production of white Pekin duck broilers. Poultry Science 2000; 79, 1548-1556.

[141] Scott ML., Dean WF. In: Nutrition and Management of Ducks. M.&. Scott, Ithaca, NY; 1991. 150-166.

[142] Vanyi A, Bata A, Kovacs F. Effects of T-2 toxin treatment on the egg yield and hatchability in geese. Acta Veterinaria Hungarica 1994; 42, 1, 79-85.

[143] Langseth W., Hqie R. Gullord M. The influence of cultivars, location and climate on deoxynivalenol contamination in Norwegian oats (1985-1990). Acta Agriculture Scandinavica. Section B: Soil and Plant Science, 1995 45: 63-67.

[144] Ma H., Zhon M., Liu Z. Liu W. Progress on genetic improvement for resistance to wheat scab in KLA. Journal of Applied Genetics, 2002; 43: 259-266.

[145] Negedu A., Atawodi SE. Ameh JB., Umoh VJ., Tanko HY. Economic and health perspectives of mycotoxins: a review. Continental Journal of Biomedical Sciences 2011; 5 (1): 5 – 26.

[146] Gbodi TA., Makun HA., Kabiru YA., Ogbadoyi E., Tijani SA., Lawal SA., Bayero RA. Effect of local processing methods on aflatoxin contents of some common Nigerian foods prepared from artificially contaminated maize, rice and sorghum. Journal of Agricultural Science. Mansoura University. 2001; 26: 3759 -3769.

[147] Desjardins AE., Manandhar GG., Plattner RD., Maragos CM., Shrestha K.. McCormick SP. (2000). Occurrence of Fusarium species and mycotoxins in Nepalese maize and wheat and the effect of traditional processing methods on mycotoxin levels. Journal of Agricultural food Chemistry. 2000; 48:1377 – 1383.

[148] Scott PM. Mycotoxins transmitted into beer from contaminated grains during brewing. Journal of the Association of Official Analytical Chemists International. 1996; 79:675.

[149] Diaz DE., Hopkins BA., Leonard LM. Hagler WM. and Whitlow LW. Effects of fumonisin on lactating dairy cattle. J ournal Dairly Science. 2000. 83 (Abstract): 1171.

[150] Fanelli C., Taddei F., Jestoi M. and Visconti A. Use of resvertrol and BHA to control fungal growth and mycotoxin production in wheat and maize seeds. Aspect of Applied Biology. 2003. 68: 63-71.

[151] Duvick J., Rood TA., Maddox JR., and Gilliam J. Advances in ochratoxin A biosynthesis. Book of Abstracts, International Conference on "Advances on genomics, biodiversity and rapid systems for detection of toxigenic fungi and mycotooxins" September 26-29, 2006. Monopoli (Bari), Italy Pp.39 Retrieved from http://www.Ispa.onr.n/mycoglobe-2006. 1998.

[152] Leggot NL and Shephard G. Patulin in South African commercial apple products. Food Control. 2001. 12 (2) 73-76

[153] Diaz DE., and Smith TK. Mycotoxin sequestering agents: Practical tools for the neutralization of mycotoxins in the mycotoxin Blue Book. D. Diaz, ed. Nottingham Univ. Press, Nottingham, U. K. 2005.Pp. 313-339

[154] Park JW., Scott PM., Lau BPY., and Levis D A. Analysis of heat processed corn foods for fumonisins and bound fumonisns. Food Additives and Contaminants. 2004; 21:1168-1178.

Section 3

Prevention and Control of Mycotoxins

Chapter 5

Strategies for the Prevention and Reduction of Mycotoxins in Developing Countries

Gabriel O. Adegoke and Puleng Letuma

Additional information is available at the end of the chapter

http://dx.doi.org/10.5772/52542

1. Introduction

According to the Fod and Agricultural Organization (FAO) of the United Nations, up to 25% of the world's food crops have been estimated to be significantly contaminated with mycotoxins (WHO, 1999). Significant losses due to mycotoxins and their impact on human and animal health have been linked with national economic implications and all these factors have combined to make mycotoxins important worldwide (Bhat and Vashanti (1999). According to Plancinta *et al.* (1999), surveillance studies showed that world-wide contamination of cereal grains and other feeds with *Fusarium* mycotoxins is a global problem. Thus, in recognition of the global public health importance of food borne diseases and in order to promote economic growth and development, the World Health Organization (WHO) commissioned the Foodborne Disease Burden Epidemiology Reference Group (FERG) to undertake the systematic reviews of some chemicals and toxins like cyanide in cassava, aflatoxin, dioxins and peanut allergens (Hird *et al.* 2009).

In order to understand the mechanisms that can be adopted for controlling mycotoxins, it is essential to have relevant information on the prevailing climatic conditions in the agricultural zones where the crops are being produced. Thus Bhat and Vasanthi (2003) noted that in developing countries of the world, tropical conditions like high temperatures and moisture, monsoons, unseasonal rains during harvest and flash floods can lead to fungal proliferation and production of mycotoxin. In temperate climates, the most important toxins are deoxynivanelol, (DON), zearalenone, diacetoxyscirpenol (DAS), T-2 toxin and fumonisins (Balazs and Schepers, 2007) and in Europe, the most frequent toxigenic fungi are *Aspergillus, Penicillium* and *Fusarium* species (Creppy, 2002).

In cereals grown in temperate regions of America, Europe and Asia, *Fusarium* spp have been reported to be the most prevalent toxin-producing fungi (Gajecki, 2002). In Africa and other developing countries, the World Health Organization (WHO, 2006) noted that fumonisins and aflatoxins are likely to be of significance. However, ochratoxin A (OTA) has been reported in food commodities in Africa, for example, Adegoke *et al* (2007) found OTA in *kunu-zaki* (a non-alcoholic beverage); Bonvehi (2004) detected OTA of up to 4 mg/kg –higher than the EU regulatory level- in cocoa powder from Ivory Coast, Guinea, Nigeria and Cameroon. Aroyeun and Adegoke (2007) reported over 50% occurrence of *Aspergillus ochraceus* and *A.niger* in cocoa beans in Nigeria with a corresponding 40-60 ppb OTA concentration.

Consumption of commodities contaminated with mycotoxins according to Bathnagar and Garcia (2001) leads to chronic mycotoxicoses which results in acute poisoning resulting in death. Therefore, as the global occurrence and importance of mycotoxins cannot be overemphasized, methods for preventing and reducing them before entering the food chain must be given continuous attention as 40% of the productivity lost to diseases in developing countries has been associated with diseases exacerbated by aflatoxins (Miller,1996).

2. Foodborne mycotoxins

There are over 300 mycotoxins that have been isolated and characterized (Adegoke, 2004). From the standpoints of health and trade, important mycotoxins are aflatoxins, ochratoxins, deoxynivalenol, zearalenone, fumonisin, T-2 and T-2 like toxins

(trichothecenes) and alternariol. Thomson and Henke (2000) noted that crops in tropical and subtropical areas are more susceptible to mycotoxin contamination than those in temperate zones because the high humidity and temperatures in tropical areas provide optimal conditions for toxin formation. Furthermore, it has been reported that drought conditions can stress plants and render them susceptible to contamination by *Aspergillus* spp (Holbrook *et al.* 2004; Robertson, 2005). With respect to some fruits, under warm and humid weather, fruit rots in blueberries are of concern as post-harvest rot can occur on berries that look fine at harvest but carry fungal spores that can infect and develop in the fruits during storage and processing (Schilder *et al.* 2006). Thus it is important to identify fungal contaminants in fresh fruits because moulds can grow and produce mycotoxins on these commodities (Tournas and Katsoudas, 2005).

3. Factors that affect mycotoxin production

In the food chain, there are some 'time-bound' factors that are important in the production of mycotoxins during pre-harvest and post-harvest handling of agricultural products like:

- **a.** intrinsic factors: moisture content, water activity, substrate type, plant type and nutrient composition;
- **b.** extrinsic factors: climate, temperature, oxygen level;
- **c.** processing factors: drying, blending, addition of preservatives, handling of grains
- **d.** implicit factors: insect interactions, fungal strain, microbiological ecosystem (Magan *et al.* 2004).

4. Prevention and reduction of mycotoxins

Generally, mycotoxin contamination of agricultural products can be prevented using

1. pre-harvest methods:
   - **a.** using resistant varieties;
   - **b.** field management;
   - **c.** use of biological and chemical agents;
   - **d.** harvest management and
2. post-harvest methods:
   - **a.** improved drying methods;
   - **b.** good storage conditions;
   - **c.** use of natural and chemical agents
   - **d.** irradiation (Kabab *et al.* 2006).

The inclusion of sorbent materials in feed or addition of enzymes or microorganisms capable of detoxifying mycotoxins have been reported to be reliable methods for mycotoxin prevention in feeds (Jard *et al.* 2011). However, while bentonite and aluminosilicate clays have been used as binding agents for reducing aflatoxin intoxication in pigs (Schell *et al.* 1993), cattle (Diaz *et al.* 1997) and poultry (Scheideler, 1993) without causing digestive problems when mixed with aflatoxin-contaminated feed, care must be taken as the clays can alter nutritional value by binding trace minerals and vitamins and reducing their bioavailability and even produce dioxins (Devegowda and Castaldo, 2000). Preference for esterified glucomannan (a naturally-occurring organic compound in yeast) over clay in reducing the toxicity of aflatoxin has been reported. Devegowda and Castaldo (2000) found that using glucomannan supplementation at 0.05% of diet of dairy cows that consumed aflatoxin-contaminated feed, there was a reduction of 58% in aflatoxin in the cow's milk. While in developing countries prevention of mycotoxins from entering the food chain may not currently be receiving sustainable attention or focus as in developed countries because of different food systems, financial constraints, availability of food policies, levels of food safety education and technological development, nonetheless, the following specific mycotoxins can be prevented from developing in agricultural products:

a. Aflatoxins

Aflatoxins may be produced by three species of *Aspergillus-A.flavus, A.parasiticus* and the rare *A.nomius* which according to Creppy (2002) contaminate plants and plant products like peanut, corn, cotton seed and tree nuts (Diener *et al.* 1987; Horn, 2005). According to Holmes *et al.* (2008), aflatoxins can be produced (in addition to *A.flavus, A.parasiticus* and *A. nomius*) by *Aspergillus toxicarius* and *A. parvisclerotigens* on crops like corn, peanuts, cotton seeds and coffee beans. Aflatoxin B_1 according to IARC (1993), is the most carcinogenic, mutagenic and teratogenic substance occurring naturally in foods and feeds. There are reports of the association of aflatoxin contamination of plant foods particularly cereals with liver cancer in Africa and China (Bababunmi, 1978; Oettle, 1964; Li *et al.* 2001). To prevent aflatoxin contamination of commodities in the farm or during storage of farm products, understanding of the prevailing environmental conditions must be considered. Environmental factors that favour *Aspergillus flavus* infection include high soil or air temperature, drought stress, nitrogen stress, crowding of plants and conditions that aid dispersal of conidia during silking (CAST, 1989; Robens, 1990). The growth of *A. flavus* and *A. parasiticus* and subsequent aflatoxin production in storage are favoured by high humidity (>85%), high temperature (25 ^{0}C) and insect or rodent activity (CAST, 1989). The most important insects that spread *A.flavus* in postharvest maize are lepidopteran ear borer, *Mussidia nigrivenella, Sitophilus zeamais* and *Carpophilus dimidiatus* (Setamou *et al.* 1998; Hell *et al.* 2000b). Thus, early harvesting and adequate drying of crops can help in reducing contamination of crops. In several developing countries however, early harvesting, unpredictable weather, labour constraint, need for cash, threat of thieves, rodents and other animals compel farmers to harvest at inappropriate time (Amyot, 1983).

With thorough drying and proper storage of groundnuts in Guinea, Turner *et al* (2005) reported that there was a 60% reduction in the mean aflatoxin levels of groundnuts in villages used for the survey. When it is realized that major portion (80%) of aflatoxin is often associated with small and shrivelled (Davidson *et al.* 1982) and mouldy and stained peanut (Fandohan *et al.* 2005; Turner *et al.* 2005), there are reports of possibility of using physical separation of apparently contaminated cereals from the bulk samples. In Benin, West Africa, Fandohan *et al.* (2005) used some unit operations like sorting, winnowing, washing, crushing and dehulling to remove significant amounts of aflatoxins and fumonisins in maize and maize products. Park (2002) also noted the effects of processing on aflatoxin.

Employing food safety practices like hazard analysis critical control point (HACCP) system can be useful in preventing and reducing aflatoxin contamination in agricultural products. Hell *et al.* (2000a) thus noted that cleaning stores before loading new produce correlated with reduced aflatoxin levels. Preharvest HACCP programmes (FAO/IAEA,2001) are available for controlling aflatoxin in corn and coconuts in South east Asia, peanuts, peanut products in Africa, nuts in West Africa, patulin in apple juice and pistachio nuts in South America. While Aldred and Magan (2004) suggested some HACCP approaches for wheat-based commodities, Lopez-Garcia *et al.* (1999) gave some useful guidance for the development of an integrated mycotoxin management.

Application of potential bio-control agents like atoxigenic strains of *Aspergillus flavus* and *A. parasiticus* which when introduced into the soil of growing crops have been reported to produce 74.3 to 99.9 % reduction in aflatoxin in peanuts in the USA (Dorner *et al.* 1998). The ability of dietary factors to counteract the effects of aflatoxins has been studied. Rompelberg *et al.* (1996) noted that phenolic compounds can metabolically enhance aflatoxin B_1 conjugation and elimination. Galvano *et al.* (2001) also noted that food components like fructose, phenolic compounds, coumarins, chlorophyll and food additives like piperine, aspartame, cyproheptadine and allyl sulfides can reduce the toxicity of mycotoxins by decreasing toxin formation and enhancing metabolism. The antioxidant, ethoxyquin has been reported to be effective as a chemo preventive agent against the carcinogenic effects of aflatoxin B_1 in humans (Bammler *et al.* 2000).

Spices and herbs and their bioactive components have been found useful for the reduction of aflatoxins. Olojede *et al.* (1993) found that when *Garcinia kola* was used at 0.32% (w/v), aflatoxin was effectively reduced from 97 to 23 μg/ml. The bioactive components or volatiles of some plants have been explored in the control of fungal growth and production of aflatoxins, for example, Norton (1999) found that anthocyanins and related flavonoids affect aflatoxin biosynthesis and Juglal *et al.* (2002) found that spice oil was effective in the control of some mycotoxin producing fungi.

In other studies conducted in a developing country, processing was found to reduce aflatoxins in cereal pastes boiled for 30 and 60 minutes by 68% and 80.8% respectively (Adegoke, *et al.* 1994). During the processing of cassava bread- a cassava-based product, while the initial raw material had aflatoxin level of 1.91μg /kg, however, after processing, the final concentration of aflatoxin in the final product, cassava bread, was found to be 0.03μg/kg (Adegoke *et al.* 1993). Roasting of peanuts has been reported to have more effect on reducing chemically detectable aflatoxins than boiling (Njapau *et al.* 1996). Scott (1991) noted that fermentation of wheat flour dough reduced detectable aflatoxin by approximately 50% while baking of the dough produced less effect.

Camou-Arriola and Price (1989) found that using 121^{0}C and alkaline treatment of naturally contaminated corn prior to frying resulted in very low levels of chemically detectable aflatoxin. Wet, dry milling processes and heat during cooking processes have been found to be effective in reducing levels of aflatoxin in foods (Scott, 1984). Conway *et al.* (1978); Hale and Wilson (1979) also found significant decreases in aflatoxin content arising from heating and roasting of corn.The use of traditional processing for reducing aflatoxin has also been examined, for example, Hwang *et al.* (2006) found that processing of traditional Korean foods like 'sujebi' (a soup with wheat flakes) and steamed bread caused 71% and 43 % decrease respectively in AFB_1 levels.

Detoxification using ozone has been found by some workers to be useful in reducing aflatoxins in food commodities for example de Alencar *et al.* (2012) noted reductions of 30 % and 25 % for total aflatoxins and aflatoxin B_1 when peanuts were exposed to 21 mg L^{-1} of ozone. McKenzie *et al.* (1997) found that ozone destroyed aflatoxins B_1 and G_1 in aqueous model systems. Prudent and King (2002) reported a 92 % degradation (reduction) in aflatoxin in ozonized contaminated corn. Exposure to sunlight has also been found effective in reducing aflatoxin levels in some food products, for example, Adegoke *et al.* (1996) found that sun drying of pepper (*Capsicum annum*) had some significant effects on aflatoxin levels.

b. Ochratoxins

Benford *et al.* (2001) noted that *Aspergillus ochraceus, A. carbonarius, A. melleus, A.sclerotium* and *Penicillium verrucosum* are the main producers of OTA. Ochratoxins have been detected in several agricultural products from temperate and tropical zones. Weidenborner (2001) found OTA in cassava flour, cereals, fish, peanuts, dried fruits, wine, eggs, milk coffee and cocoa beans. Cereals, wine, grape juice, coffee and pork are the major sources of human ochratoxin exposure (JECFA, 2001). Aish *et al.* (2004) also noted that ochratoxin A (OTA) is found in wheat, corn and oats having fungal infection and in cheese and meat products of animal consuming ochratoxin-contaminated grains.

Post-harvest measures for preventing OTA from entering the food chain have been documented. Magan and Aldred (2007) suggested the following post-harvest critical control points-that can be equally adopted in developing countries:

1. regular and accurate moisture content measurements;
2. efficient and prompt drying of wet cereal grains for safe moisture levels (maize, 14%; rice, 13-14 %; barley, 14-14.5 % and canola or rapeseed, 7-8 %);
3. infrastructure for quick response including provision for segregation and appropriate transport conditions;
4. appropriate storage conditions at all stages in terms of moisture and temperature control, general maintenance and effective hygiene of storage facilities for prevention of pests and water ingress.

Modifying the gases in atmospheres where cereals are stored can be used in the prevention of OTA production. Paster *et al.* (1983), found that OTA production by *A.ochraceus* was completely inhibited by 30% CO_2. Thus atmospheres greater than 30 % (for example, 30-60 % CO_2) can be used for preventing OTA production during storage or transportation of grains. This technique can be adopted in developing countries.

Using a combination of cleaning, scouring and removal of the bran and offal fraction, Scudamore *et al.* (2003) observed an overall reduction of about 75% of OTA in white bread. Wet- milling, according to Wood (1982), produced 96 % and 49 % reductions of OTA in the germ and grits of corn respectively. The influence of roasting on the reduction of OTA levels has been examined. Van der Stegen *et al.* (2001) noted that although OTA was relatively stable during heat processing, reductions of OTA of up to 90% was found during coffee bean roasting. Nehad *et al.* (2005) found that roasting reduced to 30µg/kg of OTA by 31% and filtering reduced OTA by 72%. Using final coffee temperature of 204 ^{0}C (dark roast), Romani *et al* (2003) obtained reductions of more than 90 % of OTA. Direct removal of damaged coffee has also been found to reduce OTA contamination (CIRAD, http://www.cirad.fr, accessed on 27-03-2012). In Europe, maximum level for OTA in roasted coffee is fixed at 5µg/kg.

In grossly contaminated samples of cocoa beans, the essential oils of some plants can be used to reduce OTA contamination, for example, Aroyeun and Adegoke (2007) used the essential oils of *Aframomum danielli* to reduce OTA levels in spiked cocoa powder and obtained a reduction efficiency of 64-95 %. Aroyeun *et al.* (2011) described the potentials of, *Aframomum danielli* spice in reducing OTA in cocoa powder as the authors found that the powder of *A. danielli* can be used as a biopreservative (maximum concentration of 60,000 ppm) in cocoa powder contaminated with OTA. Adegoke *et al.* (2007) reported that during processing, Daniellin™ completely reduced the OTA level in a non-alcoholic beverage.

c. Fumonisins

Fumonisins are produced by *Fusarium verticillioides* (Sacc.) Nirenberg (=*F.moniliforme* (Sheldon) and the related *F. proliferatum* (Matsushima) Nirenberg. Fumonisins occur in sorghum, asparagus, rice, beer and beans (Creppy, 2002). Fumonisins can also be found on asparagus and garlic (Seefelder *et al.* 2002). In Africa and several other parts of the world, *Fusarium* spp. are very important field fungi of maize as the fungi produce over 100 secondary metabolites that affect adversely human and animal health (Visconti, 2001). In fact, reports have linked maize consumption with high levels of *F. verticillioides* and fumonisins and high incidence of human oesophageal carcinoma in some parts of South Africa and China (Yoshizawa *et al.* 1994; IPCS, 2000). Fumonisins are classified as possible human carcinogens (IARC, 1993).

In developing countries and other countries where fumonisins occur in maize, useful pre- and post-harvest preventive strategies have been suggested by Maga and Aldred (2007):

a. **pre-harvest measures**:
   1. proper selection of maize hybrids, prevention of use of soft kernel hybrids;
   2. no late sowing dates and avoiding high cropping density;
   3. good and balanced fertilization;
   4. avoiding late harvesting;
   5. effective control of pests for example corn borer.

b. **post-harvest measures**:
   1. minimizing periods between harvesting and drying
   2. effective cleaning of maize prior to storage;
   3. efficient drying to less than 14 % moisture content;
   4. effective hygiene and management of silos;
   5. absence of pests in store-pests can provide metabolic water and initiate heating. Insect damage of maize is a good prediction of *Fusarium* mycotoxin contamination which can serve as a warning signal of fumonisin contamination (Avantaggio *et al.* 2002). Furthermore, the spores of *Fusarium* spp. can be carried by insects from plant surfaces to the interior of the stalk or kernels or create infection wounds due to the feeding of insect larvae on stalks or kernels (Munkvold and Hellminch. 2000).
   6. clear specifications and traceability from field to store.

While these pre-and post-harvest techniques for fumonisin management are not difficult to practise in developing countries, use of solar energy has been found useful elsewhere. Ahmad and Ghaffan (2007) in Pakistan noted that soil solarization was useful in reducing the incidence of corn ear rots and consequently fumonisins and aflatoxins in fields and stored corns. Processing can also be used for reducing fumonisins in food commodities as Jackson *et al* (1997) noted that when corn-based batter (for making muffins) was baked at 175^{0}C and 200 ^{0} C for 20 minutes, reductions of 15 % to 30 % respectively were found with increasing losses as the temperature increased. Voss *et al* (2001) found a reduction of up to 80 % in fumonisin in fried corn chips - a reduction which was attributed to nixtamilization and rinsing. Combination of agronomic techniques –seed time, seed density, N fertilization and control of corn borer have been reported to be useful in reducing fumonisin contamination in maize (Blandino *et al*. 2007).

c. **Patulin**

Food commodities commonly affected by pathogens that produce patulin are apple, grape, pear, apricots and peaches (Speijers, 2004). The most important aspect of handling patulin is by controlling the quality of fruit before it enters the food chain as patulin is not found in intact fruit because it is the damage done to the surface of the fruit which makes the fruit susceptible to infection by *Penicillium* spp (Sewram *et al.* 2000). During the clarification of apple juice and concentrates, Bissessur *et al.* (2001) found patulin reduction of up to 40% and using pasteurization or evaporation at 70-100 ^{0}C, Kadalal and Nas (2003) found a 25 % loss in naturally contaminated apple juice.

5. Conclusions

In reducing mycotoxin accumulation, it must be realized that the concentrations of aflatoxins, deoxynivalenol or fumonisins are greater in symptomatic than in non-symptomatic maize ears or kernels, thus, prevention or reduction in pre-and post-harvest infection is a critical factor (Scott and Zumno 1995; Reid *et al.* 1996; Desjardin *et al.* 1998). While some techniques for the management of mycotoxin contamination may be in practice in developed countries, however, in order to reduce or eliminate rejection of agricultural produce meant for export and at local levels as well as protect consumers from the harmful effects of mycotoxins, developing countries can adopt some of these methods described herein. Harris (1997) also suggested some practical methods for preventing mycotoxin contamination of feeds, for example, keeping grain bins clean and storage at less that 14 % moisture, use of dry feed ingredients that are oxygen-free, fermented or treated with mould growth inhibitors.

For sustained management of mycotoxins along the food chain, the following procedures are recommended:

a. HACCP-compliance: good agronomic practices through transportation and up to consumption;
b. best practices for harvesting, drying and storage of agricultural products coupled with effective insect management;
c. adoption and sustainability of relevant food safety education;
d. careful and systematic enforcement of legislation on food safety.
e. screening in developing countries where fruits and berries are grown and exported for alternariol, alternariol methylether and tenuazonic acid-mycotoxins produced by *Alternaria* spp (Greco *et al*. 2012).
f. adoption and utilization of sensitive and reliable methods for detection of mycotoxins. For public health protection and international trade, sensitive and accurate analytical methods are needed for mycotoxins (Rahmani *et al.* 2009).
g. sustained examination of agricultural commodities under different prevailing climatic conditions.

Author details

Gabriel O. Adegoke*
Department of Animal Science, National University of Lesotho, Lesotho

Puleng Letuma
Department of Crop Science, National University of Lesotho, Lesotho

6. References

Adegoke, G.O. (2004). Understanding Food Microbiology, Alleluia Ventures Ltd, Ibadan, Nigeria. ISBN 978-36676-1-0 216pp.

Adegoke, G.O; Akinnuoye, O.F.A. and Akanni, A.O. (1993). Effect of processing on the mycoflora and aflatoxin B1 level of a cassava-based product. Plant Foods Hum. Nutrit. 43, 191-196.

Adegoke, G.O; Otumu, F.J. and Akanni, A.O. (1994). Influence of grain quality, heat and processing time on the reduction of aflatoxin B_1 levels in tuwo and ogi-two cereal-based products. Plant Foods for Human Nutrition 43, 113-117.

Adegoke, G.O; Allamu, A.E; Akingbala, J.O. and Akanni, A.O. (1996). Influence of sundrying on the chemical composition, aflatoxin content and fungal counts of two pepper varities-*Capsicum annum* and *Capsicum frutescens*. Plant Foods Hum. Nutrit. 49, 113-117.

Adegoke, G.O; Odeyemi, A.O; Hussein, O. and Ikheorah, J. (2007). Control of ochratoxin A in *kunu zaki* (a non-alcoholic beverage) using Daniellin ™. African Journal of Agricultural Research 2, 200-202.

Ahmad, Y. and Ghaffar, A. (2007). Soil solarization: a management practice for mycotoxins in corn. Pakistan Journal of Botany 39, 2215-2223.

Aish, J.J; Rippon, E.H; Barlow, T. and Hattersley, S.J. (2004). Ochratoxin A. In: Magan, N. and Olsen, S. (Eds), Mycotoxins in Food.: Detection and control, CRC Press, Boca Raton, FL. pp 307-338.

Aldred, D. and Magan, N. (2004). The use of HACCP in the control of mycotoxins: the case of cereals. In: Magan, N, and Olsen, M. (Eds), Mycotoxins in Food: Detection and Control, CRC Press, Boca Raton, FL., pp 139-173.

Alencar, E.R; Faroni, L.R.D; Soares, N.F.F; Silva, W.A. and Carvalho, M.C.S. (2012). Efficacy of ozone as a fungicidal and detoxifying agent of aflatoxins in peanuts. Journal of Science of Food and Agriculture 92, 899-905.

Amyot, J. (1983). Social and economic aspects of dryer use for paddy and other agricultural produce in Thailand. Chualongkorn University Social Research Institute and International Development Research Center, Bangkok, Thailand.

Aroyeun, S.O. and Adegoke, G.O. (2007). Reduction of ochratoxin A (OTA) in spiked cocoa powder and beverage using aqueous extracts and essential oils of *Aframomum danielli.* African Journal of Biotechnology 6, 612-616.

Aroyeun, S.O; Adegoke, G.O; Varga, J; Teren, J; Karolyi, P; Kuscbe, S. and Valgvolgyi, C,. (2011). Potential of *Aframomum danielli* spice powder in reducing ochratoxin A in cocoa powder. American Journal of Food and Nutrition 1, 155-165.

---

* Present address: Faculty of Agriculture, National University of Lesotho, Lesotho

Avantaggio, G; Quaranta, F; Desidero, E. and Visconti, A. (2002). Fumonisin contamination of maize hybrids visibly damaged by Sesamia. Journal of Science of Food and Agriculture 83, 13-18

Bababunmi, E.A; Uwaifo, A.O. and Bassir, O. (1976). Hepatocarcinogens in Nigerian foodstuffs. World Review of Nutrition and Dietetics 28, 188-209.

Balazs, E. and Schepers, J.S. (2007). The mycotoxin threat to food safety. International Journal of Food Microbiology 119,1-2.

Bammler, T.K; Slone, D.H. and Eaton, D.L. (2000). Effects of dietary olipratz and ethoxyquin on aflatoxin B_1 biotransformation in non-human primates. Toxicol. Sci. 54, 30-41.

Bathnagar, D. and Garcia, S. (2001). *Aspergillus.* In: Guide to Foodborne Pathogens, Labbe, R.G. and Garcia, S. (Eds), John Wiley and Sons, New York, pp 35-49.

Bhat, R.V. and Vashanti, S. (1999). Occurrence of aflatoxins and its economic impact on human nutrition and animal feed. The New Regulation Agric. Development No 23, 50-56.

Bhat, R.V. and Vasanthi, S. (2003). Mycotoxin food safety risks in developing countries. Food Safety in Food Security and Food Trade, Vision 2020 for Food, Agriculture and Environment, Focus 10, brief 3 of 17, pp 1-2.

Benford, D; Boyle, C; Dekant, W; Fuchs, E; Gaylor, D.W; Hard, G; McGregory, D.B; Pitt, J.I; Plestina, R; Shephard, G; Solfrizzo, M and Verger, P.J.P. (2001). Ochratoxin A. Safety evaluation of certain mycotoxins in food. WHO, Geneva, WHO Food Additives Series 47, FAO Food and Nutrition Paper vol. 47, pp 281-415.

Blandino, M; Reyneri, A. and Vanara, F. (2007). Strategy for the fumonisin reduction in maize kernel in Italy. Mycotoximes fusariennes des cereals. Areachon, 11-13 sept 2007. www.symposcience.com accessed 09-04-2012.

Bissessur, J., Permaul, K and Odhav, B. (2001). Reduction of patulin during apple juice clarification. Journal of Food Protection 64, 1216-1219.

Bonvehi, J.R. (2004). Occurrence of ochratoxin A in coca products and chocolate. Journal of Agriculture and Food Chemistry 52, 6347-6352.

Camoou-Arriola, J.P. and Price, R. I. (1989). Destruction of aflatoxin and reduction of mutagenicity of naturally-contaminated corn during the production of a corn snack. Journal of Food Protection 52, 814-817.

CAST (1989). Mycotoxins: Economic and Health Risks. United States Council for Agricultural Science and Technology (CAST), Ames, Iowa, Report No 116, pp 1-91.

Conway, H.F; Anderson, R.A. and Bagley, E.B. (1978). Detoxification of aflatoxin contaminated corn by roasting. Cereal Chemistry 55, 115-118.

Creppy, E.E. (2002). Update of survey, regulation and toxic effects of mycotoxins in Europe. Toxicology Letters 127, 19-28.

Davidson, Jr. J.I; Whitaker, T.B. and Dickens, J.W. (1982). Grading, cleaning, storage, shelling, and marketing peanuts in the United States, Patee, H.E; Young, C.T. and Yoakum, T.X. (Eds), American Peanut Research and Education Society, pp 571-623.

de Alencar E.R; Faroni, L.R.R; Soares, N.F.F; Silva, W.A. and Carvalho, M.C.S. (2012). Efficacy of ozone as a fungicidal and detoxifying agent of aflatoxins in peanuts. Journal of Science of Food and Agriculture 92, 899-905.

Desjardin, A.E; Plattner, R.D; Lu, M. and Claflin, L.E. (1998). Distribution of fuminosins in maize ears infected with strains of *Fusarium moniliforme* that differ in fumonisin production. Plant Diseases 82, 953-958.

Devegouida, G. and Castaldo, D. (2000). Mycotoxins: hidden killers in pet foods. Is there a solution?. In: Technical Symposium on Mycotoxins, Altech Inc., Nicholasville, KY, USA.

Diaz, D.E; Blackwelder, J.T; Hagler, W.M.Jr; Hopkins, B.A; Jones, F.T; Anderson, K.L. and Whitlow, L.W. (1997). The potential of dietary clay products to reduce aflatoxin transmission to the milk of dairy cows. Journal of Dairy Science 80, 265.

Diener, U.L; Cole, R.J; Sanders, T.H; Payne, G.A; Lee, L.S. and Klich, M.A. (1987). Epidemiology of aflatoxin formation by *Aspergillus flavus*. Annual Review of Phytopathology 25, 249-270.

Dorner, J.W; Cole, R.J. and and Blakenship, P.D. (1998). Effect of inoculum rate of biological agents on preharvest contamination of peanuts. Biological Control 12,171-176

Fandohan, P; Gnonlonfin, B; Hell, K; Marasas, W.F.O. and Wingfield, M.J. (2005). Natural occurrence of *Fusarium* and subsequent fumonisin contamination in preharvest and stored maize in Benin, West Africa. International Journal of Food Microbiology 99, 173-183.

FAO/IAEA (2001). Manual on the Application of the HACCP System in Mycotoxin Prevention and Control. Food and Agriculture Organization/ International Atomic Energy Agency, FAO Food and Nutrition Paper 73.

Gajecki, M. (2002). Zearalenone-undesirable substances in feed. Polish Journal of Veterinary Science 5, 117-122.

Galvano, F; Piva, A; Ritieni, A. and Galvano, G. (2001). Dietary strategies to counteract the effects of mycotoxins: a review. Journal of Food Protection 64, 120-131.

Greco, M; Patriarca, A; Terminiello, L; Pinto, V.F. and Pose, G. (2012). Toxigenic *Alternaria* species form Argentinean blueberries. International Journal of Food Microbiology 154, 187-191.

Hale, G.M. and Wilson, D. M. (1979). Performance of pigs on diets containing heated or unheated corn with or without aflatoxin. Journal of Animal Science 48, 1394-1400.

Harris, B. Jr. (1997). Minimizing mycotoxin problems. Journal of Food Protection 41, 489-492.

Hell, K; Cardwell, K.F; Setamou, M. and Poehling, H.M. (2000a). The influence of storage practices on aflatoxin contamination in maize in four agroecological zones of Benin, West Africa. Journal of Stored Products Research 36, 365-382.

Hell, K; Cardwell, K.F; Setamou, M. and Schulthess, F. (2000b). Influence of insect infestation on aflatoxin contamination of stored maize in four agroecological zones regions in Benin. Afr. Entomol. 6, 169-177.

Hird, S; Stien, C; Kuchenmuller, T. and Green, R. (2009). Meeting report.: second annual meeting of the World Health Organization initiative to estimate the global burden of foodborne diseases. International Journal of Food Microbiology 133, 210-212.

Holbrook,C.C; Guo, B.Z; Wilson, D.M. and Kvien, C. (2004). Effect of drought tolerance on preharvest aflatoxin contamination in peanuts. Proceedings, 4th International Crop Science Congress, Brisbane, Australia, 26th sept- 1st oct. 2004.

IARC (1993). Monograph on the Evaluation of carcinogenic Risk to Humans, International Agency for Research on Cancer, Lyon, Volume 56, pp 257-263.

IPCS (2000). Environmental Health Criteria 219-Fumonisin B1. International Program on Chemical Safety, WHO, Geneva, 150 pp.

Jackson, L.S; Katta, S. K; Fingerhut, D.D; DeVries, J.W. and Bullerman, L.b. (1997). Effects of baking and frying on the fumonisin B1 content of corn-based foods. Journal of Agricultural. Food Chemistry 45, 4800-4805.

Jard, G; Liboz, T; Mathieu, F; Guyonvarch'h, A. and Lebrihi, A. (2011). Review of mycotoxin reduction in food and feed: from prevention in the field to detoxification by adsorption or transformation. Food Addit. Contamination Part A. Chem. Anal. Exposure Risk Assessment 28, 1590-1609.

JECFA (2001). Ochratoxin A. Joint Food and Agriculture Organization/World Health Organization Expert Committee on Food Additives. http://www.inchem.org/documents/jecfa/jecmono/v47je04.htm accessed on 27-07-2012

Juglal, S; Govinden, R. and Odhav, B. (2002). Spice oil for the control of the co-occurring mycotoxin producing fungi. Journal of Food Production 65, 683-687.

Kabak, B; Dobson, A.D. and Var, I. (2006). Strategies to prevent mycotoxin contamination of food and animal feed. Critical Review of Food Science and Nutrition 46, 593-619.

Kadakal, C. and Nas, S. (2003). Effect of heat treatment and evaporation on patulin and some other properties of apple juice. Journal of the Science of. Food and Agriculture 83, 987-990.

Li, F; Yoshizawa, T; Kawamura, O; Luo, X. and Li, Y. (2001). Aflatoxins and fumonisins in corn from high incidence area of human hepatocellular carcinoma in Guangi, China. Journal of Agricultural and Food Chemistry 49, 4122-4126.

Magan, N. and Aldred, D. (2007). Post-harvest control strategies: minimizing mycotoxicosis in the food chain. International Journal of Food Microbiology 119, 131-139.

Magan, N; Sachis, V. and Aldred, D. (2004). Role of spoilage fungi in seed deterioration. In: Fungal Biotechnology in Agricultural, Food and Environmental Applications, Aurora, D.K. (Ed.), Marcell Dekker, New York, Ch 28, pp 311-323.

McKenzie, K.S; Sarr, A; Mayra, K; Bailey, R.H; Miller, D.R; Rogers, T.D; Norred, W.P; Voss, K.A; Plattner, R.D. and Phillips, T.D. (1997). Chemical degradation of diverse mycotoxins using a novel method of ozone production. Food Chemistry and Toxicology 35, 807-820.

Miller, J.D. (1996). Mycotoxins. In: Proceedings of the Workshop on Mycotoxins in Food in Africa, November, 6-10, 1995, Cardwell, K.F. (Ed.), International Institute of Tropical Agriculture, Cotonou, Benin, pp 18-22.

Munkvold, G.P. and Hellminch, R.L. (2000). Genetically modified, insect resistant maize, implications for management of ear and stalk diseases. Plant Health Program, http://www.planthealthprogress.com /current/reviews/maize/article/htm.

Nehad, E.A; Farag, M.M; Kawther, M.S; Abdel-Samed, A.K.M. and Naguib, K. (2005). Stability of ochratoxin A (OTA) duringprocessing and decaffeination in commercial roasted coffee beans. Food Additives and Contaminants 22, 761-767.

Njapau, H; Muzungaile, E.M. and Changa, R. C. (1998). The effect of village processing techniques on the content of aflatoxins in corn and peanuts in Zambia. Journal of the Science of Food and Agriculture 76., 450-456.

Norton, R.A. (1999). Inhibition of aflatoxin B_1 biosynthesis in *Aspergillus flavus* by anthocyandins and related flavonoids. Journal of Agricultural Chemistry 47, 1230-1240.

Oettle, A.G. (1964). Cancer in Africa, especially in regions South of the Sahara. J. Nat. Cancer Inst. 33, 383-439.

Olojede, F; Engelhardt, G; Wallnofer, P.R. and Adegoke, G.O. (1993). Decrease of growth and aflatoxin production in *Aspergillus parasiticus* by spices. World Journal of Microbiology and Biotechnology 9, 605-606.

Park, D.L. (2002). Effect of processing on aflatoxin. Advances in Experimental Medicine and Biology 504, 173-179.

Paster, N; Lisker, N. and Chet, I. (1983). Ochratoxin production by *Aspergillus flavus* Wilhen grown under controlled atmospheres. Applied and Environmental Microbiology 45, 1136-1139.

Plancinta, C. M; D'Mello, J.P.F. and MacDonald, A.M.C. (1999). A review of worldwide contamination of cereal grains and animal feed with *Fusarium* mycotoxins. Animal Feed Science and Technology 78, 21-37.

Prudente, A.D. and King, J.M. (2002). Efficacy and safety: evaluation of ozonation to degrade aflatoxin in corn. Journal of Food Science 67, 2866-2872.

Rahmani, A; Jinap, S. and Soleimany, F. (2009). Qualitative and quantitative analysis of mycotoxins. Comprehensive Review in Food Science and Food Safety 8, 202-251.

Reid, L.M; Mather, D.E. and Hamilton, R.I. (1996). Distribution of deoxynivanelenol in Fusarium graminearium-infected maize ears. Phytopathology 86, 110-114.

Robens, J.F. (1990). A perspective on aflatoxins in field crops and animal food products in the United States: A Symposium, United States Department of Agriculture, Agriculture Research Service (USDA-ARS), Peoria, IL, ARS-83, pp 135.

Robertson, A. (2005). Risk of aflatoxin contamination increases with hot and dry growing conditions. Integrated Crop Management, IC -494 (23), pp185-186.
http://www.ipm.iastate.edu/ipm/icm/2005/9-19/aflatoxin.html accessed on 10-04-2012.

Romani, S; Pinnavaia, G.G. and Rosa, M.D. (2003). Influence of roasting levels on ochratoxin A content in coffee. Journal of Agricultural and Food Chemistry 51, 5168-5171.

Rompelberg, C.J; Evertz, S.J; Bruijntes-Rozier, G.C; van den Heuvel, P.D. and Verhagen, H. (1996). Effect of eugenol on the genotoxicity of established mutagens in the liver. Food Chemistry and Toxicology 34, 33-42.

Scheideler, S.E. (1993). Effects of various types of aluminosilicates and aflatoxin B1 on aflatoxin toxicity, chick performance and mineral status. Poultry Science 282-288.

Schell, T.C; Lindemann, M.D; Kornegay, E.T. and Blodgett, D.J. (1993). Effects of feeding aflatoxin-contaminated diets with and without clay to weanling and growing pigs performance, liver function and mineral metabolism. Journal of Animal Science 71, 1209-1218.

Schilder, A; Hancock, J. and Hanson, E. (2006). An integrated approach to disease control in blueberries in Michigan. Acta Horticulturae 715, 481-488.

Scott, P. M. (1984). Effects of processing on mycotoxins. Journal of Food Protection 41, 489-492.

Scott, P.M. (1991). Possibilities of reduction or elimination of mycotoxins present in cereal grains. In: Cereal grain: Mycotoxin, Fungi and Quality in Drying and Storage, Chelkowski, J. (Ed.), Elsievier, New York, pp 529-572.

Scott, G.E. and Zumno, N. (1995). Size of maize sample needed to determine percent of kernel infection by *Aspergillus flavus*. Plant Diseases 79, 861-864.

Scudamore, K.A; Banks, J. and MacDonald, S.J. (2003). Fate of ochratoxin A in the processing of whole wheat grains during milling and bread production. Food Addit. Contamination 20, 1153-1163.

Seefelder, W; Gossmann, M. and Humpf, H.U. (2002). Analysis of fumonisin B_1 in *Fusarium proliferatum*-infected asparagus spears and garlic bulbs from Germany by liquid chromatography-electrospray ionization mass spectrometry. Journal of Agricultural and Food Chemistry 50, 2778-2781.

Setamou, M; Cardwell, K.F; Schulthess, F. and Hell, K. (1998). Effect of insect damage to maize ears, with special reference to *Mussidia nigrivenella* on *Aspergillus flavus* infection and aflatoxin production in maize before harvest in the Republic of Benin. Journal of Econ. Entomology 91, 433-438.

Sewram, V; Nair, J.J; Nieuwouldt, T.W; Leggort, N.I. and Shephard, G.S. (2000). Determination of patulin in apple juice by high-performance liquid chromatography-atmospheric pressure chemical ionization mass spectrometry. Journal of Chromatography A 897: 365-374.

Speijers, G.A. (2004). Patulin, In: Magan, N. and Olsen, M. (Eds), Mycotoxins in Foods, Detection and Control, CRC Press, Boca Raton, FL. pp 339-392.

Thomson, C. and Henke, S.E. (2000). Effects of climate and type of storage container on aflatoxin production in corn and its associated risks to wildlife species. Journal of Wildlife Diseases 36, 172-176.

Tournas, V.H. and Katsoudas, E. (2005). Mould and yeast flora in fresh berries, grapes, and citrus fruits. International Journal of Food Microbiology 105, 11-17.

Turner, P; Sylla, A; Gong, Y; Diallo, M; Sutcliffe, A; Hall, A. and Wild, C. (2005). Reduction of exposure to carcinogenic aflatoxins by postharvest intervention measures in West Africa: a community-based study. Lancet 365, 1950-1959.

Van der Stegen, G.H; Essens, P.J. and van der Lijn, J. (2001). Effects of roasting conditions on reduction of ochratoxin A in coffee. Journal of Agricultural and Food Chemistry 49, 4713-4715.

Visconti, A. (2001). Problems associated with *Fusarium* mycotoxins in cereals. Bulletin of the Institute for Comprehensive Agricultural Sciences, Kinki University No 9, 39-55.

Voss, K. A; Poling, S.M; Meredith, F.I; Bacon, C.W. and Saunders, D.S. (2001). Fate of fumonisins during the production of fried tortilla chips. Journal of Agricultural and Food Chemistry 49, 3120-3126.

Weidenborner, M. (2001). Encyclopedia of Food Mycotoxins. Springer-Verlag, Berlin, Germany.

WHO (1999). Basic Food Safety for Health Workers. World Health Organization, Geneva, Switzerland.

WHO (2006). Mycotoxins in African foods: Implications to Food Safety and Health. AFRO Food safety Newsletter. World Health Organization Food Safety (FOS)., Issue No. July, 2006. www.afro.who.int./des.

Wood, G.M. (1982). Effects of processing on mycotoxin in maize. Chem. Ind. 972-974.

Yoshida, T; Yamashita, A.and Luo, Y. (1994). Fumonisin occurrence in corn from high and low -risk areas for human esophageal cancer in China. Applied and Environmental Microbiology 60, 1626-1629.

Chapter 6

Sustainability and Effectiveness of Artisanal Approach to Control Mycotoxins Associated with Sorghum Grains and Sorghum Based Food in Sahelian Zone of Cameroon

Roger Djoulde Darman

Additional information is available at the end of the chapter

http://dx.doi.org/10.5772/54789

1. Introduction

In Cameroon, the production of sorghum is mostly done in the soudano-sahelian zone on approximately 300.000 hectares for an average production of 100.000 tons [1]. This places the northern region of Cameroun on the first rank for cereal production within the sub region of Central African countries. Sorghum also occupies an essential place as food for millions of Cameroonians [2]. The good image of the sorghum in the region lead to the diversification of the food and feed, in particular in urban zone, through more attractive forms at the culinary, nutritional and economic levels: flour, grits, blown products, rolled, ...etc [3]. Grains are harvested during the rainy season, a best period for yeast and mould which favors contamination by fungi and subsequent mycotoxin contamination. It was shown that maize grain for example is contaminated by *Fusarium sp., Aspergillus sp., Penicillium sp., Acremonium sp. and Diplodia sp.* [4,5]. The contamination of maize by these fungi and their toxic metabolites has been associated with several human and animal diseases including liver and oesophageal cancer, particularly in Africa [4]. In the region, postharvest techniques for cereals are alike both for grain processing and food and feed products. It is possible that sorghum and sorghum by products are also contaminated by fungi thus potential presence of associated mycotoxins. Considering the broad use and the large quantities of sorghum produced and consumed by local population for their daily need in the soudano-sahelian region of Cameroon, it is curious that public health problems related to mycotoxins seems not relevant in the region. Are sorghum and sorghum products exempted from mycotoxin contamination or are local populations' postharvest practices quite effective against mycotoxins? The objective of this chapter is to present and discuss data from investigation on potential mycotoxin contamination and relate them to the efficacy of local artisanal practices against mycotoxins contamination of sorghum as well as some sorghum by-products by moulds in the Sahelian zone of Cameroon.

2. Methods

2.1. Field work

Designing a research on mycotoxins for artisanal technologies with very little information on these processes is not easy. Reliability of information from the popular or unscientific methods of information is sometimes questionable. This information could be the product of preconceived notions of individual observations. The experimental study of the process was thus necessary despite the fact that it incurred significant costs, without direct effects on work. It was also difficult to objectively describe a method developed by people without reference to reliable scientific data to interpret and understand the principles related to this. In addition to the compilation of bibliographic data, data collection was completed by a cross-sectional and descriptive study including two types of surveys:

- A qualitative survey in connection with the opinions, attitudes and practices of people in terms of postharvest technologies applied to sorghum by stakeholders;
- A quantitative survey, by cluster sampling at one level, on the degree of uses of these products.
- Information on post-harvest techniques used for sorghum was collected through the organization of:
- Focus Group (FG) with groups of sorghum processors;
- Depth interviews (DI) with consumers, sellers and producers identified, recruited from the focus groups, in their respective activities related to transformation of sorghum grains.

The survey was conducted using pre-tested materials. Once obtained the consent of participants, the DI and FG were conducted at locations far from all external disturbances to ensure a good animation and therefore the quality of data collection.

During the survey, information was collected from households and producers, their opinions, attitudes and practices relating to mycotoxin associated with sorghum, any changes in the manufacturing processes, source of other major ingredients, improving production conditions, and storage conditions.

3. Laboratory work

3.1. Sampling

A total of 120 samples of sorghum grains from 5 varieties and 6 different locally produced artisanal sorghum by-products (Beer, flour, babies beverage, and cake) were randomly collected from traditional breweries in the cities of Garoua, Maroua and Ngaoundere in the northern part of Cameroon.

3.2. Mycotoxins extraction

Raw grains and cake were crushed and mixed with equal quantity of distilled water prior to the extraction process. Opaque beer and baby beverage were gently shake and degassed using a vacuum pump. Prepared samples were then subjected to solid phase extraction using extraction columns C18 (Perkin Elmer, Norwalk, USA), mounted on a solid-phase extraction manifold (Vacmaster®). The C18 columns were equilibrated by passing 10 ml of methanol: water (10:90) solvent. 20 ml of degassed samples was then passed through the column and the column washed by passing through 20 ml of distilled water, followed by drying with air. The mycotoxins in the column were eluted with 2 ml of methanol, which was diluted 1:10 with phosphate buffered saline (PBS) solution, before analysis by the ELISA procedure.

3.3. Mycotoxin analysis

All analyses were performed using direct competitive microplate enzyme-linked immunosorbent assays (ELISA) as previously described by Usleber, *et al.*[6,7]. The microtitre plate wells were coated with antimycotoxin antibody solution in 0.1M sodium bicarbonate buffer and incubated 18hours at room temperature. The wells were then washed three times with NaCl-Tween (8.5 g NaCl and 250 µL of Tween-20 in 1 litre of water) solution after the free protein binding sites were coated with 3% fetal calf serum in phosphate buffer solution (200 µL/well) for 20 min. Aliquots (50 µL) of diluted sample extracts (sorghum grain, sorghum beer, sorghum based food) and respective mycotoxin standards were added into the well, followed by addition of aliquots (50 µL) of the respective mycotoxin horse radish peroxidase conjugate. The plates were incubated for two hours at room temperature, washed, and an enzyme substrate solution (100 µL) added. The absorbance was read at 450 nm using an ELISA reader reaction after the reaction was stopped by addition of 1M sulfuric acid (100 µL). Absorbance values were analyzed with competitive ELISA software [8], and the data statistically analyzed for variability and association using the SPlus 2000.

4. Results and discussion

4.1. Mycotoxins in raw sorghum grains

In northern Cameroon, there are two types of sorghum production: the rainy season production and the dry season production. Sorghum varieties are thus classified according to season. This includes:

- The *muskuwaari* group which is composed of dry season varieties namely *safraari, majeeri, burguuri* and *ajagamaari, Muskuwaari* in fulfuldé. The fulani language is used to describe all dry season varieties which are sow at the end of the wet season on argils soils called karal. Those varieties have the ability to accomplish their vegetative cycle during drying season from water reserve of those argils soils. The seedlings are prepared in August and sown in the field from September to November (winter). They're generally harvested few months later from April to March.

- The raining season varieties *Madjeri* with two principal groups: *Damougari* and *Djigari*.

All analyzed samples presented no evidence of Aflatoxin B_1, Ochratoxin, Deoxynivalenol (DON) and Fumonisin B_1 contamination in muskwari group while some raining season varieties were contaminated only by Aflatoxin B_1(Table 1). This indicates clearly that there is no incidence of mycotoxins in collected and analyzed muskwari group grains. This may be due primarily to the nature of different varieties and their vegetative cycle which includes development phase in dry season. We can also mention their relatively low moisture content [9] and the availability of grain storages and adequate facilities in rural zone [10].

	Sorghum varieties cultivated in raining season				*Sorghum varieties cultivated in dry season (Muskwari group)*					
Variety	*Damugari*		*Djigari*		*safraari*		*majeeri*		*burguuri*	
	Inci-dence	levels	Inci-dence	levels	Incide nce	levels	Inci-dence	levels	Inci-dence	levels
Aflatoxin B_1	75%	0.0-230 ng/g	45%	0.0-145 ng/g	0%	nd	0%	nd	0%	nd
Ochratoxin A	0%	nd	nd	nd	0%	nd	0%	nd	0%	nd
Deoxynivalenol (DON)	0%	nd	nd	nd	0%	nd	0%	nd	0%	nd
Fumonisin B_1 (FB_1)	0%	nd	nd	nd	0%	nd	0%	nd	0%	nd

nd: not detected

Table 1. Mycotoxins in Sorghum grains varieties from Savannah zones of Cameroon

4.2. Influence of artisanal harvesting on mycotoxin contamination

As mentioned earlier harvesting period and harvesting method may have impact on sorghum quality. In fact depending on season and scale of production most farmers use artisanal hand harvesting methods. The sorghum panicles are cut from the stalks either by hand or using a knife, placed into sacks and taken to the threshing platform where they are placed on racks or spread on the platform for drying. Proper drying is considered to be one of the greatest factors in determining whether grains will be effectively stored without damage, thus avoiding mycotoxins associated mold to growth. In the rainy season when there's not enough sun, the grains are piled on racks or heaps to dry. In this way there is lack of air movement, leading to sprouting, discoloration and microbial damage. This may explain the presence of Aflatoxin B_1 in some analyzed samples (Table1). In addition mycotoxin contamination may occur due to rats, birds, insects etc. To avoid this, dry grains are stored in granaries till they're pounded. Abarca *et al.* [12] indicate that ochratoxin A contaminates a variety of plant and animal products but is most often found in stored cereal grains. But as shown in table 1, no traces of Ochratoxin A were recorded during our study in all samples. The absence of mycotoxins in grains maybe linked to good postharvest techniques applied by local populations like mastering of the agri-calendar leading to harvesting of grains at right time[1], availability of artisanal granaries and finally agro climatic conditions which are favorable for grains storage (hot and dry air, sandy soils…). As mentioned by Van Egmon [13] mycotoxin contamination of foods and feeds depends highly on environmental conditions that lead to mould growth and toxin production. Moore-Landecker, [14]; Wilson and Payne, [15] notice that environmental conditions and some key factors such as moisture, temperature, rats, insects, human manipulation of crops are particularly important factors determining the occurrence of mycotoxins within the seeds or grains.

The observed low incidence levels of mycotoxins in raw dry sorghum grains from northern Cameroon could be link to a pre- and post-harvest strategies to prevent crop contamination which include yearly crop rotation, irrigation in hot and dry weather, use of pesticides to reduce insect population, drying crops to a safe moisture level, and providing protective storage are mastered by local rural population, managing sorghum grains in the field. Makun *et al.*,[16] indicate that although the optimum temperature and moisture content for growth and toxin production for the various aflatoxigenic fungi varies, and considering that these conditions approximate the ambient climatic conditions in most parts of Africa, this author predicts that climate change might exacerbate the aflatoxin crisis in Africa. Althought this assumption seems verified for East Africa, the situation may be different in the northern Cameroon which has a hot and dry sudano sahelian climate compared to the hot and humid climate of eastern African regions. This can also be one of the key factors associated to the high quality of sorghum from Northern Cameroon. In addition to this, the broad use of pesticides to reduce insect population, the mastering of agricultural calendar leading to right harvesting time and availability of artisanal storage facilities in rural area may explain the non-detection of targeted mycotoxins in the analyzed samples despite the none application of complicated HACCP methods.

4.3. Mycotoxins in some commonly used Sorghum derived products from the savannah zones of Cameroon

As shown in table 2 and 3, some sorghum by products, contrary to sorghum grains are contaminated by either one or more types of mycotoxin. Sorghum beer is contaminated by aflatoxin B_1, ochratoxin A and deoxynivalenol. No fumonisin were detected in beer. Sorghum balls were contaminated by ochratoxin only. Three of the fourth types of mycotoxin checked, were recorded in Sorghum porridge namely: aflatoxin B_1, ochratoxin and deoxynivalenol (DON). Aflatoxin B_1 and deoxynivalenol were detected in *dakkere*, a mixture of sorghum and maize flour baked in hot water and sundried.

	Sorghum derived product			
	Bil-Bil	*Sorghum porridge*	*dakkere*	*naakia*
Aflatoxin B_1	86%	73%	82%	nd
Ochratoxin	27%	nd	nd	76%
Deoxynivalenol (DON)	12%	16%	45%	55%
Fumonisins B_1 (FB_1)	nd	nd	nd	nd

Table 2. Incidence of mycotoxins in some commonly used Sorghum derived product of the savannah zones of Cameroon

	Sorghum derived product			
	Bil-Bil	*Sorghum porridge*	*dakkere*	*naakia*
Aflatoxin B_1(mg/kg)	0.0-245	0.0-250	0.0-178	nd
Ochratoxin A (mg/kg)	0.0-45	nd	nd	0.0-33
Deoxynivalenol (DON) (μg/kg)	0.0-120	0.00-500	0.00-423	0.0-538
Fumonisins B_1 (FB_1)(μg/kg)	nd	nd	nd	nd

Table 3. Levels of mycotoxins in some commonly used Sorghum derived product of the savannah zones of Cameroon

It is obvious from the results that despite the good quality of sorghum grains as shown in table 1, most of processed sorghum based foods are contaminated (Table 2 and 3). It is thus likely that processing may be one of the key factor in favor of mycotoxins occurrence in sorghum products. Most of the analyzed derived products contain mycotoxins at levels far above accepted values in foods and feeds.

Legal limits for aflatoxins require that food for human consumption should contain less than 10 μg/kg (parts per billion) of which only 5 ppb may be Aflatoxin B_1 and these limits are based largely on research results [17]. Legal limits for fumonisins have not yet been introduced locally and vary from one region to another. Locally a provisional tolerance level of 100-200 ppb total fumonisins has been suggested for maize/sorghum and maize/sorghum based products intended for human consumption. This lower tolerance level is based on the high human consumption of cereal within the northern part of Cameroon. Limits for deoxynivalenol have been implemented locally by some foreign non-governmental organisation (NGO) especially for trade purpose and vary from 500 to 1 000 ppb in foods and 1 000 ppb to 10 000 ppb in animal feed. Although there are no yet legal limits in Cameroon for ochratoxins in food some international NGOs working in the area have proposed a maximum limit of 5μg/kg in sorghum based products for direct human consumption. The local regional health adviser has therefore advised withdrawal of sorghum found to contain more than 1000μg/kg. At present there is no requirement to recall product, and the local government considers that occasional consumption of affected sorghum meal is unlikely to pose a risk to the consumer. However retailers and manufacturers are advised to withdraw affected batches from shelves. Despite efforts to implement these regulatory measures, there are no adequate facilities for mycotoxins detection as the ones for universities are only for educational and research purposes. We thus think that the best way to tackle the problem is to avoid contaminations during processing. In the following paragraph, we will discuss the risk of mycotoxins occurrence in relation to the processing methods applied to sorghum.

4.4. Artisanal postharvest techniques and risk of mycotoxin contamination of Sorghum grain

Data on local post-harvest techniques used for handling grains by local rural populations were collected during the survey. Processing methods for first transformation product were also screened to determine mycotoxins critical control points in the process. Collected data from focus group discussions following information were drawn from sorghum postharvest techniques to sorghum grain transformation.

4.5. Primary processing

Sorghum grain requires the removal of the outer layer before any further processing could be done. The outer layers of some sorghum varieties contain tannins, which have a bitter taste. For this reason it is normally dehulled and then pounded into flour [3]. Traditionally the processing of sorghum in northern Cameroon is carried out by pounding grain using a pestle and mortar. Grain are then winnowed to remove the bran. Pounding and winnowing are repeated several times before good quality flour is obtained. The objective of hand pounding is thus twofold, the first is to remove the bran and the second is to produce the flour, but this is time consuming and backbreaking. The removal of the bran is one of the key factors reducing the risk of mycotoxin occurrence. The processing of sorghum grain into quality flour is presented in fig 1.

4.6. Dehusking and grinding grains

Grinding and husking are essential steps for sorghum processing in rural sahelian zone of Cameroon. First, grains are spread on mats, plastic sheets or on the floor in monolayer form for sun drying with constant spreading. Dried grains are then stored in paddy forms inside granaries. At this level we had critical points which are laying and threshing. These two steps of the processing which allowed hot air to flow easily through grains may have an effect by avoiding potential mold contamination. Sometimes plastic sheets are colored black to absorb more heat, and the constant stirring contributes to distribute heat in between grains thus may reduce water activity which is an important factor for mycotoxin occurrence [5, 18].

Artisanal grain processing operations for polishing sorghum paddy are generally performed by women and usually start with cleaning of coarse paddy grain using screens. The one with large mesh is used to remove larger particles (straws, other grains ...) and a second with smaller mesh is used to remove dust, dirt or immature grains. At this level risk of contamination of sorghum by mold is reduce by about 20% as it's likely that most strains of mold originate from those larger particles.

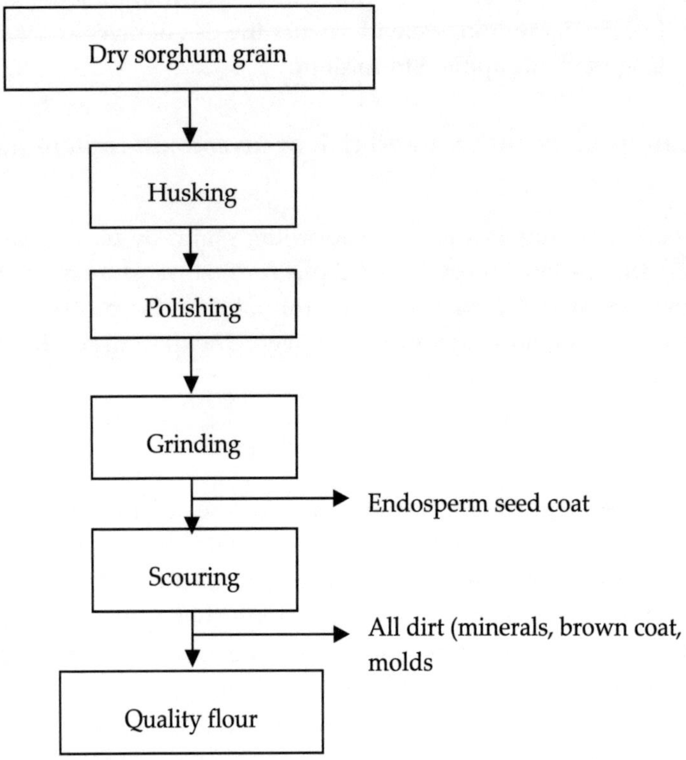

Figure 1. First transformation of sorghum grain: Quality flour production

Dehusking and polishing are carried out simultaneously in mortars and pestles. Five successive pounding, each followed by winnowing are made to separate pericarp and germ from the grain until perfect of polish. The fourth-pounding matches the winnowing stage when the grain is fed to a modern milling machine. The corresponding percentage yields of paddy are about 60-68% complete after polishing. As main mold are in pericarp we can deduce that 38-40% of contamination risk is reduced.

After the last pounding, the polished sorghum is washed. The grain are immersed in a large calabash of water and stirred by hand; dirty water containing dust and bran is continuously eliminated. This operation is repeated several times depending on the nature and color of the predominant variety (housewives often use a mixture of several varieties). Women then proceed to a step leading to removal of total sand. To do this, they dip a gourd containing the washed sorghum grain in a basin of clean water and start with slow swings to bring down gradually the grain in water until only sand settles at the bottom of the gourd. This is reproduced as many times as necessary. It can be expected at this level the removal of sand spores of yeast, and mold which are potential mycotoxins producers. Table 4 presents each operation with levels of reduction of mycotoxins contamination risk.

Step in the process	Reduce levels of risk of mycotoxin contamination
Winnowing	15%
Laying and threshing	10%
Husking and polishing	38%
cleaning of coarse paddy grain	20%
Washing	4%
Removal of sandy spores of yeast and mold, potential mycotoxins producers	5%
Grinding	20%

Table 4. Levels of mycotoxin contamination as % risk according to the steps in the sorghum artisanal processing.

Grinding is performed once the grains are washed and sometimes shelled, using a gasoline mill. When power supply is available, electric mill is used. Scouring is done to improve the quality of the flour. This is performed to remove the seed coat (bran) covering the endosperm. The operation removes all "dirt" from the pericarp (minerals, brown coat, molds ...), to give a best quality flour for preparations [3, 19]. This operation is also one of the best practices to avoid growth of molds responsible for mycotoxins production. According to interviewed women, this operation helps to reduce the bitter taste of grain, but it causes weight losses. The husking performance depends on the hardness of the grain, character related to the glassiness of the endosperm (relative importance of the vitreous and floury parts). Women also noticed poor ability to shell *muskwary* varieties. Their grain flour with brown layer mostly tends to crash during the operation and a fraction of the flour is lost in the sorghum bran. In the contrary the seed coat comes off more easily for raining season's varieties, for which vitreousness seems higher [9]. Women sometimes perform this operation manually using a mortar and pestle after moistening the grains. The operation can also be done mechanically. Nearly 75% of surveyed women, prefer to systematically wash the grains and then let the grain dry in the sun to reduce the bitterness of the grains coat before grinding. This practice may explain the observed high incidence of mycotoxins contamination of food based product (Table 2).

4.7. Risk of mycotoxin contamination during artisanal Sorghum grain processing

4.7.1. Porridge preparation

Sorghum flour is primarily used to prepare porridge, locally called couscous, the main staple of people in northern Cameroon. This preparation is made by mixing sorghum flour to boiling water and stirring vigorously until the dough has a firm and smooth consistency. The porridge is eaten by dipping rolled small cuts inside sauce. The surveyed indigenous peoples of the region are unanimous: *Muskwari sorghum* gives the best balls not only in regard with sensory properties, but also in technological point of view as it is said that "*the porridge from those sorghum varieties take well.* » This may be due to the quality of starch and low moisture content of the grains grow in dry conditions [3]. The light bitterness observed is said to be due to the pericarp. When the grain is dehusked this bitterness disappears during storage.

Interviewed women say to rarely have opportunity to mix some varieties in order to improve the quality of the ball because the grain are opened one by one. However, used varieties may vary depending on the season. During hard field work, women cook the porridge from *safraari* varieties because *it is said to give strength,* and they keep *majeeri* for a longer time as it's mainly used during the dry season. The majeeri variety is said to be less subject to alteration than other varieties, thus less susceptible to carries yeast and molds. Surveys show that some flours like *majeeri* stick least to the pot than *safraari varieties:* for the same amount of water, more *majeeri* flour is added comparing to *safraari* flour for the same desired consistency. These observations must be correlated to changes in grain composition according to the types of sorghum. The composition of the endosperm (starch solubility, amylose content ...) plays a direct role on the texture of the ball [20]. This may also explain the ability of those varieties to be moistened during cooking of porridge. The cooking temperature and reduce water absorption of flour together with some key activities during processing like mixing sorghum flour to boiling water , vigorously stirring the mixture and the dough firm and smooth consistency may be correlated to observed low mycotoxin contamination of porridge

4.7.2. The slurry

Sorghum slurry is similar to sorghum porridge but with a lesser consistency. It is mainly prepared for children. The preparation of sorghum slurry is done by incorporating flour in hot water and continuously stirs the mixture until a thick and homogeneous liquid is obtained after cooking. There are different types of slurry according to the ingredients added at the end of preparation. It's locally called *gaari Kossam* when milk and sugar are added, *gaari biriiji* when peanut butter is added, *gaari kilburi* when sodium powder is added ... The *kilburi* slurry look yellowish as it is made with flour from *safraari* sorghum varieties only. It is often taken to treat digestive disorders. But generally *majeeri* sorghums are favored by women for the preparation of the slurry. The *majeeri ranwanyaande* (white glumes) are the most popular, because even without shelling, grain flour gives a uniform color. During fasting (Ramadan period) Muslims eat pap, a soft porridge made from shelled and flour from *majeeri majeeri* whose grains are systematically shelled. Despite the fact that we did not analyse these types of sorghum slurry, it is predictable that since groundnuts, susceptible to be contaminated by mycotoxin the risk of mycotoxin contamination may be enhanced.

4.8. The *Bil Bil* (traditional beer)

Non-Muslims in villages especially in the foothills and plains of Kaélé, *muskuwaari* brew traditional sorghum beer, *bil bil.*. The process of production of *bil-bil* can be described as follows (Fig 2):

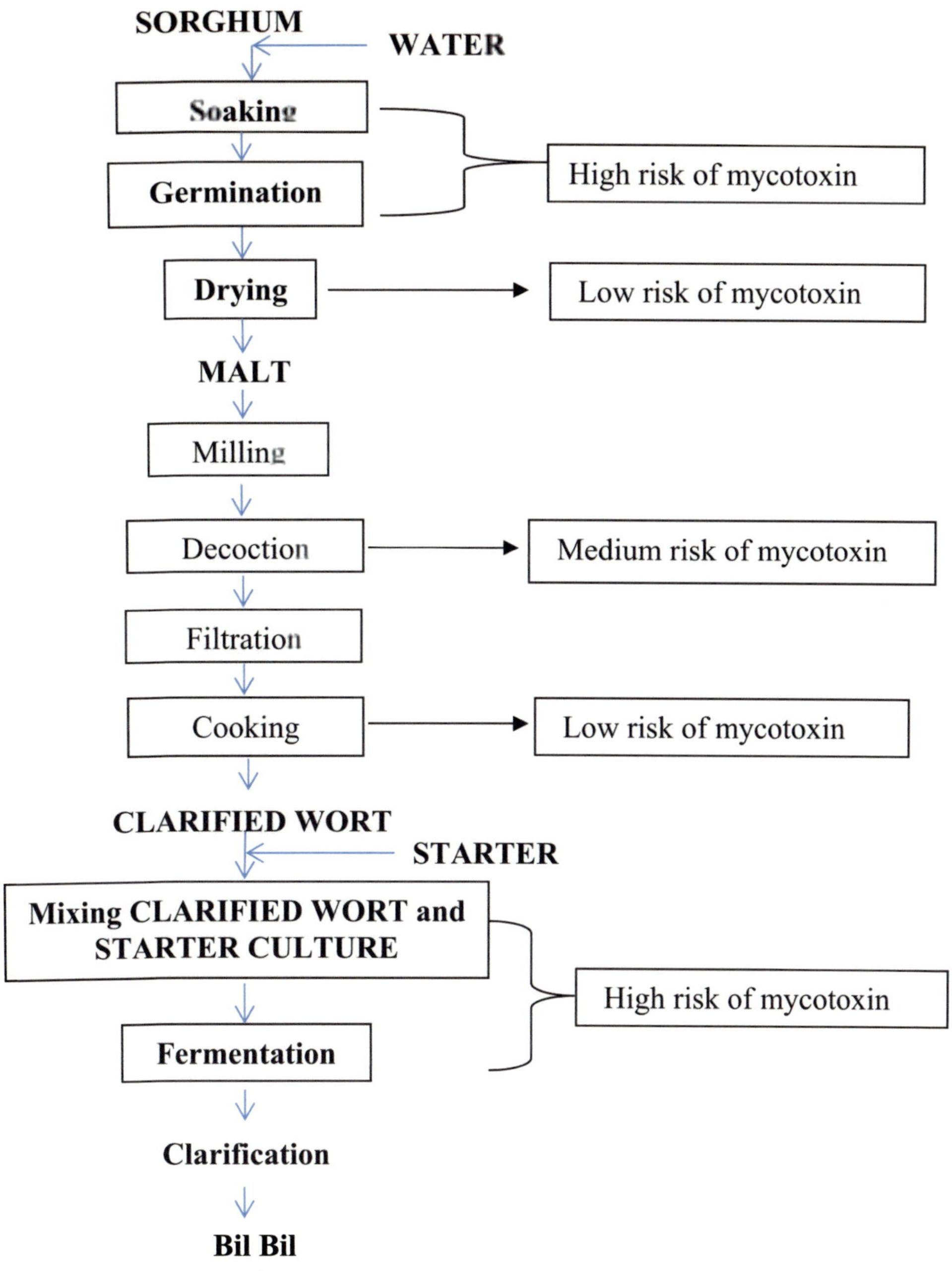

Figure 2. Mycotoxin risk assessment during the process production of *bil-bil*

This operation starts with malting. Most often populations choose a sorghum variety locally known as "mouskouari" [9]. After washing, sorghum grains are soaked in water for 72 hours to obtain a water content varying from 35% to 40 % (w/w). This soaking is required for the germination process. Information from the discussion groups revealed that water temperature is very important for soaking process. Soaking is done at high temperature so that the soaking process is rapid (20±4 hours). This high temperature close to 45°C may reduce risk of yeast and mold growth thus mycotoxin contamination. The next step is germination. Wet grains are placed on burlap bags for 24 to 36 hours or the grains are left in the tin used for soaking, usually in a container until the rootlets appear and/or grain spades. On burlap bags, the grains are sprayed with water on daily basis. At this stage the risk of yeast and mold growth is increased. The disposal of grains in heaps on burlap bags allows a rise of the temperature during the process, which facilitates the germination. This process can be the genesis of mycotoxin occurrence in the final beer.

However, many women do not follow this step, especially in the arid and hot areas and immediately after soaking, they place grains over a clean area (wood sheet, clay, rock). The grains are laid in 3±0.2 cm layers, covered with leaves that keep the grains in darkness and maintain adequate humidity. All these operations are clearly favorable conditions for yeast and mold growth. Thus increase risk of mycotoxin contamination of the final beer. Sometimes women say the soaking and germination processes can be conducted in jars in the dark but emphasize that in this case, molds are more frequent and the germination process is slow. This may be explained by the low ventilation and higher humidity inside the jars. Again at this level the risk of mycotoxin production may be high.

After germination, the grains are piled: the temperature rises, the amylase levels increase and eventually stop increasing when the temperature is too high. The next step is drying. This operation corresponds to kilning and brings moisture of the malt to 18±5% [10] to prevent from the growth of molds. The malt is dried in the sun for one day or more, sometimes less before it goes straight to the brewing. If at this stage the growth of mold is reduce, mycotoxin eventually produced during previous stages may not be destroyed. Then we have the brewing stage. The malt is crushed in a mortar or on a flat stone. In urban areas, malt is ground in a motorized mill to obtain coarse flour. The ground malt is mixed with water with a gelatinous or mucilaginous agent (okra or sap of various trees, especially *Triumfetta sp.*, which is said by women to enhance flocculation and filtration of insoluble materials. This step is like "bonding" for clarification in "high gravity" fermentation beer process [21]. At this stage there is risk of yeast and mold contamination as the use of *Triumfetta sp.* leaves are susceptible to bring spores of molds. The next stage is decoction. Here the lower phase containing the undissolved malt flour is cooked slowly to boil in order to obtain a "cooked starch "" with porridge consistency. The cooking process can be extended over an hour but the upper phase liquid is then mixed with the slurry to be saccharified more easily than if it had not been cooked [22]. Cooking of the mixture is around 65°C to 70°C which is close to the destruction temperature of some mycotoxin and mold. Thus the risk of mycotoxin production is low. At the brewing stage of "bil-bil" production, some women add a mucilaginous agent to promote emulsion. This action can also enable yeast and mold contamination. The next step is fermentation. The wort is cooled either spontaneously or by successive decanting operations. When the temperature of wort is around 30°C it is mixed with an ongoing "affouk" fermentation used as starter culture. It is also common to use an old fermentation tank containing remaining beer from previous fermentation. This operation can bring some natural pathogenic molds. Some women said, that the starter culture can also be recovered from the bottom of fermentation tanks. The cake is sun dried and kept as starter culture for new production. The risk of contamination by pathogenic mold may rise here.

According to some women Mofu Mowo, beer brewed only with *njiigari* gives headaches. Good *bil bil* is obtained by mixing in equal proportion *muskuwaari (safraari, mandoweyri yaawu* and preferentially) and rained sorghum but the proportions depend especially on the types available and the market prices. In mundangs and guizigas communities, some women also use a *corn-muskuwaari* in their preparation. The proportion is then quite variable, ranging from less than 1/6 to 1/3 corn.

4.9. Other sorghum derived product

The donuts: There are other Sorghum by product often prepared from flour of white *majeeri, tolo tolo balwanyaande, ajagamaari,* and sometimes skinned *safraari.* The main ingredients used for this are: sorghum flour, wheat flour, sugar, oil, eggs, orange, raisins, ground fennel seeds, honey, baking powder, sesame seeds, blanched almonds, baking soda. Even most of the used fruits may be source of mold contamination thus mycotoxin contamination

The *dakkere*. Typically Fulani, this is a dish prepared with the *majeeri* varieties only. The flour is moistened in a gourd into small balls. These are then steamed and eaten with yogurt. The main risk here is that during fermentation and conservation of final product pathogenic yeast and mold can grow with concomittant mycotoxin contamination. As shown in table 3 mycotoxins were detected in some of the analyzed samples

The *naakia* or *ndondooje* is a delicacy prepared by Fulani or similar. Women melt sugar in oil, and then add flour *safraari, suukkataari usuku* or *allah.* This mixture is rolled into a ball consumed especially during festivals. Again most of the steps of the production process may present risk as mycotoxins were detected in some of analyzed samples.

4.10. Social implication and sustainability

In socio economic point of view, this work involved collaboration amongst stakeholders, professionals, women, community health and other opinion leaders in the community. Thus there increased a chance capacity building for sorghum post-harvest handling techniques. The work was implemented at community level and project research assistants, community members were trained and developed HACCP practices to avoid mycotoxin in sorghum grain and by products. They may continue to train Community members or peer volunteers and other collaborating organizations, without help of trainers and thus remaining sustainable. The multi-sectoral team/ task force and community members that participated in the project, based on evidences found across the main results of the project, facilitate development of a sustainable program integrating sorghum post handling techniques in the existing community based development/health programs through participatory approaches. Promotional campaigns at the community, district, and provincial levels during the project, based on evidences found across the main results of the project, facilitate widespread acceptance of improved post-harvest practices centred on the use of locally developed HACCP.

5. Conclusion

Enduring food-safety solutions to sorghum generates good health and improved productivity within the region. Mycotoxins associated consequences, acute intoxication and cancer development which causes irreparable damage to livelihoods in the area, thereby reducing self-sufficiency of local rural population, can be reduced by relying on local artisanal approach to control mycotoxins associated with sorghum grains and sorghum based food. As this is part of the process leading to food security. This will directly contribute to livelihoods amelioration in the long term.

Author details

Roger Djoulde Darman
The higher Institute of Sahel, Maroua, Cameroon

6. References

[1] Djamen P N., Djonnéwa A., Havard M., Legile A., 2003. Former et conseiller les agriculteurs du Nord-Cameroun pour renforcer leurs capacités de prise de décision, Cahiers d'études et de recherches francophones / Agricultures. Volume 12, Numéro 4, 241-5, Juillet 2003

[2] Faure, J. (1992). Pâtes alimentaires à base de sorgho et de maïs et produits extrudés. In Utilization of sorghum and millets (Gomez, M.I., House, L.R., Rooney, L.W., et Dendy, D.A.V., éd.). Patancheru 502 324, Andhra Pradesh, Inde: ICRISAT.

[3] Fliedel, G. 1996. Caractérisation et valorisation du sorgho. Le grain et sa transformation pour l'alimentation humaine. Montpellier, France: Laboratoire de technologie des céréales, IRAT-CIRAD

[4] Marasas WFO, 2001. Discovery and occurrence of the fumonisins: a historical perspective. *Environmental Health Perspective*, 109: 239-243.

[5] Ngoko Z, Marasas WFO, Rheeder JP, Sherphard GS, Wingfield MJ, 2001. Fungal infection and mycotoxin contamination of maize in the Humid Forest and the Western Highlands of Cameroon. *Phytoparasitica* 29 (4): 352-360.

[6] Usleber, E., Renz, V., Märtlbauer, E. and Terplan, G. 1992. Studies on the application of enzyme immunoassays for the *Fusarium* mycotoxins deoxynivalenol, 3-acetyldeoxynivalenol and zearalenone, *Journal of Veterinary Medicine*. 39: 617–627

[7] Usleber, E., Straka, M. and Terplan, G. 1994. Enzyme immunoassay for fumonisin B_1 applied to corn-based food. *Journal of Agriculture and Food Chemistry*. 42: 1392–1396.

[8] Märtlbauer, E., 1993. Computerprogramm zur Auswendung kompetitiver Enzymimmuntests; Enzymimmuntests für antimikrobiell wirksame Stoffe. Ferdinand Enke Verlag: Stuttgart, pp. 206–222.

[9] Djoulde Darman Roger, Kenga Richard, Etoa Franc¸ois-Xavier, (2008). Evaluation of Technological Characteristics of Some Varieties of Sorghum (Sorghum Bicolor) Cultivated in the Soudanosahelian Zone of Cameroon, International Journal of Food Engineering, *Volume* 4, *Issue* 1 2008 *Article* 7 Published by The Berkeley Electronic Press, 2008

[10] Seignobos C., Iyebi-Mandjek O., 2000. *Atlas de la province Extrême-Nord Cameroun*, Minrest, INC, IRD, Paris, 171 p.

[11] DjouldeDarman Roger (2011). Deoxynivanol (DON) and fumonisins B_1 (FB_1) in artisanal sorghum opaque beer brewed in north Cameroon, *African Journal of Microbiology Research* Vol. 5(12), pp. 1565-1567, 18 June, 2011. Available online http://www.academicjournals.org/ajmr ISSN 1996-0808 ©2011 Academic Journals

[12] Abarca, M. L., Braugulat, M. R., Castella, G. and Cabanes, F. J. 1994. Ochratoxin A production by strains of *Aspergillus niger* var.*niger*. App. Env. Microbiol. 60:2650-2652.

[13] Van Egmond, H. P. 1989. Mycotoxins in Dairy Products. Elsevier Applied Science, London and New York.

[14] Moore-Landecker, E. 1996. Fundamentals of the Fungi. Prentice Hall International Inc., New Jersey.

[15] Moore-Landecker, E. 1996. Fundamentals of the Fungi. Prentice Hall International Inc., New Jersey.

[16] Wilson, D.M. and Payne, G. A. 1994. Factors affecting *Aspergillus flavus* group infection and aflatoxin contamination of crops. In David L. Eaton and John D. Groopman (ed.), The Toxicology of Aflatoxins. Human Health, Veterinary, and Agricultural Significance, Academic Press, Inc., San Diego, pp. 383-406.

[17] Makun Hussaini Anthony, Dutton Michael Francis, Njobeh Patrick Berka, Gbodi Timothy Ayinla and Ogbadu Godwin Haruna (2011) Aflatoxin Contamination in Foods and Feeds:A Special Focus on Africa in Trends in Vital Food and Control Engineering,

[18] Whitaker, T. B., A. B. Slate and A. S. Johansson. 2005. Sampling Feeds for Mycotoxin Analysis. The Mycotoxin Blue Book, Edited by Duerte Diaz, 1-25, Nottingham University Press.

[19] Santin, E. 2005. Mould Growth and Mycotoxin Production. The Mycotoxin Blue Book, Edited by Duerte Diaz, 225-234, Nottingham University Press.

[20] Jeffrey P. Wilson (2008) Technology for Post-harvest Processing of Pearl Millet and Sorghum in Africa, Evaluation of prototype devices developed by Compatible Technology International, USDA-ARS Crop Genetics & Breeding Research Unit Tifton, GA jeff.wilson@ars.usda.gov 21 pages

[21] Trouche G., Fliedel G., Chantereau J ., Barro C., 1999. Productivité et qualité des grains de sorgho pour le tô en Afrique de l'Ouest: les nouvelles voies d'amélioration. Agriculture et développement n°23, septembre 1999, pp 94-107.

[22] BvochoraJ.M ZvauyaR (2001) Biochemical changes occurring during the application of high gravity fermentation technology to the brewing of Zimbabwean traditional opaque beer,Volume 37, Issue 4, 10 December, Pages 365–370
[23] Taylor J. R.N., Tilman J., Schober, Scott R. B. (2006). Novel food and non-food uses for sorghum and millets; *Journal of Cereal Science* 44 252–271

Chapter 7

Nigerian Indigenous Fermented Foods: Processes and Prospects

Egwim Evans, Amanabo Musa, Yahaya Abubakar and Bello Mainuna

Additional information is available at the end of the chapter

http://dx.doi.org/10.5772/52877

1. Introduction

The deliberate fermentation of foods by man predates written history and is possibly the oldest method of preserving perishable foods. Evidence suggests that fermented foods were consumed 7,000 years ago in Babylon (Battcock and Aza-Ali, 1998). Scientist speculates that our ancestors possibly discovered fermentation by accident and continued to use the process out of preference or necessity. Preserving by fermentation not only made foods available for future use, but more digestible and flavourful. The nutritional value produced by fermenting is another benefit of fermenting.

Fermented foods are generally produced using plant or animal ingredients in combination with fungi or bacteria which are either sourced from the environment, or carefully kept in cultures maintained by humans. Just as living organisms cover the surface of the earth, fermentation microbes cover the surface of the organisms. Wild yeasts are found living on grapes (Chamberlain et al. 1997), and bacteria line the human digestive tract.

Fermented foods, whether from plant or animal origin, are an intricate part of the diet of people in all parts of the world. Fermented food plays a very important role in the socio-economics of developing countries. Each nation has its own types of fermented food, representing the staple diet and the raw ingredients available in that particular place. It makes major contributions to the protein requirements of the rural population. The preparation of many indigenous or "traditional" fermented foods and beverages remains a household art today.

2. Purpose and benefits of food fermentation

The primary benefit of fermentation is the conversion of sugars and other carbohydrates to usable end products. According to Steinkraus (1995), the traditional fermentation of foods serves several functions, which includes: enhancement of diet through development of flavour, aroma, and texture in food substrates, preservation and shelf-life extension through lactic acid, alcohol, acetic acid and alkaline fermentation, enhancement of food quality with protein, essential amino acids, essential fatty acids and vitamins, improving digestibility and nutrient availability, detoxification of anti-nutrient through food fermentation processes, and a decrease in cooking time and fuel requirement.

2.1. Nutritional benefits

Fermentation can produce important nutrients or eliminate anti- nutrients. Food can be preserved by fermentation, since fermentation uses up food energy and creates conditions unsuitable for spoilage microorganisms. For instance, in pickling, the acid produced by the dominant organism inhibits the growth of all other microorganisms.

Fermenting makes foods more edible by changing chemical compounds, or predigesting, the foods for us. There are extreme examples of poisonous plants like cassava that are converted to edible products by fermenting. Some coffee beans are hulled by a wet fermenting process, as opposed to a dry process (Battcock and Aza-Ali, 1998).

Reduction in anti-nutritional and toxic components in plant foods by fermentation was observed in a research which showed " Cereals, legumes, and tubers that are used for the production of fermented foods may contain significant amounts of antinutritional or toxic components such as phytates, tannins, cyanogenic glycosides, oxalates, saponins, lectins, and inhibitors of enzymes such as alpha-amylase, trypsin, and chymotrypsin.

- These substances reduce the nutritional value of foods by interfering with the mineral bioavailability and digestibility of proteins and carbohydrates. In natural or pure mixed-culture fermentations of plant foods by yeasts, molds, and bacteria, antinutritional components (e.g. phytate in whole wheat breads) can be reduced by up to 50%; toxic components, such as lectins in tempe and other fermented foods made from beans, can be reduced up to 95%. (Larsson and Sandberg, 1991)

Fermentation increases nutritional values of foods, and allows us to live healthier lives. Here are a few examples:

- The sprouting of grains, seeds, and nuts, multiplies the amino acid, vitamin, and mineral content and antioxidant qualities of the starting product (Wigmore, 1986).
- Fermented beans are easier for the bodies to digest, like the proteins found in soy beans that are nearly indigestible until fermented (Katz, 2003).
- Fermented dairy products, like, cheese, yogurt, and kifir, can be consumed by those not able to digest the raw milk, and aid the digestion and well-being for those with lactose intolerance and autism.
- Porridge made from grains allowed to ferment increases the nutritional values so much that it reduces the risk of disease in children (Battcock and Aza-Ali, 1998).
- Probotic supplements (beneficial bacterial cultures for microbial balance in the body) are capable of fighting cancer and other diseases.

- Vinegar is used to leach out certain flavours and compounds from plant materials to make healthy and tasty additions to the meals.

2.2. Health benefits

Fermented food, enjoyed across the globe, conveys health benefits through lactic acid fermentation. The fermentation process can transform the flavour of food from the plain and mundane to a mouth-puckering sourness enlivened by colonies of beneficial bacteria and enhanced micronutrients.

- Studies have revealed that *Lactobacillus rhamnosus* and *L. reuteri* which are common organisms in Nigerian fermented foods like ogi and kunun- zaki could colonize the vagina, kill viruses, and reduce the risk of infections, including bacterial vaginosis (Reid *et al.*, 2001a; Cadieux *et al.*, 2002). The potential therapeutic effects of Lactic Acid Bacteria (LAB) and *ogi*, including their immunostimulatory effect, are due primarily to changes in the gastrointestinal (GI) microflora to suppress the growth of pathogens. Increase in population of LAB in the intestinal or vagina reduces the cause of bacterial vaginosis, which is a major risk factor for the contraction of HIV (Reid, 2002a). It also reduces the occurrence of gonorrhoea, chlamydia, and other sexually transmitted diseases (Reid *et al.*, 2001b) and diarrhoea (Adebolu *et al.*, 2007).
- All lactic acid producing bacteria (E.g*Lactobacillus acidophilus, L.bulgaricus, L. plantarum, L. caret, L. pentoaceticus, L. brevis and L. themophilus*) produces high acidity during fermentation. The lactic acid they produce is effective in inhibiting the growth of other bacteria that may decompose or spoil the food. Despite their complexity, the whole basis of lactic acid fermentation centres on the ability of lactic acid bacteria to produce acid, which then inhibits the growth of other non desirable organisms. Other compounds are important as they improve particular testes and aromas to the final products. The *L. mesenteroides* initiates growth in vegetables more rapidly over a range of temperatures and salt concentrations than any other lactic acid bacteria. It produces carbon dioxide and acids which rapidly lower the pH and inhibit the development of undesirable micro organism.
- Over 200 species of bacteria live in gut of humans. These microbes help break down food in the intestines, aid in the digestion process, help fight off disease, and boost the immune system. A good balance of intestinal flora is very important to the overall health. If we eat nothing but overly processed and hard to digest foods, then the fermentation process occurs within the GIT resulting into gas, bloating, diarrhoea, and constipation might possibly lead to other diseases like cancer. However, providing the body with predigested foods such as fermented foods will help the existing microbes within to do the job they need to do.
- Fermentation is not only a way to preserve certain foods, in some cases it actually adds to the nutrient value of it. Fermented vegetables contain more vitamin C and fermented milk products have ample amounts of B vitamins. The bioavailability of these vitamins also increases with fermentation. Probiotics, or "good bacteria" are also formed through the process of fermentation. Fermented soy products contain more vitamin B_{12} (Chung et al, 2010)

- The desirable bacteria cause less deterioration of the food by inhibiting the growth of the spoiling types of bacteria. Some fermenting processes lower the pH of foods preventing harmful microorganisms to live with too acidic an environment. Controlled fermentation processes encourage the growth of good bacteria which starves, or fights off, the bad microbes.
- The fermentation process can be stopped by other means of preserving, such as, canning (heating), drying, or freezing. Heat (pasteurization, 63°C), and low temperatures (freezing, 0°C or below) stops the fermenting process by slowing, or killing, the preferred microorganisms, and other bacteria. A few undesirable bacteria are not killed by either means, and continue to grow. When the beneficial bacteria are gone, the unfavorable bacteria take over, growing exponentially! This causes rotting, disease, illness, and inedible foods. When the good guys are present and happy, the food remains edible.
- Phytates (phytic acid) are the storage form of phosphorus [a mineral] bound to inositol [a B vitamin] in foods high in fiber (all plant foods), and particularly the fiber of raw whole grains, legumes, seeds, and nuts. Although these foods have high phosphorus content, the phosphates in phytates are not released by human digestion. Phytates, particularly in such raw foods as bran, are a concern because they can bind a portion of the iron, zinc, and calcium in foods, making the minerals unavailable for absorption. When bread is leavened (fermented) by yeast, enzymes degrade phytic acid, and phytates pose no problem. Enzymes, called phytases, destroy phytates during fermentation processes such as: the yeast-raising of dough, Even a small amount of phytates in food can reduce iron absorption by half (by 50%), but the effect is less marked if a meal is supplemented with ascorbic acid (Vitamin C) which also helps the absorption of zinc and calcium.
- Fermented food, enjoyed across the globe, conveys health benefits through lactic acid fermentation. The fermentation process can transform the flavor of food from the plain and mundane to a mouth-puckering sourness enlivened by colonies of beneficial bacteria and enhanced micronutrients. While fermented food like yogurt, sauerkraut and kefir are well-known many other lesser-known foods also benefit from the lactic acid fermentation process. Indeed, virtually every food with a complex or simple sugar content can be successfully fermented.
- Born of both necessity and practicality, lactic acid fermentation proved to be not only an efficient method of preserving food for our ancestors, but also a critical one. Indeed, fermented food like sauerkraut, cheese, wine, kvass, soured grain porridge and breads often sustained tribes and villages during harsh winters when fresh food simply wasn't available let alone plentiful.
- In many societies including our own where yogurt has been heralded as a health food since the 19th century, fermented food has gained a reputation for its beneficial effects on immunity, intestinal health and general well-being. Modern researchers are just beginning to understand what the sages of old were tuned in to: fermented food conveys clear and calculable health benefits to the human diet. Lactic acid fermentation in and of itself enhances the micronutrient profile of several foods.

2.3. Detoxification

Detoxification of anti-nutrients through food fermentation processes. The renewal of anti-nutrient from the Nigerian fermented food is an important step in ensuring that the fermented food is safe to eat. Many fermentation foods contain naturally accruing toxins and anti-nutritional compounds. These can be removed or detoxified by the action of micro-organism during fermentation for instance, the fermentation process that produces the Sudanese product, kawal, removes the toxins from the leaves of *Cassia obtusitfolia* and fermentation is an important step in insuring that the fermentation foods are safe to eat.

Removing cyanide by fermentation: Cassava contains naturally occurring chemicals, cyanogenic glycoside. When eaten raw or improperly processed, this substances releases cyanide into the body, which can be fatal, correct processing removers this chemicals. The cassava is first peeled (as about 60-70% of the poison is in the peel) and then soaked in stagnant water or fermented in sacks for about three days. It is sometimes grated or rasped as this helps to speed up the fermentation process. At the beginning of the fermentation, *Geotricum candidia* acts on the cassava. This helps to make the product acidic, which finally kills off the microorganisms as they cannot exist in such a medium. A second strain of microorganisms (*corynebacteriumlactis*) which can tolerate the acidic environment then take over and by the third day 90-95% of the dangerous chemicals would have been hydrolyzed. The cassava also develops its characteristic flavour. The product is then sieved and the fine starch particles are fried in an iron pan over aflame or with some oil. During this process most, if not all the remaining toxins are given off. The liquor from a previous fermentation is used as a starter, thereby reducing the period of fermentation to about 6-8hours.

3. Nigerian fermented foods

3.1. Fermented tubers

These include mainly cassava and yam used in the production of foods such as garri, fufu, lafun and elubo etc.

Nigeria is one of the leading producers of cassava in the world with an annual production of 35-40 million metric tons. Over 40 varieties of cassava are grown in Nigeria and cassava is the most important dietary staple in the country accounting for over 209 of all food crops consumed in Nigeria (IITA, 2004). Cassava tubers are rich in starch [20-30%] and with possible exception of sugar cane; cassava is considered the highest producer of carbohydrates among crop plants. Despite its vast potentials, the presence of the two gynogenic glycosides, lineman calculating for 93% of total content (Okafor *et al.*, 1984) and lotaustralin or methyl linamarin, hydrolysis by the enzymes linamarase to release toxic HCN, is the most important problem limiting cassava utilization. Generally cassava contains 10-500 mg HCN/KG of root depending on the variety, although much higher levels, exceeding 1000 mg HCN/kg, may be present in unusual cases. Cassava varieties are frequently described as sweet or bitter. Sweet cassava varieties are low in cyanogens with most of the cyanogens present in the peels. Bitter cassava varieties are high in cyanogens that tend to be evenly distributed throughout the roots. Environmental (soil, moisture, temperature) and other factors also influence the cyanide content of cassava. Low rainfall or drought increase cyanide level in cassava tools due to water stress on plant. Apart from acute toxicity that may result in death, consumption of sub-lethal dose of cyanide from cassava production over a long period of time results in chronic cyanide toxicity. That increases the prevalence of goiter and cretinism in iodine deficient area. Symptoms of cyanide poisoning from consumption of cassava with high level of cyanogens include vomiting, stomach pains, dizziness, headache, weakness and charkha. Chronic cyanide toxicity is also associated with several pathological conditions including konzo, an irresistible paralysis of the legs reported in eastern, central and southern Africa. And tropical ataxic neuropathy, reported in west Africa, characterized by lesion of the skin, mucous membranes, optics and auditory nerves, spinal cord and peripheral nerves and other symptoms. Without the benefits of modem science, a process for detoxifying cassava roots by canvassing potentially toxic roots into garriand fufu was developed, presumably empirically in West Africa.

a. Gari

Gari is a creamy-white, granular flour with fermented flavour and a slightly sour taste made from fermented, gelatinized fresh cassava tubers. Gari is widely known in Nigeria and other West African countries. It is commonly consumed either by being soaked in cold water with sugar, coconut, roasted groundnuts, dry fish, or boiled cowpea as complements or as a paste made with hot water and eaten with vegetable sauce. There are basically three types of gari

1. Rough-sour gari which is preferred for soaking with sugar and sometimes roasted peanut or coconut.
2. Medium gari is usually cooked by adding to boiling water and stirred. This is usually eaten with stew or soup.
3. Smooth gari which could be mixed with pepper and other spicy ingredients. A small amount of warm water and palm oil is added and mixed with the hand to soften. This type of gari is served with fried fish.

b. Fufu

Fufu is a fermented white paste made from cassava it is ranked next to gari as an indigenous food of most Nigerians in the South. Fufu is made by sleeping whole or cut peeled cassava roots in water to ferment for maximum of three days, during the steeping, fermentation decrease the pH, softens the roots and help to reduces the potentially toxic cyanogenic compound (Agbor-Egbe and Lape Mbome, 2006)

c. Lafun

Lafun is a fibrous powdery form of cassava similar to fufu in Nigeria. The method of producing lafun is different from that of fufu in the traditional preparation; fresh cassava roots are cut into chucks and steeped for 3-4 days or until the roots become soft. The fermented roots are peeled, broken up into small pieces and sun dried on mats, flat rocks, cineol flours, or the roots of houses. The dried pieces are milled into flour. Alternatively, chips are made directly from fresh roots, cut into chucks and sun dried. Drying takes 2-4 days, depending on weather. Unlike fufu, the fiber is the related root for lafun are dried along with the mash and later sieved out. The flour is made into dough with boiling water before consumption. When properly stored, it has a shelf life of six months or more.

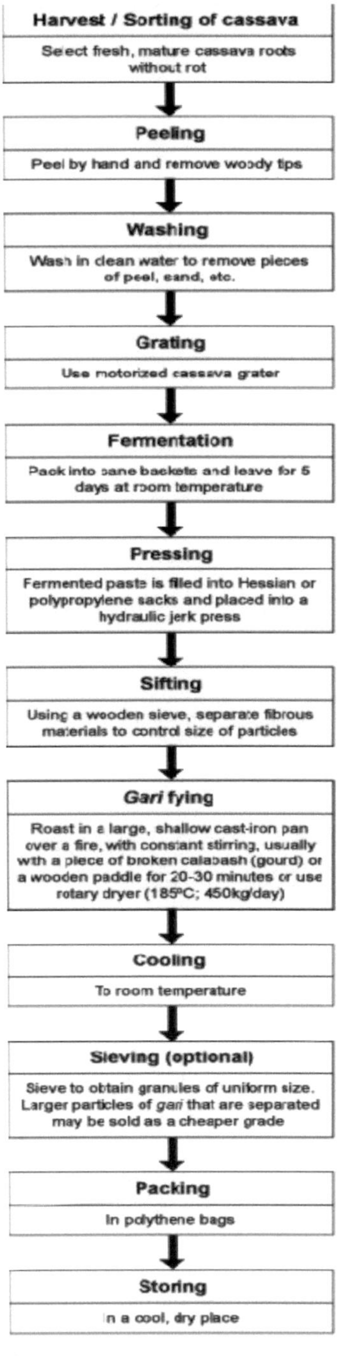

Figure 1. Process flow chart for Gari.

Matured cassava roots without rot

↓

Peel and remove skin

↓

Wash in clean water to remove sand

↓

Soak roots in water in a bowl for 48-72 hours.

↓

Fufu mash is allowed to be concentrated before decaling

↓

Fermented paste is filled into polypropylene sacks and placed in a jerk press.

↓

Motorized grater is used to pulverize cake into smaller particle and increases surface area for easy drying.

↓

Dry, using rotary dryer (184^{0}C, 450kg/day)

↓

Cool at room temperature

↓

Mill to obtain powder and pack in polyether bags

↓

Store in a cool, dry place

Figure 2. Process flow chart for fufu.

Fresh cassava roots without rots

↓

Peel Cassava roots by hand and remove the woody tips

↓

Cut into chunks of tiny pieces

↓

Wash chunks in clean water in a bowl

↓

Soak Cassava chunks in a bowl of water for 3-4 days at room temperature

↓

Crush soaked chunks by hand

↓

Fill fermented parse into hessian or polypropylene sacs and place in a hydrated jack press

Figure 3. Process flowchart for the production of lafun.

3.2. Fermented cereals

Cereals which include maize (*Zea mays*), Sorghum (*Sorghum bicolor*), millet (*Peninselum americarum*) and acha etc. are used in the production of gruels which is used as complementary food for babies and serves as breakfast for adults.

Maize, millet, rice and sorghum cereals provide mainly carbohydrates and low quality protein. The generation and fermentation of cereals enhance the availability of elemental iron, the deficiency of which is responsible for the high incidence of anaemia in tropical countries. It is estimated that about 50% of perishable food commodities including fruits, vegetables, roots and tubers and about 30% of food commodities including maize, sorghum millet, rice and cowpeas are lost after harvest in Nigeria. Nigerian in fact experience a slower growth rate and weight gain during the weaning period than during breastfeeding, due primarily to the poor nutritional qualities of traditional Nigerian complementary food such as "Ogi" which are mainly produced from cereal fermentation. Apart from their poor nutritional qualities, traditional Nigerian cereal based gruels used as complementary foods have high paste viscosity and require considerable dilution before feeding; a factor that further reduces energy and nutrient density.

Although nutritious and safe complementary foods produced by food multinationals are available in Nigeria, they are far, too expensive for most families. The economic situation in these country necessitate the adoption of simple, inexpressive processing techniques that result in quality improvement and that can be carried out at household and community levels for the production of nutritious, safe and affordable complementary foods which is the leading cause of protein-energy malnutrition in infants and preschool children in Nigeria.

a. Ogi

This is an example of traditional fermented food, it is a staple cereal of Yorubas of Nigeria and is the first native food given to babies at wearing. It is produced generally by soaking corn grains in warm water for one to two days followed by wet milling and sieving through a screen mesh. The sieved material is allowed to sediment and fermented, and is marketed as wet cake wrapped in leaves. Various food dishes are made from the fermented cakes or ogi. During the steeping corn, *Corynebacterium* spp. become prominent and appears to be responsible for the diastolic action necessary for the growth of yeast and lactic acid bacteria. Along with the corn in bacteria, *S. cerevisiae, Enterobacter cloacae* and *L.plantarum* have been found to be prominent in traditional ogi fermentation.

In Nigeria, the first weaning food is called pap, akamu, ogi, or koko and it is made from maize (zea mays), millet (*Pennisetum americanum*), or guinea corn (*Sorghum spacers*). In Anambra state most mothers introduce the thin gruel at three to six months of age. The baby is fed on demand with a spoon or a few mothers used the traditional forced hand-feeding method. After the successful introduction the thin gruel, other staple foods in the family menu are given to the child. These food include yam (*Dioscoria spp*) rice (*oriza sativa*) gari (fermented cassava grit) and cocoyam (*xanthosoma sagitifolum*), which may be eaten with soup. These foods are usually mashed thinned or pre-chewed. As soon as a child can chew, he or she is given pieces of from the family pot.

Maize, millet or sorghum

↓

Wash

↓

Sleep/ferment for 24-72 hours

↓

Drain

↓

Wet mill

↓

Ferment further for 24-72 hours (optional).

↓

Decant

↓

Ogi slurry

↓

Boil

↓

Ogi porridge

Figure 4. Process flow chart for ogi.

b. Masa

Masa (waina) is a fermented puff batter of rice, millet, maize, or sorghum cooked in a pan with individual cup like depressions. It resembles the Indian idli in shape and dosa in test. Masa is consumed in various forms by all groups in the northern States of Nigeria and other North African countries (Mali, Burkina Faso, Niger and Chad.) It is the principal ingredients of a variety of cereal-based foods and is a good source of income for the women who prepare the traditional product for sale. Though, masa is as popular as a Nigeria ogi, it has received very little attention. The problem of masa, apart from the short shelf keeping quality, is that of low protein content and inconsistence in the use of varied cereals and spices has resulted in variation in the quality of the products.

The addition of cowpea, groundnut or soybeans flour into masa during preparations improves the nutritional quality of masa. Groundnut-maize enriched masa could be a source of protein to the consumer particularly in developing countries like Nigeria where cost of feeding on animal sourced protein is unaffordable. The high calorie content of groundnut-maize masa could be due to the high fat content of the added paste. The decrease in the weight of masa with addition of groundnut paste could be due to increase in the oil content in the paste which has been proofed to be relatively lighter. Masa formulation containing millet or rice blended with cowpea or groundnut was prepared and sodium concentrations were high. Significant improvements in lysine (9-75%), threonine (16-25%) and Isoleucine(10-28%) were observed from masa samples. The biological value (81-93%), apparent digestibility (82-88%) and net protein utilization (74-79%) of all masa samples showed improved nutritional qualities. Supplementedmasa was nutritionally better than masa made from millet or rice alone.

Maize (dehulled) / rice (used directly).

↓

Wash and steep for twelve hours.

↓

Dry and mill (disc attrition mill)

↓

The ground maize / rice millet is sieved to produce flour and grits.

↓

The grifts are added to the boiling water and cooked to gelatinization and allowed to cool before mixing with raw flour in the ratio of 1:4.

↓

The resulting batter is inoculated with baker's yeast and allowed to ferment overnight.

↓

Salt and sugar are added to the inoculums.

↓

The fairly thick batter is then diluted with 5% potash solution and the batter is stirred.

↓

The batter is fried in a cup-like depression in which oil has been added to masa.

Figure 5. Process flow chart for the production of masa.

c. Pito

Pito is the traditional beverage drink of the Benins in the Mid- West part of Nigeria. It is however popularly consumed throughout Nigeria owing to its refreshing nature and low price. Pito is also widely consumed in Ghana. The preparation of pito involves soaking the cereal grains (maize, sorghum, or combinations of both) in water for two days, followed by malting and allowing them to sit for five days in basket lined with moistened banana leaves. The malted grains are ground mixed with water and boiled. The resulting mash is allowed to cool and later filtered through a fine mash, allowed to cool and later filtered through a fine mesh basket. The filterate thus obtained is allowed to stand overnight or until it assumes a slightly sour flavour, following which it is boiled to concentrate.

A starter from the previous brew is added to the cool concentrate which is again allowed to ferment overnight. Pito, the product obtained thus is dark brown liquid which varies in taste from sweat to bitter. It contains lactic acid, sugars and amino acids and has an alcoholic content of about 3%. Organisms responsible for souring include *Geotricum candidum, and Lactobacillus species,* while *Candida species* are responsible for the alcoholic fermentation.

Maize grains are soaked for 2 days.

↓

Malt (germinate) for five days and grind.

↓

Mix mash with cold water and boil for twelve hours.

↓

Filter and cool.

↓

Ferment overnight (mixed natural inoculum).

↓

Cool concentrate and add starter (sediment from previous brew).

↓

Ferment for twelve to twenty four hours.

↓

Pito.

Figure 6. Process flowchart for production of pito.

d. Burukutu

This is a popular alcoholic beverage of vinegar-like flavour, consumed in Northern Guinea Savannah region of Nigeria, in the republic of Benin and Ghana. The preparation of burukutu involves steeping sorghum grains in water overnight, following which excess water drained. The grains are then spread out onto a mat or tray, covered with banana leave and allowed to germinate. During the germination processes, the grains were watered on alternate days and turned over at intervals. Germination continues for four to five days until the plumule attain a certain length. The malted grains are spread out in the sun to dry for one to two days, following which the dried malt is ground to powder. Garri (a farinaecious fermented cassava product) is added to the mixture of the ground malt and six parts water. The resulting mixture is allowed to ferment for two days, following which it is boiled for two days. The resulting product is cloudy alcoholic beverage.

The pH of the fermenting mixture decreases from about 6.4 to 4.2 within 24 hours of fermentation and decreases further to 3.7 after 48 hours. At the termination of the 2-days maturing period, *Acetobacter species and Candida species* are dominant microorganisms. Boiling prior to maturation eliminates lactic acids and other yeast. Fully matured burukutu beer has an acetic acid content which varies between 0.4 to 0.6%.

Maize and sorghum.

↓

Soak for two days

↓

Malt(germinate) for five days.

↓

Grind or sun- dry and hold until used.

↓

Adjunct (gari) is added.

↓

Mix mash with cold water and boil for six to twelve hours

↓

Filter through a fine marsh.

↓

Cool filter.

↓

Ferment overnight (mixed natural inoculum).

↓

Boil for twelve hours.

↓

Cool concentrate and add starter (sediment from previous brew).

↓

Ferment for twelve to twenty four hours.

↓

Burukutu

Figure 7. Process flowchart for production of burukutu.

e. Kunun-zaki.

Kunun-zaki is a non-alcoholic fermented beverage widely consumed in Northern part of Nigeria. This beverage is however becoming more widely consumed in southern Nigeria,owing to its refreshing qualities. Kunun-zaki is consumed anytime of the day by both adult and children as breakfast drink, food supplement. It is a refreshing drink usually used to entertain visitors, appetizers and is commonly used / served at social gathering. Although, there are various types of kunun processed and consumed in Nigeria which include; kunun-zaki, kunun-gyada, kunun-jiko, and amshau and kunun-gayamba. However, kunun-zaki is mostely consumed. The traditional process for the manufacture of kunun-zaki involves the steeping of millet grains, wet milling with spices (ginger, cloves and pepper) ,wet sieving and partial gelatinization of the slurry, followed by the addition of sugar and bottling.

The fermentation which occurs briefly during steeping of the grains in water for 8 to 48 hours period involves mainly lactic acid bacteria and yeast. Storage studies revealed that the product has a shelf-life of about 24hours at ambient temperature, which was extended to 8 days by pasteurization at 60 °C for 1 hour and stored under refrigeration conditions.

Cereal (millet)

↓

Cleaning and washing.

↓

Steep in water.

↓

Draining.

↓

Spread on a layer of sack.

↓

Germinate for 3 to 4 days at 25 to 30 degrees centigrade with intermittent sprinkling of water.

↓

Paste milling.

↓

Uncooked past + malted paste.

↓

Fermentation for appropriate time.

↓

Sieve using cheese cloth.

↓

Kunun-zaki.

Figure 8. Flowchart for the traditional processes of kunun-zaki.

4. Fruits and vegetables

a. Ogiri

This is a condiments gotten from the fermentation of castor oil seeds. The raw castor oil seed are boiled for two hours until the seed changes colour to brown. The seeds are dehaulled, rinsed in clean water. The boiled seeds are boiled again for one more hour. It is then cooled and wrapped with enough banana leaves, which is then packed in a clean container with cover to ferment at room temperature.

Castor oil seed.
↓
Boil for two to three hours.
↓
Dehaul
↓
Rinse in clean water.
↓
Boil for one hour.
↓
Allow to cool.
↓
Wrap with enough banana leaves.
↓
Pack in clean containers, ferment for four days.
↓
Ogiri

Figure 9. Flow chart for the production of ogiri.

5. Legumes (locust-beans,african oil beans, soya beans) iru, dadawa ugba, afiyo, dangwua)

a. Dadawa/Iru

This is one of the most important food condiments in Nigeria and many countries of West and Central Africa. It is used in much the same way as bouillon cubes are used in the Western world as nutritious flavouring additives along with cereal grains sauce and may serve as meat substitute. Dadawa (Iru) is prepared from the seeds of African locust beans, thus are rich in fat (39 to 40%) and protein (31 to 40%) (Achi, 2005) and contributes significantly to the energy intake, protein and vitamins, especially riboflavin, in many countries of West and Central Africa. Dadawa or iru is made from locust-bean (*Parkia biglobosa*) seed, a leguminous tree found in the Savannah region of Africa, Southeast Asia and South America. Dadawa is produced by a natural un-inoculated solid –substrate fermentation of the boiled and dehaulled cotyledon, the major fermenting organisms are the *Bacillus* and *Staphylococcus*. The beans mass after fermentation is sun-dried and moulded into round balls or flattened cakes. Due to the high protein content, it has a great potential as a key protein source and basic ingredient for food supplement.

Dadawa fermentation is very similar to that of okpehe prepared from the seeds of *Prosopis africana*, ogiri prepared from melon seeds (*Citrullus vulgaria*) and castor oil bean (*Ricinus cummunis*). Although, the organisms involved in the fermentation of these foods condiments and others have been identified, this has marginal effects as the industrial or commercial production is concerned. Traditionally fermentation of African locust beans involves boiling the beans for twelve hours in excess water, until they are very soft to allow for hand dehaulling after which the separated cotyledon is boiled for another two hours to soften it. The cotyledon is then wrapped with enough banana leaves (*Musa saplentum*) and packed with cover to ferment at room temperature.

African locust beans.

↓

Boil for two hours.

↓

Allow to cool.

↓

Dehaul

↓

Boil for another two hours.

↓

Spread on a sack bag to cool.

↓

Wrap with enough banana leaves.

↓

Pack in a clean container, ferment for five days in warm place.

↓

Dadawa

Figure 10. A Flow chart for the production processes of dadawa.

Other biochemical changes that occur during dadawa fermentation include the hydrolysis of indigestible oligosaccharide present in African locust beans notably stachyose and raffinose, to simple sugars by alpha and beta galactosidase, the synthesis of B-vitamins (thiamin and riboflavin),vitamin C and the reduction of anti-nutritional factors(oxalates and phytates). An improved process for industrial production of dadawa involves dehaulling African locust bean with ball(disc) mill, cooking in a pressure retort for one hour inoculating with *Bacillus subtilis* culture, drying the fermented beans and milling into a powder. Cadbury Nigeria Plc. In 1991 introduced cubed dadawa but it failed to make the desired market impact and it is withdrawn. It would appear that consumers preferred the granular product to the cubed product.

b. Ugba

Fermented African Oil bean seed, (*Panthaclethra macrophylla benth*) *Ugba,* is an indigenous fermented food and a popular staple among the eastern part of Nigeria. It is rich in protein and other minerals and is obtained by solid-state fermentation of the African Oil bean seed.

It is gotten traditionally from the fermentation of oil bean seed. It contains up to 44% protein, which comprise of at least 17 of the 20 amino and protein digestibility and utilization increases with fermentation (Okechukwu *et al*, 2012). The oil bean seeds are boiled for three hours, dehaulled and cooked, the cooked seeds are then sliced (0.5 to 1mm thickness) and boiled again for two hours, drained, rinsed thrice in water and steeped in cold water for four hours so as to eliminate the bitter taste. The sliced beans are wrapped with enough banana leaves (*Musca sapientum*), packed in a clean container and covered to ferment at room temperature.

African oil bean seed.

↓

Allow to cool.

↓

Dehaull the seeds.

↓

Discard seed coats.

↓

Slice the cotyledon.

↓

Boil for two hours.

↓

Drain and rinse thrice with water.

↓

Steep in water for four hours.

↓

Drain

↓

Wrap with enough banana leaves.

↓

Pack in a clean container and ferment for three or four days in warm place(30 degrees).

↓

Ugba

Figure 11. A flow chart for the production process of ugba.

c. Afiyo (Okpehe)

Afiyo as is called by the Hausas or Okpehe as known by the Idomas in Benue state is a fermented food flavouring condiment most popular in the middle belt of Nigeria. It is produced from *Prosopis Africana,* which is a leguminous oil seed, fermented in most part of Benue, Niger, Kaduna states and northern parts of Kwara state. This fermented product of *Prosopis Africa* is a strong smelling mash of sticky browned seed and fermentation is moist solid state by chance inoculation, supposedly by various species of micro-organisms.

Various fermented foods have been recorded and these are highly placed condiments while some serve as main meals. Of the thousands of legumes, less than twenty are used extensively in use. Those in common use include peanuts, soy beans, locust beans, oil beans, cowpea and lentils etc.

Prosopis Africana seeds.

↓

Boil for one to two days (on a kerosene stove)

↓

Dehaull by pressing with fingertips or pounding in the mortar with a pestle

↓

Wash seed coats removed

↓

Wrap Cotyledon with pawpaw leaves traditionally

↓

Packwrapped cotyledon in nylon.

↓

Ferment for five to six days.

↓

Afiyo(okpehe)

Figure 12. Flow chart for the traditional preparation of okpehe.

Generally, the concentration of amino acids increases during the production of condiments (dadawa, ogiri, ugba) as the fermentation day increases, and it reaches a peak at day four, day three, and day two respectively. This progressive increase in concentration of amino acids in condiments is due to the decrease in total protein as fermentation progresses, which may be attributed to the effect of protease enzymes which result in the hydrolysis of protein molecules to small molecules such as amino acids, such protease activities in the fermenting oil seed increases digestibility than the seed.

Reducing sugar concentration increases with days of fermentation and reaches a peak at the day five, day four, day three for African locust bean, African oil bean seed and castor oil seed respectively. The increase in reducing sugar is due to the hydrolysis of carbohydrates in the presence of certain enzymes such as amylases and galactase. This phenomenon is expected since microbial amylase hydrolyses higher carbohydrates (polysaccharides and disaccharides) to reducing sugars which are then readily digestible by humans. Similarly, galactose softens the texture of the seeds and liberates sugar for digestion. The reduction in the amino acids and the reducing sugar concentration may be due to the presence of some micro-organism that feed on amino acids and reducing sugars.

6. Animal products (milk, meat) nono, cheese, kilishi

a. Nono

Nono is a fermented food drink derivatives gotten from cow milk. As a general practice among Fulani Herdsmen, the milking is done between the third and sixth months of lactation. Until the third month, the calves are left to consume milk. Cows are only milked at night and since no milking is possible during the day calves roam with the dam. Milk, if left untreated, spoils within a short time due to microbial activity; thus, processing of milk improves its storage and diversifies its use.

Traditionally, nono is prepared by inoculating freshly drawn cow milk with a little of the leftover as starter and then is allowed to ferment for twenty four hours at room temperature. During fermentation, some of the lactose is converted to the lactic acid. At the end of the fermentation period, the milk butter is removed by churning for further use and the remaining sour milk, nono is a delicious and refreshing beverage. Most of the organisms involved in the fermentation process are usually of three main groups; bacteria, yeast, and mould. Of these, *Lactobacilli* (*L. acidophilus and L.bulgaris*), *Lactococci species* (*L. cremoni, and L.lactis*), *Streptococcus thermophilus, Leuconostoc species and Saccharomyces species* seems to be the most prominent, each giving the product a characteristic flavour.

Nono has yoghurt-like taste (sharp acid taste), and is therefore usually taken with sugar, and fura which is made up of millet flour compressed in balls and cooked for about twenty to forty minutes. The cooked fura is crumbled in a bowl of nono (now called fura de nunu). Nono is an excellent source of protein, rich in essential amino acids and a good source of calcium, phosphorus and vitamin A, B, C, E and B complex. However, like other milk products, it is poor in ascorbic acid and iron. Wives of pastorialist usually process fresh milk into various traditional milk product. These include nono, (sour milk), kindirimo (sour yoghurt), maishanu (local butter), cuku (Fulani cheese) and wara (Yoruba cheese). These products are usually hawked around the local markets in certain towns. These products are usually only available within the walking distance of Fulani settlement. For the same reason, these products are also more readily available in the northern states of the country.

b. Production of kilishi and other processed meats of interest.

Suya (esire or balangu), banda (kundi) and kilishi are the most important traditional processed meats in Nigeria and other West African countries including Chad, Niger and Mali.

Banda is a salted, smoke-dried meat product made from chunks of cheap, low quality meat from various types of livestock including donkeys, horses, camel, buffallo and wild life. The meat chunk is pre-cooked before smoking/ kiln drying or sun-drying. The traditional smoking/ kiln for banda, usually an open top. Fifty-gallon of oil drum fitted with layers of wire mesh that hold the product, and fired from the bottom. Banda is a poor product, stone-hard and dark I and n colour. Unlike banda, suya, and kilishi are made by roasting, spiced, salted, slices,/ strips of meat (usually beef).

Kilishiis is different from suya in that a two stage sun-drying process proceeds to roasting. Consequently, kilishi has a low moisture content (6-14%) than suya (25-35%) and a longer shelf- life. A variety of spices and other dried ingredients are used in kilishi processing including ginger (*Zingiberofficnale*), chillies (*Capsicufrtescens*), melegueta pepper (*Aframomum melegueya*), onion (*Allium cepa*) and defatted peanut (*Arachis hypogea*), cake powder, kilishi consist of about 46% meat and 54% non-meat ingredients with defatted powder accounting for about 35% of the ingredients formulation. Other traditional processed meat products in Nigeria include ndariko and jirge.

The summary of micro organism associated with Nigerian fermented foods is shown in table 1

SUBSTRATE	MICROORGANISM	PRODUCT
Cassava	*Leuconostoc sp Geotrichum candidum Pseudomonas* sp. *Scolecotrichum graminisBacteriodes* sp. *Tallospora asperaActinomyces* sp. *Passalora bacilligera Corynebacterium* sp. *Varicosporium species Lactobacillus* sp. *Culicidospora gravida Diplococcium spicatum*	Gari
Yam	*Streptococcus* sp. *Articulospora inflate* *Lactobacillus* sp. *Aspergillus niger* *Listeria* sp. *Aspergillus rapens* *Aspergillus flavus* *Lemonniera aquatic*	Elubo-isu
African locust beans *Parkia filicoida*	*Lactobacillus* sp. *Rhizopus stolonifer Streptococcus* sp. *Aspergillus fumigatus Pediococcus* sp. *Triscelophorus monosporus Bacillus* sp., *Coryneform bacteria*	Iru
Castor seed *Ricinus communis*	*Bacillus* spp., *Pseudomonas* spp. *Micrococcuss* spp., *Streptococcus*	Ogiri-igbo
Fluted pumpkin seeds *Telferia ocidentalis*	*Bacillus* spp., *E. coli, Staphylococcus* Spp., *Pseudomonas*	Ogiri ugu

SUBSTRATE	MICROORGANISM	PRODUCT
African oil beans *Pentaclethra macrophylla*	*Bacillus subtilis, Staphylococcus* spp., *Micrococcus* spp., *Corynebacterium* spp.	Ugba / Ukpaka
Soya bean	*B. subtilis, B. Iicheniformis, B.megaterium,* *Staphylococcus epidermidis,* *Micrococcus* spp.	Okpiye/Okphehe
African yam beans *Stenophylis stenocarpa*	*Bacillius subtilis, B. licheniformis, B. pumilis,* *Staphylococcus* sp.	Owoh
Melon seed *Citrulus vulgaris*	*Bacillus subtilis, B. megateruim, B. firmus E.coli,. Proteus, Pediococcus,* *Alcaligenes* spp., *Pseudomonas aeruginosa*	Ogiri-egusi
Cereals: maize, sorghum, millet	*Saccharomyces cerevisiae,* *Lactobacillus spp., Fusarium spp.*	Ogi Agidi
Milk	*Lactobacillus spp.* *Lactococcus spp.* *Streptococcus spp.* *Pediococcus spp.* *Leuconostoc spp.* *Propionibacter spp.*	Wara (Nigerian cheese)
Grain flour	*Saccaromyces cerevisiae*	Bread
Cereals (Millet, sorghum, maize, rice)	*Lactobacillius plantarum,* *L. fermentum and Lactococcus lactis*	Kunun-zaki

Ijabadeniyi(2007), Achi (2005) Agarry, et.al.,(2010) Osho, et, al.,(2010)

Table 1. Role of fermented food in detoxification.

6.1. Mycotoxin detoxification

Food and feeds are often contaminated with a number of toxins either naturally or through infestation by micro-organisms such as moulds, bacteria and virus. Certain moulds often produce secondary toxic metabolites called mycotoxins. These include fumonisins, ochratoxins A, zearalenone and aflatoxins. Several methods are available for degrading toxins from contaminated food. For example, using alkaline ammonia treatment to remove mycotoxins from food. However, these methods are harsh to food as they involve the use of chemicals which are potentially harmful to health or may impair or reduce the nutritional value of foods. Cooking foods does not remove mycotoxins either as most of them are heat stable. Detoxification of mycotoxins in foods through LAB fermentation has been demonstrated over the years (Biernasiak et.al. 2006). Using LAB fermentation for detoxification is more advantageous in that it is a milder method, which preserve the nutritive value and flavour of de-contaminated food. In addition to this, LAB fermentation irreversibly degrades mycotoxins without leaving any toxic residues. The detoxifying effect is believed to be through toxin binding effect.

In mycotoxin detoxification, LAB fermentation has also been successfully used to detoxify cassava toxins (cyanogens) following fermentation of cassava food product. In addition to cyanogens detoxification, cassava fermentation contributes to the preservation and improvement of flavour and aroma of cassava ferment. Although cooking has been used as a method of cyanogens detoxification, it has a number of problems as it leaves residual cyanogens in processed cassava, which exist as glucosides, cyanohydrins or free cyanide which are equally toxic as their parent compounds in uncooked food.

In a review, Bankole and Adebanjo (2003), found that the level of aflatoxin B_1, B_2 and

G_1 were significantly higher in corn from the high incidence area for human hepatocellular carcinoma and the average daily intake of aflatoxin B1 from the high risk area was 184.1 g/kg aflatoxin. Udoh *et al* (2000) reported 33% of maize sample from ecological zones of Nigeria contaminated with aflatoxins.

Fermented maize (Ogi) is a staple cereal in Nigeria and it is a popular weaning food in most rural communities in Nigeria. Oluwafemi and Ikeowa (2005) have reported that in fermenting maize to ogi, aflatoxin B1 was reduced by about 50% after 72hours of fermentation. Maize as well as other Nigerian cereals are also important raw materials for both local and commercial beer brewing. Oluwafemi and Taiwo (2003) have shown that the role of *S. cerevisiae* in reducing the pH from 5.2 to 3.7 during fermentation is important in detoxifying aflatoxin B during beer fermentation.

6.2. Cyanide detoxification

Processing of cassava roots improves palatability, reduces or eliminates potential toxicity, transforms raw cassava into other preservable forms which are more beneficial to man. Fermentation is by far the most common method of processing the cassava crop in Africa (Okafor *et al.*, 1984). The rate of detoxification of cyanide by traditional fermentation is shown in figure 13. Fermentation is a very effective way for detoxification of cyanide in cassava with r^2 of 98%.

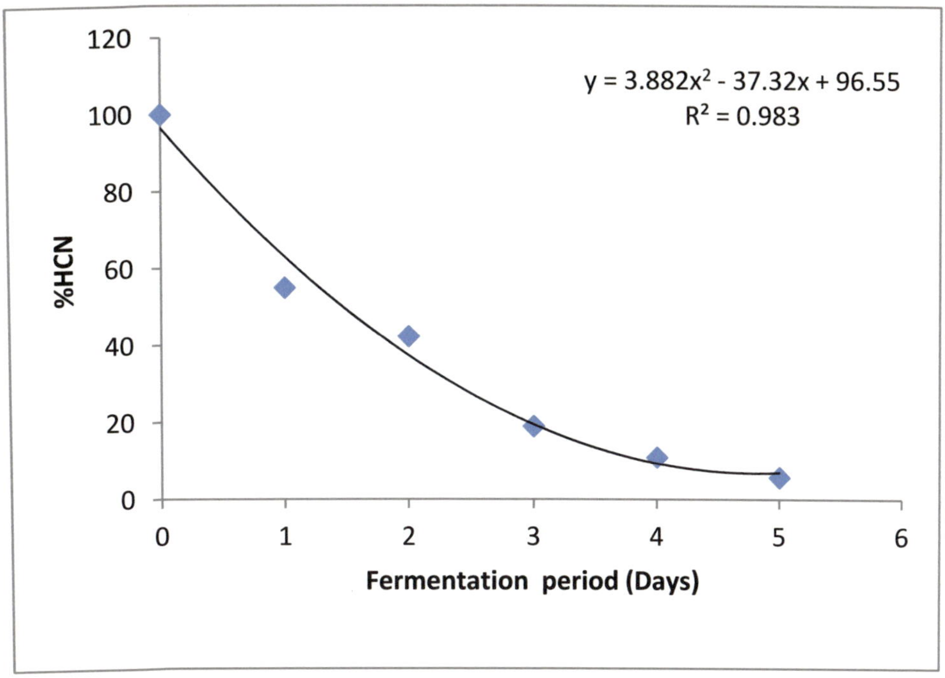

Figure 13. Effect of fermatation on %HCN.

6.3. Loop fermentation

Loop fermentation is achieved by using starter culture from already fermented product to inoculate a fresh barge of fermentation process. Ohenhen and Ikenebomeh (2007) have shown that that loop fermentation can prolong the shelf-life of ogi from about 40days, obtained by traditional fermentation method to well over 60days. We have observed in our laboratory that by using loop fermentation technique in gari processing, fermentation was completed in three days as against five days by the conventional traditional fermentation. Cyanide content also reduced to about 3% with loop fermentation. With a second loop (double loop) ie using products of a first loop fermentation to inoculate a fresh process, fermentation in gari production was completed in 2day with only about 2.6% cyanide remaining. The explanation is that the organisms are "trained" to better utilize the compounds in the fermenting substrate When the fermenting substrate in the double loop was acidified by squeezing some limes (citrus) juice into it before inoculating, cyanide content was 0% after 3days. The summary is shown in Fig. 14.

6.4. Detoxification of phytates, tannins and oxalates

The anti-nutrients including Phytates, tannins and oxalates interferes with mineral absorption and palatability of the cereals so detoxification is vital to enhance their nutrient value and organoleptic properties. Several detoxification methods are available, including decortication, malting, fermentation and alkali treatment (Osuntogun *et al.*, 1989; Banda-Nyirenda and Vohra, 1990). Yeast fermentationhas proved very effective in the detoxification of antinutrients. The table below summarizes the effectiveness of yeast in detoxification of different anti-nutrient.

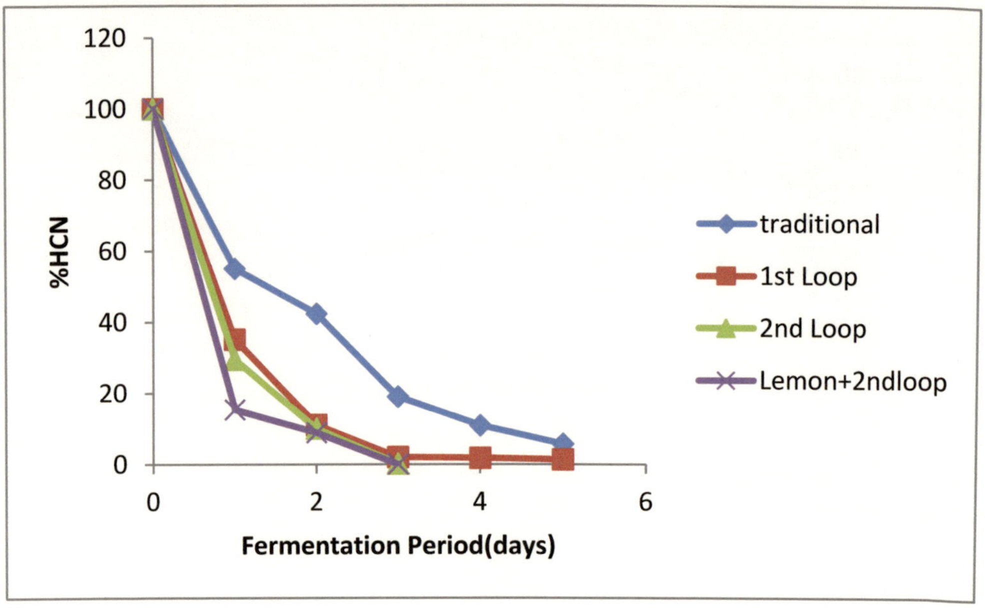

Figure 14. Effect of fermentation loop on Percentage residual HCN

Onyesom *et al*(2008) have also shown that fermentation of cassava to fufu with lemon grass reduces cyanide to less than 1% after 5days.

Phytic acid is well documented to block absorption of not only of phosphorus, but also other minerals such as calcium, magnesium, iron and zinc. It also negatively affects the absorption of lipids and protein. One reason this is true is because phytic acid also inhibits enzymes that are needed to digest foods such as pepsin (which helps break down protein), amylases (convert starch into sugar for digestion) and trypsin (also used in protein digestion). While whole grains have a much higher mineral content than processed grains, the full benefit of that nutrition is lost if phytic acid blocks the nutrients from being absorbed. It is well known that most cereals and legumes contain high levels of these ant-nutrients. It is also common knowledge that most of the Nigerian staples as in other developing countries constitute mainly cereals and legumes. It is therefore important that these foods staples are fermented as well as improve on the traditional fermentation techniques.

Activity	Yeast species	Effects
Biodegradation of phytate	*Saccharomyces cerevisiae, Saccharomyces kluyveri, Schwanniomyces castellii, Debaryomyces castellii, Arxula adeninivorans, Pichia anomala, Pichia rhodanensis, Pichia spartinae, Cryptococcus laurentii, Rhodotorula gracilis, Torulaspora delbrueckii, Kluyveromyces lactis Candida krusei (Issatchenkia orientalis) and Candida spp.*	Nutritional importance, i.e., bioavailability of divalent minerals such as iron, zink, calcium and magnesium
Folate biofortification	*S. cerevisiae Saccharomyces bayanus, Saccharomyces paradoxus, Saccharomyces pastorianus, Metschnikowia lochheadii, Debaryomyces melissophilus, Debaryomyces vanrijiae var. vanrijiae, Debaryomyces hansenii, Pichia philogaea, Kodamaea anthophila, Wickerhamiella lipophilia, Candida cleridarum and Candida drosophilae Candida milleri and T. delbrueckii Saccharomyces exiguous and Candida lambica P. anomala and Candida glabrata Kluyveromyces marxianus and C. krusei (I. orientalis)*	Prevention of neural tube defects in the foetus, megaloblastic anaemia and reduction of the risk for cardiovascular disease, cancer and Alzheimer's disease
Degradation of mycotoxins	*. cerevisiae spp Phaffia rhodozyma and Xanthophyllomyces dendrorhous*	Antitoxic in some degree

Moslehi-Jenabian, *et al.*, 2010

Table 2. Overview of yeasts activities in degradation of anti-nutrients.

7. Conclusion

Developing countries like Nigeria require food processing technologies that are appropriate, suitable for tropical regions and affordable to rural and urban economies. Fermentation techniques are one of such technologies that have been developed indigenously for a wide range of food products. These include root crops, cereals, legumes, fruit and vegetables, dairy, fish and meat. As a unit operation in food processing, fermentation offers various advantages, including, improved food safety, improved nutritional values, enhance flavour and acceptability, reduction in anti-nutrients, detoxification of toxigenic compounds, enhanced shelf-life and improved functional properties.

The present review has shown that Nigerian fermented food and food products can be developed into medium or large scale level for standard commercial products. However, there is the need to further optimize the processes.

Author details

Evans C. Egwim, Amanabo Musa, Yahaya Abubakar and Bello Mainuna
Biochemistry Department, Federal University of Technology, Minna, Niger State, Nigeria

8. References

Achi, A.O(2005) Traditional fermented protein condiments in Nigeria. *African Journal of Biotechnology Vol. 4 (13), pp. 1612-1621*

Adebolu, T. T., Olodun, A. O. and Ihunweze, B. C. (2007). Evaluation of *ogi* liquor from different grains for antibacterial activities against some common pathogens. *Afr. J. Biotech.* 6 (9): 1140-1143.

Agarry , O. O. I. Nkama and O. Akoma (2010) Production of Kunun-zaki (A Nigerian fermented cereal beverage) using starter culture. *International Research Journal of Microbiology Vol. 1(2) pp. 018-025*

Agbor-Egbe T, Lape Mbome I. (2006) The effects of processing techniques in reducing cyanogen levels during the production of some Cameroonian cassava foods. *Journal of Food Composition and Analysis; 19: 354-363.*

Banda-Nyirenda, D.B.C. and Vohra, P. (1990).Nutritional improvement of tannin containing sorghums (Sorghum bicolor) by sodium bicarbonate. *Cereal Chem. 67: 533-537.*

Bankole, S.A., Adebanjo, A. (2003). Aflatoxin contamination of dried yam chips marketed in *Nigeria.Tropical Science* 43 (3-4).

Biernasiak, J. Piotrowska M and Libudzisz Z(2006) Detoxification of mycotoxins by probiotic preparation for broiler chickens. Mycotoxin Research 22,(4)*: 230-235.*

Cadieux, P., Burton, J, and Kang, C. Y., (2002). *Lactobacillus* strains and vaginal ecology. *JAMA;* 287:1940-1941.

Chamberlain, G., J. Husnik and R.E. Subden. (1997). Freeze-desiccation survival in wild yeasts in the bloom of icewine grapes. *Canadian Instituteof Food Science and Technology Journal* 30, 435-439.

Chung Shil Kwak, Mee Sook Lee, Se In Oh, and Sang Chul Park (2010) Discovery of Novel Sources of Vitamin B_{12} in Traditional Korean Foods from Nutritional Surveys of *Centenarians* Curr Gerontol Geriatr Res. 2010; *2010: 374897.*

Ijabadeniyi, A.O(2007) Microbiological safety of gari, lafun and ogiri in Akure metropolis, Nigeria. *African Journal of Biotechnology Vol. 6 (22), pp. 2633-2635.*

Katz, S.E.(2003). *Wild Fermentation: The Flavor, Nutrition, and Craft of Live-Culture Foods.* White River Junction, VT.: Chelsea Green Publishing Company.

Moslehi-Jenabian,S; Pedersen,LL and Jespersen,L(2010) Beneficial Effects of Probiotic and Food Borne Yeasts on Human Health. *Nutrients, 2, 449-473.*

Ohenhen RE, Ikenemoh MJ(2007) shelf stability and Enzyme Activity Studies of Ogi: A corn meal fermented product. *J. Am. Sci. 3(1): 38-42.*

Okafor, N., B. Lioma and C. Oylu, (1984). Studies on the microbiology of cassava retting for "foo-foo"production. *J. Appl. Bacteriol., 56: 1-13.*

Okechukwu R. I, Ewelike N,Ukaoma A. A, Emejulu A. A4, And Azuwike C. O (2012). Changes in the nutrient composition of the African oil bean meal "ugba" (*Pentaclethre macrophylla* Benth) subjected to solid state natural fermentation. Journal of Applied Biosciences 51: 3591– 3595

Oluwafemi, F. and Ikeowa, M.C.(2005) Fate of Aflatoxin B1 During Fermentation of Maize into "Ogi" Nigerian *Food Journal, Vol. 23(www.ajol.info/journals/nifoj)*

Oluwafemi, F., and Taiwo, V. O(2003)Reversal of toxigenic effects of aflatoxin B1 on cockerels by alcoholic extract of African nutmeg *Monodora myristica. J. Sci. Food Agric* 84: 333-340. .

Onyesom I,. Okoh P.N and O.V. Okpokunu(2008) Levels of Cyanide in Cassava Fermented with Lemon Grass (*Cymbopogon citratus*) and the Organoleptic Assessment of its Food Products. *World Applied Sciences Journal 4 (6): 860-863.*

Osho A. Mabekoje O. O. and Bello O. O (2010) Comparative study on the microbial load of Gari, Elubo- isu and Iru in Nigeria. *African Journal of Food Science Vol. 4(10), pp. 646 – 649.*

Osuntogun, B.O., Adewusi, S.R.A., Ogundiwin, J.O. and Nwasike, C.C. (1989). Effect of cultivar, steeping, and malting on tannin, total polyphenol, and cyanide content of Nigerian sorghum. *Cereal Chem. 66: 87-89.*

Reid, G, Bruce, A. W., Fraser, N., Heinemann, C., Owen, J. and Henning, B. (2001b) Oral probiotics can resolve urogenital infections. *FEMS Immunol Med Microbiol;* 30:49-52.

Reid, G. (2002a) Probiotics for urogenital health. *Nutr. Clin. Care;* 5:3-8

Reid, G., Beuerman, D., Heinemann, C. and Bruce, A. W. (2001a). Probiotic Lactobacillus dose required to restore and maintain a normal vaginal flora. *FEMS Immunol Med Nlicrobiol;* 32:37-41.

Steinkraus, K. H., Ed. (1995). Handbook of Indigenous Fermented Foods. New York, Marcel Dekker, Inc., 776 pp.

Udoh, J.M; Cardwell, K.F; and Ikotun, T.(2000). Storage structure and aflatoxin content of maize in five agroecological zones of Nigeria, *J. Stored Prod. Res* 36: 187-201.

Chapter 8

Control of Toxigenic Fungi and Mycotoxins with Phytochemicals: Potentials and Challenges

Toba Samuel Anjorin, Ezekiel Adebayo Salako and Hussaini Anthony Makun

Additional information is available at the end of the chapter

http://dx.doi.org/10.5772/53477

1. Introduction

Mycotoxin-producing fungi are significant contaminant and destroyers of agricultural products and seeds in the field, during storage, during processing and in the markets, and reduce their nutritive value (Jimoh and Kolapo, 2008). Mycotoxin contamination in foods and feedstuffs poses serious health hazard to animals and humans (Mokhles *et al.*, 2007; Iheshiulor *et al.*, 2011). Mycotoxins are commonly produced by species of *Aspergillus, Penicillium* and *Fusarium* (Chandra and Sarbhoy, 1997; Masheshwar *et al.*, 2009). Several strategies are used at controlling fungal growth and the mycotoxin biosynthesis in seeds, grains and feedstuff by chemical treatments, and food preservatives, by physical and biological methods. These methods often require sophisticated equipment and expensive chemicals or reagents. Chemical control of fungi and mycotoxins also result in environmental pollution, health hazard and affects the natural ecological balance Yassin *et al.*, 2011). Use of plant products inform of plant extracts and essential oils provides an opportunity to avoiding synthetic chemical preservatives and fungicide risks (Mohammed *et al.*, 2012).

Phytochemicals, a term given to naturally occurring, non-nutritive biologically active chemical compounds of plant origin, have some protective or disease-preventive properties. Some phytochemicals are injurious to fungi and could be used to protect crops, animals, humans, food and feeds against toxigenic fungi and mycotoxin (OMAF, 2004). Phytofungicides could be prepared or formulated from the leaves, seeds, stem bark or roots of plants of pesticidal significance and could be applied inform of extract, powders and cakes or as plant exudates (Owino and Wando, 1992; Anjorin and Salako, 2009). Phytochemicals vary in plants depending on their growing conditions, varietal differences, age at harvest, extraction methods, storage conditions and age of sample. The use of plant derivatives for fungal control is common in developing countries before the advent of synthetic fungicides and due to relatively cost implication of imported fungicides (Galvano *et al.*, 2001). Over the years, efforts have been devoted to the search for new antifungal materials from natural sources for food preservation (Juglal *et al.*, 2002; Onyeagba *et al.*, 2004; Boyraz and Ozcan, 2005). Several edible botanical extracts have been reported to have antifungal activity (Ferhout *et al.*, 1999; Pradeep *et al.*, 2003). The essential oils extracted from clove have been shown to possess significant antifungal properties. Afzal *et al.*, (2010) reported that *A. sativum* has a wide antifungal spectrum, reached about 60-82% inhibition in the growth of seed borne *Aspergillus* and *Penicillium* fungi. This was attributed to phytochemical properties of garlic plant, allicin which could decompose into several effective antimicrobial compounds such as diallyl sulphide, diallyl disulphide, diallyl trisulphide, allyl methyl trisulphide, dithiins and ajoene (Salim 2011; Tagoe, 2011).

In recent years, the need to develop fungal disease control measures using phytochemicals as alternative to synthetic chemicals has become a priority of scientists worldwide (Reddy *et al.*, 2007). Therefore, it is important to find a practical, cost effective and non-toxic method to prevent fungal contamination and mycotoxins load in stored farm produce. Use of natural plant extracts and biocontrol agents provides an opportunity to avoid chemical preservatives. A multitude of fungitoxic plant compounds (often of unreliable purity) is readily available in the fields. Today, there are strict regulations on chemical pesticide use, and there is political pressure to remove the most hazardous chemicals from the market (Pal and Gardener, 2006). However, in order to protect food quality and the environment, low persistent synthetic fungicides are still relevant at present to prevent diseases of food crops. The search for an alternative or a complement to synthetic fungicide is justified. This paper reviewed the potential of botanicals in the control of toxigenic fungi and mycotoxin, constraints in their formulation and usage or in their proper formulation. Ascertaining the quality of fungitoxic phytochemicals during the production, registration, marketing and their usage is very important.

2. Why the use of phytofungicides?

Vast fields in developing countries are blessed with abundant plants with fungicidal potential with preparation and application attracting lower capital investment than synthetic fungicides (Anjorin and Salako, 2009). Rotimi and Moens (2003) reported that botanical pesticides are locally renewable, user-friendly and environmentally safe. The knowledge and technology involved in using botanicals is embedded in folklores and tradition of the farmers (Anjorin and Salako, 2009). Among several control strategies, natural control appears to be the most promising approach for the control of mycotoxins such as aflatoxin in post-harvested crops. Though synthetic fungicides improve plant protection but most of them are hazardous to man. Health hazards from exposure to toxic chemicals and economic considerations make natural plant extracts ideal alternatives to protect food and feed from fungal contamination (Reddy *et al.*, 2007). Hence antimicrobial properties of some plant constituents are being exploited in protecting food, feed and seeds from storage moulds (Centeno *et al.*, 2010).

Antifungal action of plant extracts has great potential as they are easy to prepare and apply. Further, these are safe and effective in view of their systemic action and lack residual effect, easily biodegradable and exhibit stimulating effect on plant metabolism. Also, large number of earlier workers has reported antifungal properties of several plant species (Naganawa *et al.*, 1996; Kubo *et al.*, 1995). Efficacy of some plant phytochemicals against mycotoxin producing fungi suggests its possible use in minimizing the risk of mycotoxins as well as fungicides exposure. Varieties of secondary metabolites in plants are tannins, terpenoids, alkaloids, and flavonoids, which have been found *in vitro* to have fungitoxic properties (Table 1).

Common name	Scientific name	Compound	Class	Activity
Apple	*Malus sylvestris*	Phloretin	Flavonoid derivative	General[a]
Betel pepper	*Piper betel*	Catechols, eugenol	Essential oils	General
				Bacteria, fungi
Ceylon cinnamon	*Cinnamomum verum*	Essential oils, others	Terpenoids, tannins	General
Garlic	*Allium sativum*	Allicin, ajoene	Sulfoxide	General
Grapefruit peel	*Citrus paradise*		Terpenoid	Fungi
Green tea	*Camellia sinensis*	Catechin	Flavonoid	General
Lantana	*Lantana camara*	6,7-dimethylesculetin	alkaloid	General
Mesquite	*Prosopis juliflora*	Phenethylamine	alkaloid	General
Olive oil	*Olea europaea*	Hexanal	Aldehyde	General
Orange peel	*Citrus sinensis*	d-limonene	Terpenoid	Fungi
Peppermint	*Mentha piperita*	Menthol	Terpenoid	General
Periwinkle	*Vinca minor*	Reserpine	Alkaloid	General
Potato	*Solanum tuberosum*	Solanine		Bacteria, fungi
Snakeplant	*Rivea corymbosa*	Ergine		General
Thyme	*Thymus vulgaris*	Caffeic acid	Terpenoid	Viruses, bacteria, fungi
		Thymol	Phenolic alcohol	
		Tannins	Polyphenols	
			Flavones	
Physic nut	*Jatropha gossyphiifolia*	Curcin		General
Valerian	*Valeriana officinalis*	Essential oil	Terpenoid	General

Source: Cowan, 1999; "General" denotes activity against multiple types of microorganisms (e.g., bacteria, fungi, and protozoa)

Table 1. Plants and their phytochemicals containing antimicrobial activity

Antifungal action of plant extracts has great potential as they are easy to prepare and apply. Further, these are safe and effective in view of being systemic in their action and lack residual effect, easily biodegradable and exhibit stimulating effect on plant metabolism. Several authors have confirmed the antifungal properties of several plant parts and phytochemicals (Giridhar and Reddy, 1996; Benharref and Jana, 2006; Satish, 2007).

Plant fungicides have been reported to be safe to beneficial organisms such as pollinating insects, earthworms and to humans (Rotimi and Moens, 2002). Khalid *et al.* (2002) reported that their toxic effect is normally of an ephemeral nature disappearing within 14-21 days. Thus phytofungicides are environment-friendly. Due to very high and disproportionate monetary exchange rate, synthetic fungicides are now more expensive than they were before, thus making them unaffordable by most of the resource-poor farmers (Salako, 2002). Some synthetic fungicides such as methyl bromide are phytotoxic and often leave undesirable residues when applied on the growing crops (Anastasiah, 1997). Other deleterious effects include occupational hazards, mammalian toxicity and soil pollution. Thus, the search for an alternative or complement to synthetic fungicide is justified.

3. Toxigenic fungi and mycotoxin

Field and storage fungal contaminants of grains in Nigeria had previously been reported by Makun *et al.*, (2007) and in rice in India by Reddy *et al.*, (2004). They include *Alternaria alternata, Cladosporium cladosporioides, Curvularia* spp., *Phoma* spp., *Fusarium* spp., *Aspergillus flavus, Aspergillus niger, Aspergillus parasiticus, Aspergillus tamarii, Aspergillus nidulans, Aspergillus candidus* and *Penicillium* spp. Fungal deterioration of seeds, grains and feed stuff is a chronic problem in the developing countries field and storage system as most of them are in tropical hot and humid climate. The presence and growth of fungi may cause spoilage of food and its quality and quantity (Candlish *et al.*, 2001; Rasooli and Abyaneh, 2004).

Aspergilli are the most common fungal species that can produce mycotoxins in seeds, food and feedstuffs. Several outbreaks of mycotoxicoses diseases in humans and animals caused by various mycotoxins have been reported after the consumption of mycotoxin-contaminated food and feed (Reddy and Raghavender, 2007).

Mycotoxins occurring in food commodities are secondary metabolites of filamentous fungi, which can contaminate many types of food crops throughout the food chain (Reddy *et al.*, 2010). Fungal toxins of most concern are produced by species within the genera of *Aspergillus, Fusarium* and *Penicillium* that frequently occur in major food crops in the field and continue to contaminate them during storage, including cereals and oilseeds. Among these mycotoxins, aflatoxin B_1 (AFB_1), fumonisin B_1 (FB_1) and ochratoxin A (OTA) are the most toxic to mammals, causing a variety of toxic effects including hepatotoxicity, teratogenicity and mutagenicity, resulting in diseases such as toxic hepatitis, hemorrhage, oedema, immunosuppression, hepatic carcinoma, equine leukoencephalomalacia (LEM), esophageal cancer and kidney failure (IARC, 1993, Santos, Lopes, and Kosseki, 2001 Donmez-Altunta *et al.*, 2003; Negedu *et al.*, 2011) Aflatoxin B1 (AFB1) has been classified as a class 1 human carcinogen by the International Agency for Research on Cancer (IARC, 1993).

4. Control of mycotoxigenic fungi and mycotoxins with plant products

In this section, the potentials of using plant-derived products to reduce toxigenic fungi and mycotoxin contamination of foods with particular emphasis on aflatoxins, ochratoxins and fumonisins are discussed.

4.1. Control of aflatoxigenic fungi and aflatoxins with plant products

Aflatoxins refer to a group of four mycotoxins (B_1, B2, G_1 and G_2) produced primarily by two closely related fungi, *A. flavus* and *A. parasiticus*. Aflatoxin contamination of crops is a worldwide food safety concern. An inhibitory effect of neem extracts on biosynthesis of aflatoxins (groups B and G) in fungal mycelia was reported by Bhatnagar *et al.* (1990). More than 280 plant species have been investigated for their inhibitory effect on toxigenic *Aspergilli* and nearly 100 of these plants had some activity on growth or toxin production by fungi (Montes and Carvajal, 1998). Karapynar (1989) reported the inhibitory effect of crude extracts from mint, sage, bay, anise and ground red pepper on the growth of *A. parasiticus* NRRL 2999 and its aflatoxin production *in vitro*. Saxena and Mathela (1999) found antifungal activity of new compounds from *Nepeta leucophylla* and *N. clarkei* against *Aspergillus* sp. Mathela (1981) screened 12 terpenoids against growth of *Aspergillus* species and found thymol and carvacrol to be more active than nystatin and talsutin. In another study, aflatoxin production by *A. parasiticus* was suppressed depending on the concentration of the plant aqueous extract added to the culture media at the time of spore inoculation.

Aflatoxin production in fungal mycelia grown for 96 h in culture media containing 50% neem leaf and seed extracts was inhibited by 90 and 65%, respectively (Razzaghi-Abyaneh *et al.*, 2005). More recently Mondali *et al.* (2009) studied the efficacy of different extracts of neem leaf on seed borne fungi, *A. flavus*. In this study the growth of the fungus was inhibited significantly and controlled with both alcoholic and water extracts of all ages and of the concentrations used. Efficacy of various concentrations of four plant extracts prepared from garlic, neem leaf, ginger and onion bulb were studied on reduction of *A. flavus* on Mustard. They found that garlic extract is most effective followed by neem (Latif *et al.*, 2006). Recently, Srichana *et al.* (2009) studied the efficacy of betel leaf extract on growth of *A. flavus* and it was found that the extract at 10,000 ppm completely inhibited the growth of this fungus. Hema *et al.* (2009) evaluated some of the South Indian spices and herbs against *A. flavus* and other fungi. They found that *Psidium guajava* is more effective on all tested fungi. In an another study by Satish *et al.* (2007) aqueous extracts of fifty-two plants from different families were tested for their antifungal potential against eight important species of *Aspergillus*. Among 52, twelve extracts have recorded significant antifungal activity against one or the other *Aspergillus* species tested. Similarly Pundir and Jain (2010) studied the efficacy of 22 plant extracts against food associated fungi and found that clove and ginger are more effective than other plant extracts.

Awuah (1996) reported that the following plants *Occimum gratissimum, Cymbopogon citratus, Xylopia aethiopica, Monodera myristica, Sizygium aromaticum, Cinnamomum verum* and *Piper nigrum* are effective in inhibiting formation of non sorbic acid, a precursor in aflatoxin synthesis pathway. Leave powder of *Occimum* has been successfully used in inhibiting mould development on stored soybean for 9 months (Awuah, 1996). The powder extracts of *Cymbopogon citratus* inhibited the growth of fungi including toxigenic species such as *A. flavus* and *A. fumigatus* (Adegoke and Odesola, 1996). Awuah and Ellis (2002) reported the effective use of powders of leaves of *O. grattisimum* and cloves (*S. aromaticum)* combination with some packaging materials to protect groundnut kernels artificially inoculated with *A. parasiticus*. There have been a number of reports citing the inhibitory effects of onion extracts on *A. flavus* growth, with an ether extract of onions, thio-propanol-S-oxide, being demonstrated to inhibit growth (Fan and Chen 1999). Pepper extracts have been shown to reduce aflatoxin production in *A. parasiticus* IFO 30179 and *A. flavus* var *columnaris* S46 (Ito *et al.*, 1994). Large-scale application of different higher plant products like azadirachtin from *Azadirachta indica*, eugenol from *Syzygium aromaticum*, carvone from *Carum carvi* and allyl isothiocyanate from mustard and horseradish oil have attracted the attention of microbiologists to other plant chemicals for use as antimicrobials (Singh *et al.*, 2008). Such products from higher plants would most likely be biodegradable, renewable in nature and perhaps safer to human health (Varma and Dubey, 1999).

Plant products, especially essential oils, are recognized as one of the most promising groups of natural compounds for the development of safer antifungal agents (Varma and Dubey, 2001). Many reports are available on use of neem oil to control toxigenic fungi and their toxins. Plant essential oils from *Azadirachta indica* and *Morinda lucida* were found to inhibit the growth of a toxigenic *A. flavus* and significantly reduced aflatoxin synthesis in inoculated maize grains (Bankole *et al.*, 2006). Zeringue *et al.* (2001) observed the increase of 11-31% of dry mycelial mass along with a slight decrease (5-10%) in AFB_1 production in 5-day-old aflatoxigenic *Aspergillus* sp., submerged cultures containing either 0.5 or 1.0 mL Clarified Neem Oil (CNO) in 0.1%.

Clove oil and its major component, eugenol has been extensively used to control mycotoxigenic fungi and mycotoxins. On rice treated at 2.4 mg eugenol/g of grains, the inoculum of *A. flavus* failed to grow and thus AFB_1 biosynthesis on rice was prevented (Reddy *et al.*, 2007; Jham *et al.*, 2005; Faria *et al.*, 2006) reported antifungal activity of cinnamon bark oil against *A. flavus*. Juglal *et al.* (2002) studied the effectiveness of nine essential oils in controlling the growth of mycotoxin-producing mouslds and noted that clove, cinnamon and oregano were able to prevent the growth of *A. parasiticus* while clove (ground and essential oil) markedly reduced the aflatoxin synthesis in infected grains.. More recently, Kumar *et al.* (2010) studied the efficacy of *O. sanctum* essential oil (EO) and its major component, eugenol against the fungi causing biodeterioration of food stuffs during storage. *O. sanctum* and eugenol were found efficacious in checking growth of *A. flavus* and also inhibited the AFB_1 production completely at 0.2 and 0.1 $\mu g\ mL^{-1}$, respectively.

Apart from neem and clove oils, various plant essential oils have been used for reduction of mycotoxins. Recently, Singh *et al.* (2008) extracted essential oils from different parts of 12 plants belonging to eight angiospermic families and tested for activity against two toxigenic strains of *A. flavus*. The oil of the spice plant *Amomum subulatum* Roxb. (Fam. Zingiberaceae) was found effective against two strains of *A. flavus*, completely inhibiting their mycelial growth at 750 μg mL^{-1} and AFB_1 production at 500 μg mL^{-1}. The oil completely inhibited the mycelial growth at 100 μg mL^{-1} with significant reduction of AFB_1. From this plant extract they have identified 13 antifungal compounds. Thanaboripat *et al.* (2007) studied the effects of 16 essential oils from aromatic plants against mycelia growth of *A. flavus* IMI 242684. The results showed that the essential oil of white wood (*Melaleuca cajeputi*) gave the highest inhibition followed by the essential oils of cinnamon (*Cinnamomum cassia*) and lavender (*Lavandula officinalis*), respectively.

In addition lemon and orange oils (at concentrations of 0.05-2.0%) effected more than a 90% reduction in aflatoxin formation by *A. flavus* has been demonstrated (Hasan, 2005). Kumar *et al.* (2009) studied the efficacy of essential oil from *Mentha arvensis* L. to control storage moulds of Chickpea. The oil effectively reduced mycelial growth of *A. flavus*. During screening of essential oils for their antifungal activity against *A. flavus*, the essential oil of *Cymbopogon citratus* was found to exhibit fungitoxicity. In another extensive study, Tamil-Selvi *et al.* (2003) demonstrated that *A. flavus* growth and AFB_1 production were both inhibited by an essential oil containing mainly garcinol from the tropical shrub/tree *Garcinia indica* at 3000 ppm.

4.2. Control of ochratoxigenic fungi and ochratoxins with phytochemicals

This mycotoxin can contaminate agricultural products, including cereals, coffee, dried fruits, wine and pork. Ochratoxin A (OTA) is a nephrotoxic and carcinogenic mycotoxin produced by certain species of *Aspergillus* and *Penicillium* (Reddy *et al.*, 2010). Various studies have been conducted to reduce the ochratoxigenic fungi and ochratoxins contamination using plant extracts. The effect of *Azadirachta indica* (neem) extracts on mycelial growth, sporulation, morphology and OTA production by *P. verrucosum* and *P. brevicompactum* were studied by Mossini *et al.* (2009). In this study they observed that inhibition was mainly of fungal growth and not OTA production. The effects of four alkaloids on the biosynthesis of OTA and ochratoxin B (OTB) were examined on four OTA-producing Aspergilli: *A. auricomus*, *A. sclerotiorum* and two isolates of *A. alliaceus*. Piperine and piperlongumine, natural alkaloids of *Piper longum*, significantly inhibited OTA production at 0.001% (w/v) for all Aspergilli examined. The antitoxigenic potential of the spices was tested against OTA-producing strain of *A. ochraceus* Wilhelm. Clove completely inhibited the mycelial growth of the fungi *A. ochraceus*. Garlic and laurel completely inhibited the OTA production. Cinnamon and anis inhibited the synthesis of OTA starting from the concentration of 3% and mint starting from 4% (Bugno *et al.*, 2006). Reddy *et al.* (2010) reported the efficacy of certain plant extracts on mycelial growth of *A. ochraceus* and OTA biosynthesis.

Very few reports are available on effects of plant oils on growth of ochratoxigenic fungi and ochratoxin biosynthesis. Recently Mossini *et al.* (2009) conducted *in vitro* trials to evaluate the effect of *Azadirachta indica* (neem) oil on mycelial growth, sporulation, morphology and OTA production by *P. verrucosum* and *P. brevicompactum*. Oil extracts exhibited significant reduction of growth and sporulation of the fungi. No inhibition of OTA production was observed. Essential oils of 12 medicinal plants were tested for inhibitory activity against *A.*

ochraceus and OTA production. The oils of thyme and cinnamon completely inhibit all the test fungi and OTA at 3000 ppm (Soliman and Badea, 2002).

4.3. Control of fumonisin producing fungi and fumonisins with phytochemicals

Fungi of the genus *Fusarium* are widely found in plant debris and crop plants worldwide (Reddy *et al.*, 2010). Several species from this genus are economically relevant because, apart from their ability to infect and cause tissue destruction on important crops such as corn, wheat and other small grains on the field, they produce mycotoxins on the crops in the field and in storage grains (Makun *et al.*, 2010). Fumonisins are mycotoxins produced mainly by the fungi *F. verticillioides* and *F. proliferatum* (Dambolena *et al.*, 2010). Fumonisin B_1 (FB_1) is generally the most abundant member of the family of mycotoxins and is known to cause various animal and human diseases (Reddy *et al.*, 2007). Additionally, fumonisins are potent liver toxins in most animal species and are suspected human carcinogens (Bhat *et al.*, 2010). Very few scattered reports are available on control of *Fusarium* sp. and their mycotoxins using plant extracts. The *in vitro* efficacy of different plant extracts viz., *Azadiachta indica, Artemessia annua, Eucalyptus globules, O. sanctum* and *Rheum emodi* were tested to control *F. solani*. All plant extracts showed significant reduction of pathogen (Joseph *et al.*, 2008). Recently, Anjorin *et al.* (2008) reported the efficacy of neem extract on the control of *F. verticillioides* in Maize. In another study, Amin *et al.* (2009) reported the efficacy of garlic tablet against *Fusarium* sp., associated with cucumber and found that garlic tablet effectively inhibited all the fungi tested.

Several reports are available on use of plant essential oils against fumonisin producing fungi and fumonisins biosynthesis. Recently Sitara *et al.* (2008) evaluated essential oils extracted from the seeds of neem (*Azadirachta indica*), mustard (*Brassica campestris*), black cumin (*Nigella sativa*) and asafoetida (*Ferula assafoetida*) against seed borne fungi viz., *F. oxysporum, F. moniliforme, F. nivale, F. semitectum*. All the oils extracted except mustard, showed fungicidal activity of varying degree against test species. Kumar *et al.* (2007) extracted essential oil from the leaves of *Chenopodium ambrosioides* Linn. (Chenopodiaceae) and tested against the *F. oxysporum*. In another study, Jardim *et al.* (2008) reported antifungal activity of essential oil from the Brazilian epazote (*Chenopodium ambrosioides* L.) against postharvest deteriorating fungi *F. oxysporum* and *F. semitectum*. Growth of the fungi was completely inhibited at 0.3% concentration.

More recently Dambolena *et al.* (2010) investigated the constituents and the efficacy of essential oils of *O. basilicum* L. and *O. gratissimum* L. from different locations in Kenya against *F. verticillioides* infection and fumonisin production. All oils showed some inhibitory effects on growth of *F. verticillioides*. However, the extent of inhibition was widely dependent upon the composition and the concentration of oils. When maize was treated with *O. basilicum* oils, no effects were observed in the FB_1 biosynthesis but *O. gratissimum* essential oils were found to induce a significant inhibitory effect on FB1 production with respect to control. Fadohan *et al.* (2004) showed that *O. basilicum* essential oil of Benin possess significant inhibitory effect on growth of *F. verticillioides* and FB_1 production in corn. Juglal *et al.* (2002) reported spice oils of eugenol, cinnamon, oregano, mace, nutmeg, tumeric and aniseed displayed antifungal activity against *F. moniliforme* and 78% reductions in fumonisin B1 (FB1) formation by this fungus, when treated with 2 μL mL^{-1} clove oil.

The anti fungal effects of 75 different essential oils on *F. oxysporum* f. sp., *cicer* (FOC) were evaluated. The most active essential oils found were those of lemon grass, clove, cinnamon bark, cinnamon leaf, cassia, fennel, basil and evening primrose (Pawar and Thanker, 2007). The effect of cinnamon, clove, oregano, palmarosa and lemongrass oils on fumonisin B_1 (FB_1) accumulation by one isolate each of *F. verticillioides* and *F. proliferatum* in non-sterilised naturally contaminated maize grain at 0.995 and 0.950 a_w and at 20 and 30°C was evaluated. The concentration used was 500 mg kg^{-1} maize. Under these conditions it was shown that antimycotoxigenic ability only took place at the higher water availabilities and mostly at 20°C. Only cinnamon, lemongrass and palmarosa oils were somewhat effective. Moreover, it was suggested that competing mycoflora play an important role in FB_1 accumulation. It was concluded that the efficacy of essential oils in real substrates, such as cereals, may be much lower than in synthetic media; different essential oils may be found to be useful and at different concentrations. Their effectiveness is highly dependent on both abiotic and biotic factors involved (Marin *et al.*, 1998).

5. Challenges in the production and usage of fungicidal botanicals

The effective control by fungitoxic plant products in developing countries remains poor and seriously hampered by several factors including lack of proper legislative authority; shortage of trained personnel in natural pesticide regulatory procedures; lack of infrastructure, transportation, equipment and materials; lack of product and phyto pesticide residue analysis facilities and capabilities (Akunyili and Ivbijaro, 2006). However, the inadequate availability of raw materials, formulation of quality, potent products and their commercialization are among the constraints facing phytofungicides.

At the present time in most developing countries, research on product quality is uncoordinated, with quality research projects conducted in isolation and the results often not widely disseminated. Knowledge transfer from academia to industry and government, and information dissemination between industry members is quite limited. Fostering the development of a cohesive quality research network could make significant inroads in addressing this problem, and could generally assist in the successful execution of strategies to close quality research gaps (Anjorin, 2008).

There are relatively few standard commercialized botanical fungicides produced in developing countries despite several reports of *in vitro* fungicidal activities of several plant products. Only the resource-poor farmers are left with the usage of home-produced plant fungicides. Anjorin and Salako (2009) reported the following constraints faced by Nigerian farmers in the preparation and usage of home-produced plant fungicides:

- Collection and utilization of natural products seemed to be expensive in terms of time and labour.
- Crude and inadequate processing tools and implements such as grinding stone instead of a grinder or a blender thus making their preparation full of drudgery. However, 65%

of the farmers agreed that if sophisticated facilities are available, they might not be able to afford it.

- Scarcity of certain plant materials especially those that people compete for because of its efficacy such as *Erythrophleum suaveolens* or those that are of commercial value such as cashew nut.
- Low efficacy of most botanicals due to their brief persistence or short shelf-life as they are easily prone to microbial, thermal or photo degradation. This often leads to a repetitive or frequent application of these plant products for optimal efficacy. Thus many of the farmers indicated that if they have the cash, they would rather switch to synthetic products because of ease of handling and efficacy.
- Bulkiness of some botanical materials during collection, preparation and application, such as 10 kg of neem leaf powder required for amending 100 m^2 of tomato field per time. Thus up to 65% of farmers used plant materials exclusively as protectants of stored seeds because of the limited quantities needed while lower percentage of the farmers applied it only on small gardens not more than one-tenth of a hectare
- Washing away of extracts on foliage or leaching during rainfall which often warrant repetitive application thus increasing labour involvement. Thus addition of surfactants might be required.

These weaknesses of home-produced plant fungicides in developing countries necessitate an improvement so that natural fungicides could be standardized and commercialized. Some local pesticidal plants used by Nigerian farmers and their constraints are as shown in Table 2. Production of commercial phytofungicides is more sophisticated than the home-produced crude form. That might have been the reason why the patented natural fungicide is relatively scarce and expensive in the open-markets in developing countries. The standard procedure involved in phytofungicide production is the use of variety of solvents such as hexane, ethanol, pentane, methanol or ether singly or in a mixture for fractionating the components or extracting the active compounds in the fungicidal plants. Once the active ingredient has been extracted and purified, it has to be added to inert compounds to produce a fungicide product with a known stable plant pesticide concentration. During the process of isolating the active ingredients, it should be bioassay guided (McGuffin, 2001).

The structures of natural plant products are normally too complex, illusive and very expensive to pursue. The process of simplification and purification are often slow and cumbersome; may lead to loss of activity (Dayan *et al*., 1992). A standard of active ingredient from fungicidal plant is required for the registration of commercial fungicide and their subsequent use on a commercial scale. Most of these natural products should be subjected to rigorous mammalian toxicity testing as it is done to synthetic pesticide before it is confirmed safe to man. Nicotine has been reported to be highly toxic to man and pyrethrum and derris were toxic to fish and should not be used near water (Asogwa, 2009). The aqueous extract from Azadirachta indica leaf, neem oil from the kernel, neem cake have all been reported to cause infertility (e.g. by retarding spermatogenesis) in studies with male rats, mice, rabbits and guinea pigs. Oral administration of neem oil to female rats caused infertility or had abortive effect (Moravati, *et al*. 2008).

Name	Family	Local names	Parts used	Use	Constraints
1. Iron weed (*Blumea perotitiana)*	*Asteraceae*	Gw*: *Sinmisinmi* Ba: *Gbagbaje* Ha:*Tabataba*	Whole leaf Leaf powder	For seed dressing	Difficult to renew; scattered in the wild
2. Bush tea (*Hyptis suaveolens)*	*Lamiaceae*	Gw:*Basamsin* *Ba.:Adabwa* Ha:*Dadoya*	Whole leaf Leaf powder/ slurry	Fumigant in the farm produce store	Offensive odour produced
3. Ground star *weed (Mitracarpus villosus))*	*Rubiaceae*	Gw: *Jiji pampi* Ba: *Olugodotondo* Ha:*Gogamasu*	Leaf powder/ extract	Seed/tuber dressing at low concentration	Tiny leaves difficult to harvest
4. Lophira (*Lophira lanceolata)*	*Ochnaceae*	Gw: *Gbonrii* Ba: *Zhimya* Nu:*Gbetseti*	Leaf powder/ extract	Yam sett dressing	Difficult to processing because of the tough leaves
5. Neem (*Azadirachta indica)*	*Meliaceae*	Gw: *Sawaki* Ba: *Kunini*	Whole leaf/leaf power/extract	Used to protect foliage, seed/soil treatment	Seed collection laborious and bitter taste residue
6. Tobacco (*Nicotiana tabacum)*	*Solanaceae*	Gw: *Taba* Ba: *Taba*	Whole leaf/leaf power/extract	Seed /store treatment	Leaf has other competitive demand/market value.
7. Stinking cassia (*Senna alata)*	*Leguminosae: Caesalpinioidea*	Gw: *Wampin* Ba: *Kpe tesuusu*	Whole leaf/leaf power/extract	Store protectant	Low efficacy
8. Olax (*Olax subscorpiodea)*	*Leguminosae: Caesalpinioidea*	Gw: *Wazigege* Ba: *Ombolaawe* Ha:*Gwanonkurmi*	Leaf powder/ extract	Store pesticide	Not wide spread. Found beside stream/river or in the forest
9. Sodom apple (*Calotropis procera)*	*Asclepiadacea*	Gw: Kokekoke Ba: Obiyawae	Leaf extract	Seed treatment	Not easily available
10. Mushroom (*Amanita phaloides)*	*Amanitaceae*	Gw: Munu Ba: Tsatsigba Ha:Ganganzomo	Powder/ cap extract	Seed treatment	Cap not renewable; seasonal and sparsely distributed in the wild
11. Lippa (*Lippa multiflora)*	*Verbanaceae*	Gw: Minsin Ba: Bukamburu Ha:Agwantaaki	Leaf powder/ extract	Store protectant	Causes itching when it touches the skin.

* Gwa= Gwari languages; Ba= Bassa; Ha= Hausa

Table 2. Plant leaves locally used for crop protection and their constraints among Abuja, Nigerian farmers

It should be noted that despite the vast literature on the efficacy of plant material in controlling mycotoxigenic moulds in developing countries, there has not been any concerted effort on its commercial production for a large-scale use on farmers' field. Jaryum *et al.*, 2002 believed that botanicals are most suitable for seed protection than on the crop field or stored farm produce. They cited the complaints of farmers on the residual bitter taste on the grains treated with neem seed powder.

Udoh *et al.* (2000) were of the view that caution must be exercised in using plant materials to control mycotoxins, because some of these materials are natural media for *A. flavus* growth. Hell *et al.* (2000) found that the use of *Khaya senegalensis* bark to protect maize against insects increased the risk of aflatoxin development, and that even the farmers in Benin, West Africa were aware of the low efficiency of the indigenous products, but were being compelled to use them because of their inaccessibility to chemical products. Some toxigenic *A. flavus* have been found to grow and produce mycotoxins in herbal plants. Also *C. odorata*, which has been reported to be potent against insects, was found to be an excellent substrate for the growth of storage fungi (Efuntoye, 1996, 1999). This might be due to the fact that phytochemicals are prone to photo-, microbial- and thermal-degradation if not properly stored. For an effective control of toxigenic fungi and mycotoxins with the use of fungicidal botanicals, integrated approach by adoption of good agronomic/cultural practices is imperative. This is by reduction of insect pest, early harvesting, rapid drying of agricultural products to a safe low moisture content of about 15% and the use of improved storage structures. Other complementary methods of control could be by manually or electronically sorting out of physically damaged, discoloured and infected grains from the apparently healthy ones.

5.1. Demanding plant fungicide regulations in developing countries

The introduction and use of natural pesticides in developing countries require proper regulation. In Nigeria for instance, Section 1 of the Pesticide Registration Regulations Decree, 1996 prohibited the manufacture, formulation, import, export, advertisement, sale, and distribution of any pesticide, unless it has been registered in accordance with the provisions of these regulations. Included among the essential parts of the regulations are the following:

5.1.2. Issuance of certificate of registration

For a pesticide registration, the completed application form shall include the original certificate of analysis of the pesticide product. The form shall include product chemistry which shall state the product composition, normal concentration, physical and chemical characteristics as well as standard laboratory analytical methods for each active ingredient, and impurity or inert ingredient that is toxicologically significant (NAFDAC, 1996).

5.1.3. Reports required by the regulations agency

Other studies demanded include environmental fate (fate in air, soil, and water); mobility and distribution; persistence and bioaccumulation (half life and degradation); hazards to human or domestic animals; toxicity whether by oral, dermal, and or inhalation (acute toxicityor chronic toxicity) reproductive studies; effects on non-target flora and fauna, including birds and fishes; mutagenicity; product performance including efficacy trials in the country of usage. Other requirements include dosage and direction for use of the fungicidal natural pesticide; fields of application; and methods of application. The registration of any pesticide product shall be valid for a period of five years, thus it is subject to periodical renewal

5.1.4. *Default and penalty*

In the event of a default in compliance with the requirements of these regulations, the individual concerned may be prohibited from carrying on this business either absolutely or for a given period declared by National Agency for Food and Drug Administration and control (NAFDAC) in addition to a fine of one hundred thousand naira ($625.00).

6. Strategies for effective fungitoxic phytochemicals production and usage

In this section, some strategies for effective fungitoxic phytochemicals production and usages are discussed.

6.1. Fungicidal plant formulation and quality control

Several laboratories have found literally thousands of phytochemicals, which have inhibitory effects on most toxigenic fungus *in vitro* but have not been formulated for the protection of crops and animal produce against fungi and mycotoxin. The aspect of quality control of phytochemicals, which is practically low or non-existent in most developing countries, should be taken seriously. It would be advantageous to standardize methods of extraction, and *in vitro* testing so that the search could be more systematic and interpretation of results would be facilitated. The development and validation of relevant bioassays pose significant challenges in developing countries. There is necessity for validated biological assays with a demonstrated high correlation between *in vitro* activity and field efficacy in order to provide the most reliable laboratory measurement of product potency/ strength (Anjorin and Salako, 2009)

In the formulation of plant fungicide, biological activity and its efficacy should be stabilized and further enhanced by the addition of stabilizers, antioxidants and synergists. Certain additives could be added to increase the shelf-life and ease of handling. Sun screens such as para-amino benzoic acid (PABA) could be added to reduce the photoxidation of most active ingredient by ultra-violet light (Zubkoff, 1999). Also, as phytochemicals such as azadirachtin, the principal bioactive ingredient in neem, is heat sensitive and cold processing technology for neem seed would be needed. Dark-coloured, sterile containers with a lid are required to minimize photodegradation and microdegradation respectively.

6.2. Proper product labelling

Labeling of commercial phytofungicidal products and following label directions should be enforced in developing countries of the world just as it is being done in some developed countries. During the registration processes of botanicals, a label created should contain directions for proper use of the material labeling and package insert shall be informative, accurate and in *lingual franca* or in local language. Minimum requirements on a package label shall include name of product, brand name and common or chemical name of active ingredients, batch number, manufacture date, expiry date; precautions for storage and handling in transit; leaflet insert, giving full description for application and safe use, and pictograms. Many stores also sell whole dried plants, which have been found occasionally to be misidentified, with potentially disastrous consequences. The new rules, issued in late 1997, require products to be labeled as a botanical fungicide and carry a "fungitoxicity facts" panel with information similar to the "synthetic pesticides" panels appearing on the formulated botanical product. The rules also require that products containing botanical ingredients specify the part of the plant used (Food and Drug Admnistration (1997). This is not often done in the markets in the developing countries.

6.3. Phytochemical application techniques

Home-produced plant fungicide should be timely applied, not in a bright sunlight. Otherwise, it should also be stored appropriately. Also, improved methods of application such as mechanical mixers for uniform and bulk coating of oil on grain should be adopted. The use of slow release dispensers/sachets which could be placed at different depths in storage structures, bins or bags, could be devised for ensuring and enhancing efficacy.

The active life and efficacy of natural products in the soil is determined by factors such as soil temperature and structure, water stress, microbial action, and fertilizer applied (Breland, 1996). Combination of two or more plant parts or species could make the plant fungicides to have broad spectrum. Anjorin, *et al.* (2008) reported that combination of two plant extracts proved more effective and could reduce the risk of resistance developing by the target fungi.

6.4. Identification of phytofungitoxic plant species

Plant species and botanical characterization is very important for the sake of quality control. Proper identification of fungicidal botanicals can be achieved by using morphological differences or anatomic microscopy to show the difference between any two plants at the time of cultivation while collecting the plant material.

There should be botanical monographs that provide specific tests for identity - usually at least three tests per botanical: macroscopic identity, microscopic identity and chromatography. The personnel making the identifications of botanicals must have recognized expertise and the procedures must be stringent, with sufficient safeguards to discourage and detect falsification. Moreover, the required reference standards encompass pure chemicals, authenticated herbarium voucher specimens, raw and powdered herb samples, and prepared microscopy slides. An electronic inventory of herbal pesticide reference materials should be created. Reference texts are also indispensable resources (Jackson and Snowdon, 1990).

The main disadvantage of organoleptics and microscopy is that a significant investment in human resources is required to train personnel. Also problems associated with the selection and use of fungitoxic material standards is instability, special handling or storage requirements and shelf life (Flaster and Lassiter, 2001). Recombinant DNA analysis and gene chip technology are superior methods of identification. DNA methods for species characterization and adulterant detection have been published (Wolf *et al.*, 1999).

6.5. Collection of information

There should be databases which can supply information about plants with fungitoxic potential in each ecological zone. An example is the Grainge and Ahmed Handbook of Plants with Pest-Control Properties (1988). A database has been developed in National Pharmaceutical Institute, Idu, Abuja, Nigeria and in Zimbabwe (Elwell, pers. comm.) which could provide a valuable source for their respective region. Linking the information obtained from the database to the knowledge of the indigenous flora could draw rings on the most promising plants which deserve further studies. Important aspects to consider are not only fungitoxic properties of the plants but also their proper identification, distribution, abundance and easiness to be propagated. Cooperation with botanists at the National Herbaria and Universities would facilitate the work.

7. Summary

The potentials and constraints in controlling mycotoxigenic fungi and mycotoxins in developing countries with phytochemicals were looked into in this chapter. It was indicated from this review that natural fungicides application would result in more efficient control of toxigenic fungi and may lead to reduction of mycotoxins in the stored products. Vast fields in developing countries are blessed with abundant plants with fungicidal potential with local preparation and application attracting lower capital investment than synthetic fungicides. Plants are rich in a wide variety of secondary metabolites, such as tannins, terpenoids, alkaloids, and flavonoids, which have been found *in vitro* to have antimycotic and antimycotoxin properties. However, there are several challenges involved. These include the low fungitoxic efficacy of several phytochemicals, some are hazardous to beneficial non-target organisms and humans; while few could even support the growth of pathogens including fungi. In view of the constraints involved in the preparation and application of these botanicals and in order to enhance their efficacy, there is a need for standardizing the production, formulation, commercialization and application of these fungitoxic phytochemicals commonly used in developing countries.

8. Conclusion

The development of fungitoxic botanicals in developing countries is rather slow or it often terminates in the laboratory, in the experimental fields or locally used by rural farmers. There is yet very few or no locally produced quality marketable phytofungicide in developing countries. This situation is unsatisfactory thus commercial production of phytofungicide is strongly advocated. More research on toxigenic fungi control with natural products should be undertaken; provision of appropriate proc essing facilities and some of the marketing strategies for the products should be carefully planned. Also protocols on production of fungitoxic compounds for large scale production should be developed. Communication between researchers and extension organization should be intensified. Through this, phytofungicide research can be directed at farmers need and the knowledge concerning their use will be provided. Both vertical and horizontal information exchange on plant pesticide related issues should be intensified at local, national and international level. This is to confirm, collaborate and upgrade technical innovations toward commercializing phytofungicide as it has been in Ghana and India. Plant fungicide production could be sequentially integrated into a sustainable crop protection system in the developing countries. Integrated Disease Management strategy of prevention and control of toxigenic fungi and mycotoxins should be considered.

An ideal fungitoxic plant is expected not to compete with crop land, not act as weeds, not support crop pests and the products from it should be easily prepared. It is recommended that reliable toxigenic fungi and mycotoxin control methods that are attractive and safe should be developed. With a time perspective of four stages the following recommendations are given:

- to compile information on plants with potential fungi and mycotoxin control properties, to identify crops and target fungi and mycotoxin and to formulate projects in developing countries;
- to concentrate on some promising fungitoxic plants, including different aspects, to establish work groups focusing on one or a few plants with a key-person as a coordinator and advisor, to carry out comparative studies with emphasis on the mechanisms;
- to publish and to organize a workshop where new findings are presented and the methods are critically analysed in relation to the feedback from farmers
- and to produce extension material on fungicidal phytochemicals preferably in the form of leaflets, one for each plant, to organize workshops at the village level.

Research priorities on fungicidal plants such as investigation of the taxonomic status and agronomy of existing plants with fungicidal potentials, and initiation of a selection/breeding programme with multilocation testing of promising provenances is necessary. The use of modern genetic and molecular techniques such as cell culture, genetic engineering and biotechnology in boosting active ingredients should be considered. This could be by employing recombinant DNA technology or metabolic engineering strategies to breed plant species with higher quantity of fungitoxic bioactive compounds in them.

Author details

Toba Samuel Anjorin* and Ezekiel Adebayo Salako

Department of Crop Science, Faculty of Agriculture, University of Abuja, Abuja, Nigeria

Hussaini Anthony Makun

Department of Biochemistry, Faculty of Science, Federal University of Technology, Minna , Nigeria

9. References

Adegoke G. O, Odelusola B. .A. (1996) Storage of maize and cowpea and inhibition of microbial agents of biodeterioration using the powder and essential oil of *Cymbopogon citratus*. *Internat. Biodeter. Biodegrad.* 37: 81-84.

Afzal, R., S.M. Mughal, M. Munir, S. Kishwar, R. Qureshi, M. Arshad and Laghari, M.K. (2010) Mycoflora associated with seeds of different sunflower cultivars and its management. *Pak. J. Botany*, 42: 435-445.

Akunyili, D and Ivbijaro, M.F.A. (2006) Pesticide regulations and their implementation in Nigeria. In:). Sustainable Environmental Management in Nigeria. M.F.A. Akintola F and Okechukwu R.U. (eds.) Mattivi Production, Ibadan. Pp. 187-210.

Anjorin, S.T. and Salako, E. A. (2009) The status of pesticidal plants and materials identification in Nigeria. *Nigerian Journal of Plant Protection 23*, 25-32.

Anjorin, S.T. (2008) Quality Assessment of Botanical pesticides in Nigeria. Proceeding of the 42nd Annual Conference of the Agricultural Society of Nigeria held at Ebonyi State University Abakaliki- Nigeria. 19th-23rd, November, pp 130-135.

Anjorin, Toba Samuel, Hussaini Anthony Makun, Titilayo Adesina and Ibrahim Kudu (2008) Effects of *Fusarium verticilloides*, its metabolites and neem leaf extract on germination and vigour indices of maize (*Zea mays* L.) *African Journal of Biotechnology 7(14)* pp. 2402-2406.

Asogwa, E. U and Dongo, L. N. (2009) Problems associated with pesticide usage and application in Nigerian cocoa production: A review. *African Journal of Biotechnology* 8 (25), 7263-7270.

Awuah, R.T. and Ellis, W.O. (2002). Effects of some groundnut packaging methods and protection with *Ocimum* and *Syzygium* powders on kernel infection by fungi. Mycopathologia, 154: 29-36.

Awuah, R. T.and Kpodo, K. A. (1996) High incidence of *Aspergillus flavus* and aflatoxins in stored groundnut in Ghana and the use of microbial assay to assess the inhibitory effects of plant extracts on aflatoxin synthesis. *Mycopathologia*, 134, 109e114.

Bhatnagar, D., Zeringue, H. J. and Cormick, S. P. (1990) Neem leaf extracts inhibit aflatoxin biosynthesis in Aspergillus flavus and A. parasiticus.. In Proceedings of

* Corresponding Author

the USDA neem workshop (pp. 118–127). Beltsville, Maryland: US Department of Agriculture.

Bankole, S.A., Ogunsanwo, B.M., Osho, A., Adewuyi, G.O. (2006) Fungal contamination and aflatoxin B_1 of 'egusi' melon seeds in Nigeria. *Food Control* 17, 814-818.

Benharref, A. and Jana, M. (2006) Antimicrobial activities of the leaf extracts of two Moroccan *Cistus* L. species. *Journal of Ethnopharmacology* 104, 104-111

Boyraz, N. and Özcan, M. (2005) Antifungal effect of some spice hydrosols. *Fitoterapia* 76, 661–665.

Bugno, A., Almodovar, A.A.B. and Pereira, T.C. (2006) Occurrence of toxigenic fungi in herbal drugs. *Brazilian J ournal of Microbiology* 37 (1), 1-7.

Candlish, A. A. G., Pearson, S. M., Aidoo, K. E., Smith, J. E., Kell, B. and Irvine, H. (2001) A survey of ethnic foods for microbial quality and aflatoxin content. *Food Additives and Contaminants* 18, 129–136.

Centeno, S., M.A. Calvo, C. Adelantado and Figueroa, S. (2010) Antifungal activity of extracts of *Rosmarinus officinalis* and *Thymus vulgaris* against *Aspergillus flavus* and *A. ochraceus*. *Pak. J. Biol. Sci.*, 13: 452-455.

Chandra, R. and Sarbhoy, A.K. (1997) Production of Aflatoxins and Zearalenone by the toxigenic fungal isolates obtained from stored food grains of commercial crops. *Indian Phytopathology* 50, 458-68.

Cowan, M.M. (1999) Plant products as antimicrobial agents. *Clin Microbiol Rev*.12(4):564–582.

NAFDAC - National Agency for Food and Drug Administration and control (1996) *Pesticide Registrations*. B 303 -

Dambolena, J.S., M.P. Zunino, A.G. Lopez, H.R. Rubinstein and Zygadlo, J.A.*et al.*, (2010) Essential oils composition of *Ocimum basilicum* L. and *Ocimum gratissimum* L. from Kenya and their inhibitory effects on growth and fumonisin production by Fusarium verticillioides. Innovat. *Food Science Emergence. Technology* 11, 410-414.

Dayan, F.G.M. Tellez, A. and Duke, S (1992) Managing weeds with natural products. *Pesticide Outlook* (October):185-188.

Donmez-Altuntas, H., Z. Hamurcu, N. Imamoglu and Liman, B.C. (2003) Effects of ochratoxin A on micronucleus frequency in human lymphocytes. *Nahrung,* 47:, 33-35.

Fadohan, P., J.D. Gbenou, B. Gnonlonfin, K. Hell, W.F. Marasas and Wingfoeld, M.J. (2004) Effect of essential oils on the growth of *Fusarium verticillioides* and fumonisin contamination in corn. *Journal of Agriculture and Food Chemistry Food Chemistry* 52, 6824-6829.

Ferhout, H., Bohatier, J., Guillot, J. and Chalchat, J. C. (1999) Antifungal activity of selected essential oils, cinnamaldehyde and carvacol against Malassezia furfur and *Candida albicans*. *Journal of Essential Oil Research* 11, 119–129.

Faria, T.J., R.S. Ferreira, L. Yassumoto, J.R.P. de Souza, N.K. Ishikawa and. Barbosa, A.M (2006) Antifungal activity of essential oil isolated from *Ocimum gratissimum* L.

(eugenol chemotype) against phytopathogenic fungi. *Braz. Arch. Biol. Technol.*, 49: 867-871.

Food and Drug Admnistration (1997) .FDA talk paper: FDA publishes final dietary supplement rules, publications rules, T97-45. Press office, Food and Drug Adminisration, Washington, D.C.

Galvano, F., Piva, A., Ritieni, A., and Galvano, G. (2001) Dietary strategies to counteract the effects of mycotoxins. *Review of Journal of Food Protection* 64, 10–131.

Hasan, M.M., S.P. Chowdhury, Shahidul Alam, B. Hossain and Alam, M.S. (2005) Antifungal effects of plant extracts on seed-borne fungi of wheat seed regarding seed germination, Seedling health and vigour index. *Pak. J. Biol. Sci., 8:* 1284-1289.

Hell, K., K.F. Cardwell, M. Setamou and Poehling, H.M. (2000). The influence of storage practices on aflatoxin contamination in maize in four agroecological zones of Benin, West Africa. *J. Stored Prod. Res.*, 36: 365-382.

IARC, International Agency for Research on cancer (1993) Some naturally occurring substances: Food items and constituents, heterocyclic aromatic amines and mycotoxins. IARC monographs on the evaluation of carcinogenic risks to humans. 56th International Agency for Research on Cancer (pp. 489–521).

Iheshiulor, O.O.M., B.O. Esonu, O.K. Chuwuka, A.A. Omede, I.C. Okoli and Ogbuewu, I.P. (2011) Effects of mycotoxins in animal nutrition: A review. Asian J. Anim. Sci., 5: 19-33.

Ito, H., H. Chen and Bunnak, J. (1994) Aflatoxin production by microorganisms of the *Aspergillus flavus* group in spices and the effect of irradiation. *J. Sci. Food Agric.*, 65: 141-142.

Jackson, B. and Snowdon, D. (1990) Atlas of Microscopy of Medicinal plants, culinary herbs and spices Boca Raton: CRC press.

Jham, G.N., O.D. Dhingra, C.M. Jardim and Valente, V.M.M.(2005) Identification of major fungitoxic component of cinnamon bark oil. *Fitopatologia,* 30: 404-408.

Jimoh, K.O. and Kolapo, A.L. (2008) Mycoflora and aflatoxin production in market samples of some selected Nigerian foodstuffs. Res. J. Microbiol., 3: 169-174.

Juglal, S., Govinden, R., and Odhav, B. (2002) Spice oils for the control of co-occurring mycotoxin producing fungi. *Journal of Food Protection* 65, 683–687.

Giridhar, P and S.M. Reddy (1996) Effect of some plant extracts on citrinin production by *P. citrinum* in vitro. *Journal of Indian Botanical Science* 75, 153-154.

Khalid, S and Shad, R.A (1991) Potential advantage of recent allelochemical discoveries in agroecosystems *Programmed Farmer 11*, 30-35.

Kubo, A., C.S. Lunde and. Kubo, I. (1995) Antimicrobial activity of the olive oil flavor compounds. Journal .of Agricultural. Food Chemistry. 43: 1629-1633.

Makun, H.A, Gbodi, T.A., Akanya, H.O, Salako, A.E., Ogbadu, H.G. (2007) Fungi and some mycotoxins contaminating rice (*Oryza sativa*) in Niger state, Nigeria. *African J ournal of Biotechnology* 6 (2), 99–108

Makun, H.A., Anjorin, S.T. Moronfoye, B., Adejo, F.O., Afolabi, O. A., Fagbayibo, G., Balogun, B. O. and Surajudeen, A. A. (2010) Fungal and aflatoxin contamination of some human food commodities in Nigeria. *African Journal of Food Science* 4(4), 127-135.

Marin, S., Sanchis, V., Saenz, R., Ramos, A.J., Vinas, I., Magan, N., (1998) Ecological determinants for germination and growth of some *Aspergillus* and *Penicillium* spp. from maize grain. *Journal of Applied Microbiology 84*,25–36

Masheshwar P. K, Moharram S. A, Janardhana GR (2009) Detection of fumonisin producing *Fusarium verticillioides* in paddy (*Oryza sativa*. L) using Polymerase Chain Reaction (PCR). *Brazillian Journal of Microbiology* 40, 134-138.

McGuffin, M. (2001) Issues of quality: Analyzing herbal materials and the current status of methods validation." HerbalGram 53: 44-49.

Mohamed A. Yassin, Mohamed A. Moslem and Abd El-Rahim M.A. El-Samawaty, (2012) Mycotoxins and Non-fungicidal Control of Corn Grain Rotting Fungi. *Journal of Plant Sciences, 7:96-104.*

Mokhles, M., M.A. Abd El Wahhab, M. Tawfik, W. Ezzat, K. Gamil and. Ibrahim, M. (2007) Detection of aflatoxin among hepatocellular carcinoma patients in Egypt. *Pak. J. Biol. Sci.*, 10: 1422-1429.

Morovati, M., M Mahmoud, M. Ghazi-Khansari, A. Khalil Arial and Jabrari L. (2008). Sterility And Abortive Effects Of The Commercial Neem (*Azadirachta indica* A. Juss.) Extract Neemazal- T/S® On Female Rat (Rattus Norvegicus). Turk J Zool 32 155-162

Mossini, S.A.G., C. Carla and Kemmelmeier, C. (2009). Effect of neem leaf extract and neem oil on *Penicillium* growth, sporulation, morphology and ochratoxin A production. *Toxins* 1, 3-13.

Naganawa, R.,N. Iwata, K. Ishikawa, H. Fukuda, T. Fujino, and Suzuki A. (1996) Inhibition of microbial growth by ajoene, a sulfur-containing compound derived from garlic. *Appl. Environ. Microbiol.* 62:4238-4242

Negedu, A., Atawodi, S.E., Ameh, J.B., Umoh, V.J., and Tanko, H.Y. (2011). Economic and health perspectives of mycotoxins: A review. *Continental J. Biomedical Sciences (Wilolud Journals).* 5 (1): 5 - 26,

OMAF (2004) Pesticide storage, handling and application. Ontario Ministry of Agriculture, Food and Rural Affairs. California, United States.

Onyeagba, R. A., Ugbogu, O. C., Okeke, C. U., and Iroakasi, O. (2004) Studies on the antimicrobial effects of garlic (*Allium sativum* Linn) ginger (*Zingiber officinale* Roscoe) and lime (*Citrus aurantifolia* Linn). *African Journal of Biotechnology* 3, 552–554.

Owino, P. O and Waudo, S.W. (1992) Medicinal plants of Kenya: effects of *Meloidogyneincognita* and the growth of okra. *Afro-Asian Journal of Nematology 2*, 64 – 66.

Pal, K. K., and Gardener, B. S. (2006) Biological control of plant pathogens. *The Plant Health Instructor* 10 (1094), 1117- 02.

Pawar, V.C. and Thanker, V.S. (2007) Evaluation of the anti-*Fusarium oxysporum* f. sp *ciceri* and anti-*Alternaria porri* effects of some essential oils. *World Journal Microbiol. Biotechnol.*, 23: 1099-1106.

Pradeep, A. G., Lokesh, S. and Ravi, V. R. (2003) Efficacy of some essential oils on seed mycoflora and seedling quality of some crop species saved by farmers. *Advances in Plant Sciences* 16, 53–58.

Pundir, R.K. and Jain, P. (.2010) Antifungal activity of twenty two ethanolic plant extracts against food-associated fungi. *J. Pharmacy Res.*, 3: 506-510.

Rasooli, I. and Abyaneh, M. R. (2004) Inhibitory effects of thyme oils on growth and aflatoxin production by *Aspergillus parasiticus*. *Food Control* 15, 479–483.

Reddy, C. S., Reddy, K. R. N., Raja Kumar, N., Laha, G. S., and Muralidharan, K. (2004) Exploration of aflatoxin contamination and its management in Rice. *Journal of Mycology and Plant Pathology* 34(3), 816–820.

Reddy, K. R. N., Reddy, C. S., and Muralidharan, K. (2005) Characterization of aflatoxin B_1 produced by *Aspergillus flavus* isolated from discolored rice grains. *Journal of Mycology and Plant Pathology* 35(3), 470–474.

Reddy, C. S., Reddy, K. R. N., Prameela, M., Mangala, U. N., and Muralidharan, K. (2007) Identification of antifungal component in clove that inhibits *Aspergillus* spp. colonizing rice grains. *Journal of Mycology and Plant Pathology* 37(1), 87–94.

Reddy, B. N., and Raghavender, C. R. (2007) Outbreaks of aflatoxicoses in India. African *Journal of Food, Agriculture, Nutrition and Development* 7(5), 1–15.

Reddy K.R.N., C.R. Raghavender, B.N. Reddy and Salleh, B. (2010) Biological control of *Aspergillus flavus* growth and subsequent aflatoxin B_1 production in sorghum grains. *African Journal of Biotechnology* 9(27), 4247-4250

Rotimi, M.O. and Moens, M (2003) The use of leaf extracts of some herbs in the control of *Meloidogyne incognita. Proceedings of Nigerian Society for Plant Protection. 21*, 34-9

Salako, E. A. (2002) Plant protection for the resource-poor farmers*:* A key note address at the Nigerian Society for Plant Protection (NPSS). 30th Annual Conference held on Sept.1st – 4th, 2002 UNAAB Abeokuta. 1 – 11.

Salim, A.B. (2011) Effect of some plant extracts on fungal and aflatoxin production. *Int. J. Acad. Res.*, 3: 116-120.

Satish, S., Mohana, D.C., Ranhavendra, M.P. and Raveesha, K.A. (2007) Antifungal activity of some plant extracts against important seed borne pathogens of *Aspergillus* sp. *Journal of Agricultural Technology* 3(1), 109-119.

Saxena, J. and Mathela, C. H. (1999) Antifungal activity of new compounds from *Nepeta leucophylla* and *Nepeta clarkei*. *Applied and Environmental Microbiology*, 702–704.

Soliman, K.M. and Badea, R.I. (2002) Effect of oil extracted from some medicinal plants on different mycotoxigenic fungi. *Food and Chemical Toxicology* 40, 1669-1675.

Tagoe, D., S. Baidoo, I. Dadzie, V. Kangah and H. Nyarko, H. (2011) A comparison of the antimicrobial (Antifungal) properties of onion (*Allium* cepa), Ginger (*Zingiber officinal*) and garlic (*Allium sativum*) on *Aspergillus flavus*, *Aspergillus niger* and *Cladosporium herbarum* Using organic and water base extraction methods. *Res. J. Med. Plant*, 5: 281-287. Udoh, J. M., Cardwel K.F., Ikotun, T. (2000) Storage structures and aflatoxin content of maize in five agro-ecological zones of Nigeria. *Journal of Stored Product Reserve* 36, 187–201

Varma, J. and Dubey, N.K. (1999) Perspective of botanical and microbial products as pesticides of tomorrow. *Curriculum Science*. 76, 172-179. Varma, J. and Dubey, N.K. (2001) Efficacy of essential oils of *Caesulia axillaris* and *Mentha arvensis* against some storage pests causing biodeterioration of food commodities. *International Journal Food Microbiology*, 68: 207-210.

Wolf, H, Zundorf, I, Winckler T, Bauer R, Dingermann, T. (1999) "Characterization of Echinacea species and detection of possible adulterants by RAPD analysis. *Planta Medica* 65, 773-4.

Yassin, M.A., A.M.A. El-Samawaty, M. Moslem, A. Bahkali and. Abd-Elsalam, K.A (2011) Fungal biota and occurrence of aflatoxigenic *Aspergillus* in postharvest corn grains. *Fresenius Environ. Bull.*, 20: 903-909.

Zubkoff, P. (1999) Regulation of neem in the U. S. paper presented at the Worlds Neem Conference (1999). UBC Vancouver,Canada.

Chapter 9

Antioxidant Properties of Selected African Vegetables, Fruits and Mushrooms: A Review

R.U. Hamzah, A.A. Jigam, H.A. Makun and E.C. Egwim

Additional information is available at the end of the chapter

http://dx.doi.org/10.5772/52771

1. Introduction

Africa is blessed with vast amount of vegetables, fruits and mushrooms which are consumed for their nutrients or for their medicinal purposes. In recent years these vegetables, fruits and mushrooms have been shown to possess valuable antioxidants of great nutritional and therapeutic values. Antioxidants are substances which when present at low concentration compared to those of an oxidizable substrate [1] significantly delay or prevent the oxidation of that substrate. They are capable of preventing or attenuating damages such as lipid peroxidation, oxidative damage to membranes, glycation of proteins and inactivation of enzymes caused by free radicals. There are several evidences that show that oxidative stress resulting from reactive oxygen species including free radicals such as hydroxyl ($OH^{\cdot}$), superoxide ($O_2^{\cdot-}$), nitric oxide ($NO^{\cdot}$), nitrogen dioxide ($NO_2^{\cdot-}$), peroxyl ($ROO^{\cdot}$) and non free radical like hydrogen peroxide and singlet oxygen play an important role in the development of several pathological conditions such as lipid peroxidation, protein oxidation, DNA damage and cellular degeneration. These have been implicated in the aetiology of these pathological conditions related to cardiovascular diseases, diabetes, inflammatory diseases, cancer, Alzheimer and Parkinson disease, monogolism, ageing process and perhaps dementia [2,3-4, 5] .

Free radicals and other reactive oxygen species are constantly formed in the human body during normal cellular metabolism e. g during energy production in the mitochondria electron transport chain, phagocytosis, arachidonic acid metabolism, ovulation, fertilization and in xenobiotic metabolism [6]. They can also be produced from external sources such as food, drugs, smokes and other pollution from the environment [7]. Organisms are endowed with endogenous (catalase, superoxide dismutase, glutathione peroxidase/reductase) and exogenous (vitamin C, E, β-carorene) antioxidant defense system against reactions of free radicals. However the generation of free radicals in the body beyond its antioxidant capacity leads to oxidative stress which has been implicated in the aetiology of several pathological conditions such as lipid peroxidation, protein oxidation, DNA damage and cellular degeneration related to cardiovascular disease, diabetes, inflammatory disease, cancer and parkinson disease [8]. As a result of this much attention is been focused on the use of antioxidants especially natural antioxidant to inhibit and protect damage due to free radicals and reactive oxygen species. Synthetic antioxidant such as butylated hydroxyanisole(BHA), tert-butylated hydroxyquinone and butylated hydroxytoluene have been of utmost concern to many researcher because of their possible activity as promoters of carcinogenesis[9] Plant based antioxidant are now preferred to the synthetic ones because of their safety.

Epidemiological studies have shown that the consumption of vegetables and fruits can protect humans against oxidative damage by inhibiting or quenching free radicals and reactive oxygen species [8].Many plants including fruits and vegetables are recognized as sources of natural antioxidants that can protect against oxidative stress and thus play an important role in the chemoprevention of diseases that have their aetiology and pathophysiology in reactive oxygen species (10, 11-12]. These positive effects are believed to be attributable to the antioxidants; particularly the carotenoids, flavonoids, lycopene, phenolics and β-carotene [13] Mushrooms which have long been appreciated for their flavour and texture are now recognized as a nutritious food as well as an important source of biologically active compounds of medicinal value [14]. Mushrooms accumulate a variety of secondary metabolites, including phenolic compounds, polyketides, terpenes and steroids. Also, a mushroom phenolic compound has been found to be an excellent antioxidant and synergist that is not mutagenic [15]. Studies have shown that tropical mushrooms are highly rich in proteins, minerals, vitamins, crude fiber and carbohydrate with low fat and oil content. The protein content of mushrooms has been reported to be twice that of vegetables and four times that of oranges and significantly higher than that of wheat [16, 17]. The high level of vitamins in mushrooms particurlary vitamin C and D has been reported as responsible for its antioxidative activity [17, 18]. Mushrooms contains also an appreciable quantities of crude fibres, although, little information exist on Total Dietary Fibre (TDF) content of mushrooms. The crude fibre content values reported from many studies suggest that mushrooms are potential sources of dietary fibre [16]. Mushrooms generally contain low fat and oil content [16]. Because of the low fat and oil content, they are recommended as good source of food supplement for patients with cardiac problems or at risk with lipid induced disorders.

Also a lot had been reported on the nutrient; antinutrient and mineral composition of some edible mushrooms in Nigeria [19, 20] however there are few reported data on the antioxidant properties of commonly consumed mushrooms. This Chapter is therefore intended to discuss the antioxidant properties of selected African vegetables fruits and mushrooms.

2 Antioxidant properties of selected vegetables

2.1. *Vernonia amygdalina* (VA)

Vernonia amygdalina is a perennial shrub that belongs to the *Asteraceae* family and is popularly called bitter leaf in English a. It is known as 'Grawa' in Amharic, 'Ewuro' in

Yoruba, 'Etidot' in Ibibio, 'Onugbu' in Igbo, 'Ityuna' in Tiv, 'Ilo' in Igala 'Oriwo' in Edo and 'Chusar-doki' in Hausa.It has petiolate leaves of about 6mm diameter and ellicptic in shape. The leaves are green with a characteristic odour and bitter taste [21]. They are well distributed in tropical African and Asia and are commonly found along drainage lines and in natural forest or commercial plantation.

In most part of Africa, the leaves of VA are used as soup condiments after washing or boiled to get rid of the bitter taste. Specifically it is used to prepare the popular Nigerian bitter leaf soup, "onugbo" and as spice in the Cameroon dish called "Ndole" [22].

VA has a long history of use in folk medicine particularly among the sub Saharan African. Huffman and Seifu [23] reported the use of VA in the treatment of parasite related disease in wild chimpanzee in Tanzania. This necessitated quite a great number of researches to test the efficacy of different part of the plant in managing a wide array of ailments [22, 24]. Many traditional medicine practitioners use different parts of the plants in treating various ailments for instance the whole plant is being used as antihelminth, antimalaria and as a laxative [25]. Others use the aqueous extract of the leaves as a digestive tonic, appetizer and for treatment of wounds [26]. The decotion from leaves is used in the treatment of malaria fever in Guinea and cough in Ghana [24]. The leaf is also in Ethiopia as hops in preparing beer [27]. In Malawi and Uganda it is used by traditional birth attendants to aid expulsion of placenta after birth, aid post-pertum uterine contraction, induce lactation and control postpartum haemorrhage.

Their traditional use is not limited to human alone, in northern Nigeria it has been added to horse feed to provide a strengthening or fattening tonic *chusan Dokin* in Hausa.

Different extracts of VA has been shown to posses antioxidant properties both invitro and invivo. Ayoola et al [28] showed the invitro antioxidant properties of the ethanolic extract of leaves of VA using the diphenyl picyryl hydrazyl radical (DPHH) scavenging test. *V. amygdalina* was shown to have moderate inhibition of 77.7% thus indicating the scavenging ability of the vegetable. Also the aqueous and ethanolic extract of VA has further been shown to have potent antioxidant properties as they were able to inhibit bleaching of B-carotene, oxidation of linoleic acid and lipid peroxidation induced by $Fe^{2+/}$ ascorbate in a rat liver microsomal preparation. This study showed that the antioxidant activity of the ethanolic extracts was higher than that of the aqueous extracts, and compared favourably with synthetic antioxidant BHT and BHA [29]. However another study reported that methanol extract displayed highest antioxidant activity followed by acetone and water extract [30].

Adesanoye and Farombi [31] reported the hepatoprotective activities of the aqueous extract of *Vernonia amygdalina* leaves against carbon tetrachloride-induced hepatotoxicity and oxidative stress in mice. Administration of *Vernonia amygdalina* resulted in accelerated reversion of hepatic damage via reduction of liver marker enzymes like ALT, AST, ALP, Lactate dehydrogenase and bilirubin. Similarly antioxidant enzymes such as superoxide dismutase, glutathione S-transferase and reduced glutathione concentration and catalase activity were increased significantly at different doses of the methanolic extract of VA. This study is in agreement on previous work reported on the antioxidant properties of VA on aacetaminophen induced hepatotoxicity in mice [32]. The presence of flavonoids, phenols and other phytochemicals in this vegetable have been attributed to its antioxidant properties

Further confirmation of the antioxidant activities of VA was carried out by Oloyede and Ayila [33]. They investigated the antioxidant activity of different extracts, aqueous, methanol, hexane, ethylacetate and butanol extracts of *Vernonia amygdalina* using three methods: scavenging effect on 2,2-diphenyl-1-picryhydrazyl radical (DPPH), hydroxyl radical and peroxide oxidation by ferric thiocynate method. All fractions showed significant antioxidant activity ($p<0.05$) when compared with antioxidant standards like butylated hydroxyl anisole (BHA), ascorbic acid and α-tocopherol used in the assay. This plant contains natural antioxidants against aqueous radicals and reactive species ions [30].

Oxidative stress has been implicated in numerous human diseases including cancer, atherosclerosis, diabetes, malaria, iron overload, rheumatoid arthritis, Parkinson disease, and in HIV infection and AIDS [1]. This term actually refer to the imbalance between the generation of reactive oxygen species and the activity of the antioxidant defenses[34].Reactive oxygen comprises both free radicals such as hydroxyl (OH!), superoxide ($O_2^{\cdot-}$), nitric oxide ($NO^{\cdot}$), nitrogen dioxide ($NO_2^{\cdot-}$), peroxyl ($ROO^{\cdot}$) and lipid peroxyl ($LOO^{\cdot}$ And non free radical or oxidants like hydrogen peroxide (H_2O_2), ozone (O_3), singlet oxygen (${}_1O^{\cdot}$), hypochlorous acid (HOCl), nitrous acid (HNO_3), peroxynitrite ($ONOO^-$), dinitrogen trioxide (N_2O_3), lipid peroxide (LOOH), oxidants, although, they can easily lead to free radical reactions in living organisms [35]. Many of these ROS serve useful physiological functions but can be toxic when generated in excess or inappropriate environment thus causing oxidative damage to membranes and enhanced susceptibility to lipid peroxidation or enzyme inactivation.

Vernonia amygdalina has been used in various part of Africa for the treatment of several ailments ranging from diabetes, malaria, cancer and for general wellbeing. This local treatment has been backed up in recent times scientifically.

Nwanjo [36] reported the antidiabetic effect of the aqueous extract VA in streptozotocin induced diabetic rats. He showed in his finding that VA was capable of reducing plasma glucose, triglycerides, and LDL-cholesterol and the marker of oxidative stress malondialdehyde. These may be due to decreased oxidative stress which may be via direct scavenging of the ROS or by increasing the synthesis of antioxidant molecule [37].

Recently Akpaso et al [21] showed that the antidiabetic effect of the combined leaf extracts of *vernonia amygdalina* (bitter leaf) and *Gongronema latifolium* on the pancreatic β – cells of streptozotocin – induced diabetic rats. The extracts were observed to increase the animal body weight against the loss in weight in the diabetic group. In the same manner the serum glucose significantly decreased after 28days of treatment with the combined extract. Regeneration of islets cells was explained to be the one of the possible cause as there will be an increase in insulin production and secretion [38]. Previous studies by Ebong et al [39] reported this possible synergestic action using the extracts of Azadirachta indica and VA. It has been clearly demonstrated that *Vernonia amygdalina* extract contains active ingredients such as vernoniosides, glucosides, (VA) flavonoids and antioxidants [40] which may be responsible for their potentials in reversing pancreatic damage caused by STZ or alloxan in experimental animals. It was proposed that sesquiterpene lactones and the bitter principle of the plant may also be responsible for insulin production, stimulation and release of pancreatic islets from the beta-cells [41]. On the other hand, tannin, flavoniods glycosides and phytosterols of the plant may also act as alpha glucosidase inhibitor which contributed to the hypoglycemic effect of the plant.

Cancer has become a serious global problem. Prostate cancer and breast cancer are the most diagnosed non-skin cancers in men and women respectively. Breast cancer represents 15% of new cases of all cancers [42] while prostate cancer represents 15.3% of all cancers in men in the developed countries [43]. *V. amygdalina* Del. is increasingly becoming a strong contender for cancer management. Coumarins, flavonoids, sesquiterpene lactones and edotides may be the principles in VA that are responsible for its anticancer activity [44-46].

It was reported that the aqueous extract of VA exhibited a cytotastic action on cultured human breast tumour cells (MCF-7) growth in vitro. This implies tumour stabilization or preventive effects in vivo [46]. Fractions of *Vernonia amygdalina* extract were found to inhibit DNA synthesis. However the physiological concentrations of the water-soluble *Vernonia amygdalina* extract potently inhibited DNA synthesis in a concentration-dependent manner both in the presence and absence of serum [27]. It was also reported that fractions of hexane, chlorofrm, butanol and ethylacetate extracts of VA was capable of inhibiting the growth of human breast cancer cells even at very low concentrations of 0.1 mg/ml to concentration of 1 mg/ml, the inhibition was as high as 98% for some fractions of the extract [47]

Cold water, hot water and ethanol extract were found to induce apoptosis against acute lymphoblastic leukemia (ALL) and acute myeloid leukemia (AML) from the patients with IC50 ranging between 5 to 10 μg/ml. Ethanol extract was found to be most effective against both ALL and AML when compared to cold and hot water extract [48. Petroleum ether/ ethyl acetate leaf extract also possessed cytotoxic effect towards human hepatoblastoma (HepG2) and urinary bladder carcinoma (ECV-304) cell lines [49]. These findings establish the usefulness of *V. amygdalina* Del. in managing breast cancer.

Bioactive peptides from the aqueous extract of the plant leaves (edotides) have been shown to be potent in managing cancer by its activity on mitogen activated protein kinases and signal transduction pathways [46, 50].

Vernoninia amgdalina leaf is a vegetable with several potentials in the prevention and treatment of various ailments associated with oxidative stress.

2.2. *Telfairia occidentalis* (T.O.)

Telfairia occidentalis Hook f. commonly called fluted pumpkin occurs in the forest zone of West and Central Africa, most frequently in Benin, Nigeria and Cameroon. It is a popular vegetable all over Nigeria. It has been suggested that it originated in south-east Nigeria and was distributed by the Igbos, who have cultivated this crop since time immemorial [51]. It is a vigorous perennial vine, growing to 10m or more in length. The stems have branching tendrils and the leaves are divided into 3– 5 leaflets. The fruits are pale green, 3 – 10 kg in weight, strongly ribbed at maturity and up to 25cm in diameter. The seeds are 3– 5cm in diameter [52]. The leaf is consumed in different parts of the country because of the numerous nutritional and medicinal attributes ascribed to it. It has different traditional names; among Igbos, it is known as "Ugu", "iroko" or aporoko in Yoruba, ubong in Efik, umee in Urhobo and umeke in Edo [53]. Young succulent shoots and leaves are used as vegetables in the eastern part of Nigeria. The herbal preparation of the plant has been employed in the treatment of sudden attack of convulsion, gastrointestinal disorders, rmalaria and anaemia [54].Also the plant has agricultural and industrial importance in addition to its nutritional value [55].

Quite a number of researchers in the field of medical sciences have observed free radical scavenging ability and antioxidant property in *Telfairia occidentalis*. The darkish green leafy vegetable of *Telfairia occidentalis* and extracts (such as aqueous and ethanol extracts) from the leaves have been found to suppress or prevent the production of free radical and scavenge already produced free radical, lower lipid peroxidation status and elevates antioxidant enzymes (such as superoxide dismutase and Catalase) both in vitro and *in vivo* ([56,57-61,62]. They reported that extracts of this vegetable using various solvents were able to offer a chemopreventive and protective effects on oxidative stress induced serum and organs like kidney, liver and brain. Studies have shown that T.O. leaves are rich in antioxidants such as ascorbic acid and phenols [63, 64].

Specifically Oboh et al [57] in their study showed the antioxidant properties of T. O. by assessing their total phenolic content, reducing property and free radical scavenging properties against DPHH radical. From that study the aqueous extracts had a significantly higher total phenol content than the ethanolic extracts which clearly indicates that the phenols present in *Telfairia occidentalis* leaves are more water soluble than ethanol, consequently, the aqueous extracts could be a more potent antioxidant than the ethanolic extracts. this gives credit to the fact that aqueous extracts of the leaf is presently used in the management and prevention of anaemia and diabetes. This high phenol content in the aqueous extracts could have contributed to the prevention/ management of hemolytic anaemia [65] diabetes [66] which is associated with free radical damage.

Antioxidants may been classified into two separate groups: those that suppress the generation of reactive oxygen species and those that scavenge the reactive oxygen species generated[57] . Also in the same study it was observed that the aqueous extract had a significantly higher reducing power and higher free radical scavenging ability than the ethanolic extracts. The higher phenolic content in the aqueous extract would have accounted for the higher ability of the aqueous extract to reduce Fe (III) to Fe (II) in the FRAP test for reducing ability [67]. Also the chelating properties of phenols have been reported to have high reducing power [68] which clearly indicate that *Telfairia occidentalis* leaf antioxidant potentials will be more harness in its aqueous extraction than the ethanolic extraction and this is in accord with the form in which the plant is presently been used. Furthermore, the high reducing power and free radical scavenging ability of the extracts clearly indicate that both extracts of *Telfairia occidentalis* could suppress the generation of free radical and scavenge free radical. Protocatechiuc acid (PRA) and caffeic acid was shown to be the main polyphenolic compound present in the leaves of T.O.[69]. Cafeic acid is a phenollic compound present in the plant kingdom [70]. It is known to have a large number of physiological activities including anti-inflammatory, anti allergic and anti tumour [71, 72, 73]. They also revealed in their study the high flavonoid content, total antioxidant content, lipid peroxidation inhibition, free scavenging activity towards hydroxyl radical and superoxide scavenging abilities of *Telfairia occidentalis* amongst other vegetables. Therefore the consumption of leaves of T O will provide adequate antioxidants capable of preventing diseases arising from oxidative stress thus promoting the general well being of an individual.

The hepatoprotective properties of polyphenol extracts on T O leaves on acetaminophen induced liver damage was observed [58]. It was demonstrated that the soluble free polyphenol had a higher protective effect on the liver than bound polyphenol in this vegetable. This agrees with previous studies where correlation was reported between antioxidant properties and total polyphenolic content of some commonly consumed vegetables and fruits [56, 57, 74, 75,] Free phenolics are more readily absorbed and thus exert beneficial bioactivities in early digestion. The significance of bound phytochemicals to human health is however not clear [75, 76] and Chu et al 2002.

Telfairia occidentalis leaves have been reported to also be protective against liver damage [76, 77]. The use of the leaves in folk medicine in Nigeria in the treatment of certain diseases in which the participation of reactive oxygen species have been implicated could be as a result of the antioxidant and free radical scavenging ability [62].

Oxidative stress which have been implicated in quite a number of diseases such as anaemia, malaria, diabetes cancer and so on have been reported to be relieved by antioxidants inherent in vegetables, fruits and other plants. It is to this end that Salama *et al* [78] reported that aqueous extract of *Telfairia occidentalis* leaves reduces blood sugar and increases haematological and reproductive indices in male rats. *T. occidentalis* actually caused significant increases in packed cell volume, haemoglobin concentration, red blood cell count and white blood cell count in addition to a significant decrease in blood glucose. The increase in the hematological indices observed in this study is consistent with the observations made when rats were fed with the diet preparation of the air-dried leaves of *T. occidentalis* for four weeks [79] This study has also shown for the first time that new blood cells would have started appearing in the circulation after the fifth day of treatment with *T. occidentalis* and the increase would become significant after the seventh day of treatment and beyond. This increase is due to the chemical composition of *Telfairia occidentalis* particularly the presence of the vitamin A and C which are well known antioxidants capable of scavenging free radicals [80]. Some of these constituents are well-established haemopoietic factors that have direct influence on the production of blood in the bone marrow. For instance, iron is a well known haemopoietic factor [81]. Also the amino acids derived from *T. occidentalis* could also be used for the synthesis of the globin chains of the haemoglobin and this could also contribute to the increase in haemoglobin concentration. The significant increase observed in this study is however inconsistent with the insignificant change in haematological parameters observed when birds were fed with the dietary preparation of the sun-dried leaves of the plant [82]. The insignificant change observed with the sun-dried leaves might be due to the denaturing of the active ingredients especially proteins in the leaves during exposure to sunlight. In addition, the inconsistence may be an indication of a species variation in the responses to the effects of the plant. In the same study the leaves were observed to reduce blood sugar significantly, an indication of its hypoglycemic properties. This was confirmed in recent study on the comparative hypoglycemic properties of the ethanolic and aqueous extracts of leaves and seeds of this plant [83]. The hypoglycemic property is more in the leaves and was concluded to be better extracted with ethanol than water.

In the same way it was shown that this leave extract improve sperm motility, viability and counts generally improving sperm quality [78]. This is attributed to the actions of some of its active ingredients which have well documented spermatogenic activities. In this respect, studies have shown that nutritional therapies with zinc [84], vitamin C [85], vitamin E [86] and arginine [87] proved beneficial in treating male infertility. Therefore it may be very useful in the treatment and management of infertility especially that associated with reduction in sperm performance.

The antianaemic potentials of the aqueous extract of leaves of *Telfairia occidentalis* extracts against phenyl hydrazine-induced anaemia in rabbits was investigated [88]. Anaemia constitutes a serious health problem in many tropical countries because of the prevalence of malaria and other parasitic infections. In anaemia there is decreased level of circulating haemoglobin, less than 13 g dL^{-1} in male and 12 g dL^{-1} in females [89]. In the tropics, where malaria is endemic, between 10 to 20% of the population presents less than 10 g dL^{-1} of Haemoglobin [90]. Children are more vulnerable. The leaves are rich in iron and play a key role in the cure of anaemia, they are also noted for lactating properties and are in high demand for nursing mothers [91].

Elaboration of the therapeutic effect of *Telfairia occidentalis* on protein energy malnutrition-Induced liver damage was specifically emphasized in previous study [61]. The protein deficient diet caused a significant increase in hepatic malondialdehyde (MDA) level and the liver function enzymes alkaline phosphatase (ALP), alanine amino transferase (ALT) and aspartate amino transferase (AST) activities in the serum. It also caused a marked reduction in glutathione level, significant decrease in the antioxidant enzymes superoxide dismutase (SOD) and catalase (CAT) and significant damage to the hepatocytes. Recovery diets of protein alone and protein supplemented with *T. occidentalis* had significant effects on all the parameters. The MDA level and the serum liver function enzymes were significantly reduced while glutathione and antioxidant enzymes levels were markedly increased and a highly significant hepatocyte healing observed in the histology images.

2.3. OCIMUM

The genus ocimum is represented by over 50 species of herbs and shrubs in Africa. *Ocimum basilicum* and *Ocimum gratissimum* are known in Africa to manage different diseases. They belong to the family of plant known as Lamiaceae [92]. Local names of different species of ocimum in various ethnic groups include *Efirin* (Yoruba), *neh-anwu* (Ibo), *ntion* (Efik) and *dai-doya ta gida* (Hausa). The leaves can be petiolate or sessile, often toothed at the margin. They are erected and have characteristic pleasant aroma due to their volatile oil [92]. *Ocimum gratissimum* leaf or the whole plant is known to be popular treatment remedy for diarrhoea [93]. The plant is rich in voltile oils, which contain up to 75 percent of thymol, the antimicrobial activity of which is well known. Infact, the antimicrobial activity of the water-saturated oil had been shown to be proportional to the thymol content [94].

Ocimum gratissimum is effective in the management of upper respiratory tract infection, diarrhoea, headache, skin disease, pneumonia, fever, and conjuctivities.[95]. Traditionally *Ocimum basilicum* (basil) has been used as a medicinal plant for various ailments, such as headaches, coughs, diarrhoea, constipation, warts, worms and kidney malfunction. It is also thought to be an antispasmodic, stomachicum, carminative, antimalarial, febrifuge and stimulant [96, 97]. Ethnobotanical surveys report the traditional utilization of basil as a veterinary medicinal plant as well. Basil oil, especially the camphor containing oil, has antibacterial properties. The vapour of boiling leaves is inhaled for nasal or bron-chial catarrh and colds. The leaves may be rubbed between the palms and sniffed for colds. It cures stomach- ache and constipation. The leaves are crushed and the juice is used as vermifuge. It is further used to repel mosquitoes and as a broom to sweep chicken house in order to get rid of fleas.

Reactive oxygen species (ROS) have been implicated in some of the disorders associated with the traditional uses of some vegetables, such as malaria, anaemia, gastrointentional tract disorders, diabetes mellitus and inflammatory injury. Hence this forms the basis for the investigation of the antioxidant properties of some of these vegetables in order to validate the acclaimed traditional use.

A comparative study on the antioxidant properties of two Nigerian species of Ocimum showed that the methanolic extract of *Occimum gratissimum* posses a higher polyphenolic, flavonoid comoponent and free radical scavenging activities when compared to the methanolic extract of *O. basillicum* [98]. Thus this may be reason behind wider utilization of *O. gratissimum* in Nigerian folk medicine than *O. basillicum.*

Basil has been shown to contain *flavonoid* glycosides (0.6–1.1%) and flavonoid aglycones. A flavone, xanthomicrol (5, 4'-dihydroxy-6, 7, 8-trimethoxyflavone) was isolated from the leaves of a Nigerian *O.basilicum* [99, 100]. Basil herb *(O.basilicum)* contains apart from essential oil and flavonoids also tannins and polyphenols (2.2–2.3%)[99, 100].

The phytochemical and antioxidant activity of methanolic and aqueous extract of *Ocimum gratissimum* (OG) were investigated and the results showed the presence of flavonoids, steroids, cardiac glycosides, tannins, phlobatannins in both extract [101]. The methanoilic extract of OG was shown to exhbit a higher DPHH scavenging activity (84.6%) at 250 μg/ml and a reductive potential of 0.77 at 100 μg/ml comparable with those of gallic acid, 91.4% at 250 μg/ml and ascorbic acid, 0.79 at 60 μg/ml as standards for DPPH scavenging activity and reductive potential, respectively. Thus OG - leaf extracts possess antioxidant potential probably because of its phytochemical constituents which has also been reported in other studies [102,103-104]). Also the hepatoprotective effect of extract of leaf of OG was also reported [105].

The methanolic extract of leaf of OG was also shown to be capable of scavenging the free radiacal 2,2-diphenyl-1-picrylhydrazyl (DPPH.) radical, superoxide anion radical ($O2^{.-}$), hydroxyl radical (.OH), nitric oxide radicals (NO.), as well as inhibiing lipid peroxidation, using appropriate assay systems compared to natural and synthetic antioxidants.

The analgesic and hepatoprotective activity of the methanolic extract of *Ocimum gratissimum* (L.) leaves in carbon tetrachloride hepatoxic - albino rats was reported. A significant decrease in the liver enzmes were observed in the the hepatoxic albino rats after treatment with the methanolic extract of OG thus showing its protective effect on the damaged liver [106].

2.4. *Adansonia digitata*

Baobab (*Adansonia Digitata* L) is a tree found widely throughout Africa and known locally in African countries as the "tree of life" due to its ability to sustain life owing to its water holding capacity, as well as its many traditional medicinal and nutritional uses [107]. The baobab tree is an important food, water and shelter source in many African countries [108].). *Adansonia digitata* is commonnly called *Kukah* by the Hausa of Northern Nigeria, Niger *konian,* Kenyans *Mwambom*, Mali *sira*, Senegal, *goui* ([109]). *Adansonia digitata* is one of eight species of the *Adansonia* genus, and its name originates from the fact that the oblong leaves of the tree, often formed in groups of five, look like the fingers or digits of the human hand. It is a deciduous tree which has four growth phases and produces a fruit consisting of a yellowish-white pulp which has a floury texture and numerous hard, round seeds, enclosed in a tough shell [107].

The leaves of the baobab tree are a staple for many populations in Africa, especially the central region of the continent [110, 111]. During the rainy season when the baobab leaves are tender, the leaf is harvested fresh. During the last month of the rainy season, leaves are harvested in great abundance and are dried for domestic use and for marketing during the dry season. The leaves are typically sun-dried and either stored as whole leaved or pounded and sieved into a fine powder [112]. The Powdered leaves are used as a tonic and an anti-asthmatic and known to have antihistamine and anti-tension properties. The leaves are also used to treat insect bites, guinea worm and internal pains, dysentery, diseases of the urinary tract, opthalmia and otitis ([109].). In Indian medicine, powdered leaves are similarly used to check excessive perspiration ([109].). Baobab leaves are used medicinally as a diaphoretic, an astringent, an expectorant and as a prophylactic against fever [113].

Baobab leaves have been investigated in an attempt to identify the potential bioactives associated with this part of the plant [12,114,115-116,117. Certain bioactive compounds may be responsible for the treatment of certain ailments, as well as containing properties that can be beneficial to overall health. Examples of such bioactive compounds include tannins, phlorotannins, terpenoids, glycosides, saponins and terpenoids [116] as well as antioxidants including flavonoids and polyphenols [114]. The chemical profile of the methanolic and aqueous extracts of the leaves of the plant was also investigated [118]. They reported the presence of glycosides, phytosterols, saponins, protein and amino acid, phenolic compounds and tannins, gums, mucilage and flavanoids. Only few authors have investigated the vitamin A content of baobab leaves. Scheuring *et al.* [119] found that the simple practice of drying baobab leaves in the shade protects against deterioration of provitamin A. The selection of small leaves further increased provitamin A by 20%. The combination of small leaves and shade drying enabled the retention of the provitamin content up to 27 μg retinol equivalent per gram of dried leaf powder. Other authors mention the carotenoid content of baobab leaves [120,121].

Literature review revealed a great variation in reported values of nutrient contents of baobab part. According to Chadare *et al* [122] the causes of these variations are not well known, however they made several assumptions. The variation may be due to the quality of the sample, the provenance of the sample, the age of the sample, the treatment before analysis, the storage conditions, the processing methods, a probable genetic variation, and the soil structure and its chemical composition.

It is a known fact that the consumption of antioxidant-rich foods can contribute to the prevention of oxidation in the human cell, hence of some diseases. In addition to the general chemical composition of baobab pulp and leaves discussed previously, the antioxidant content of the aqueous extract of wild plants including *Adasonia digitata* was investigated [123]. They showed that baobab leaves have an antioxidant content of 7.7 μmol/g dw expressed as Trolox equivalents. This result is almost 1000 times lower than composition and nutritional value of baobab foods the one reported by Vertuani *et al.* (2002), who found that the water-soluble antioxidant capacity of dry baobab leaves was 6.4 mmol Trolox equivalent/g. These antioxidant activities were measured in fresh raw material and the effect of cooking and storage is not well known. Only Tarwadi and Agte [125] reported the antioxidative activity of some fruits and root vegetables before and after cooking. The antioxidant activity was measured as the inhibition of thiobarbituric acid reactive substances (TBARS), superoxide radical scavenging activity (SOSA), and ferrous iron chelating ability (FICA). They reported that there were significant cooking losses for each of the assessed antioxidant parameters.

A. digitata leaves, fruit-pulp and seeds have earlier been reported to show antiviral activity against influenza virus, herpes simplex virus and respiratory syncytial virus and polio [117]. Chemical analyses have reported the presence of various potentially bioactive ingredients including triterpenoids, flavonoids and phenolic compounds [122]. These bioactive compounds especially flavonoids and phenolic may be responsible for the nutritive and medicinal properties of this vegetable.

Karumi *et al* [125] also reported the gastro protective effect of *Adansonia digitata* leaf on ethanol induced ulceration. This study elucidated a significant dose- dependent increase both in preventive ratio and percentage ulcer reduction after pretreatment with *Adansonia digitata* leaves. Ethanol is an established ulcerogen especially in empty stomach [126]. The ulcerogenicity of ethanol is due to intracellular oxidative stress producing mitochondrial permeability, transition and mitochondrial depolarization which results to the death of cells in gastric mucosa [126,127]. This is because of its congestive inflammation and tissue injury. It is a known fact that flavonoids and anti-oxidant (Vit A, E and C) present in this plant has protective role. This view is supported by the fact that gastric mucosa is known to have certain antioxidant activity thereby reducing mucosal damage mediated by free radicals[128] which in turn attack cell membrane causing a lipid derived free radicals such as conjugated diene and lipid hydroperoxides which are extremely reactive and unstable. This study corroborate with previous report on the anti-ulcerative properties of the aqueous extract of *Adasonia digitata* leaves against ethanol induced ulceration in rats [129]. Although the precise mechanism of action of *A. digitata* is not clear, it was proposed that the gastoprotective role of this vegetable extract may be partly due to its high content of flavonoids and antioxidant [130] which are well known compounds that prevent and combat the formation of reactive oxygen species. Another possible mechanism is the fact that the leaves being an astringent may have precipitated microproteins on the site of ulcer thereby forming an impervious protective pellicle over the lining to prevent absorption of toxic substance and resist the attack of proteolytic enzymes [131].

2.5. *Corchorus olitorius*

*Corchorus olitorius (*Linn). is a leafy vegetable that belongs to the family tiliaceae and commonly called jute mallow in English and "ewedu" in the south western Nigeria. It is an animal herb with a slender stem and an important green leafy vegetable in many tropical area including Egypt, Sudan, India, Bangladesh, in tropical Asia such as Philippine and Malaysia, as well as in tropical Africa, Japan, the Caribbean and Cyprus [132]. The plant is widely grown in the tropics for the viscosity of its leaves. The leaves (either fresh or dried) are cooked into a thick viscous soup or added to stew or soup and are rich sources of vitamin and minerals [133]. Nutritionally, *C. olitorius* on the average contain 85-87 g H_2O, 0.7 g oil, 5 gcarbohydrate, 1.5 g fiber 250-266 mg Ca, 4.8 mg Fe, 1.5 mg 300010 vitamin A, 0.1 mg thiamine, 0.3 mg riboflavin, 1.5 mg nicotinamide, and 53-100 mg ascorbic acid per 100 g [134]

In West African countries including Ghana, Nigeria and Sierra Leone, the vegetable is cultivated for the stem bark which is used in the production of fibre (Jute) and for its mucilaginous leaves which are also used as food vegetable [135] The leaf extract of the plant is also employed in folklore medicine in the treatment of gonorrhea, pain, fever and tumour [136]. It is reportedly consumed as healthy, vegetable in Japan because of its rich contents of carotenoids, vitamin B_1, B_2, C and E, and minerals [137]. Its leaves and roots are eaten as herbal medicine in South East Asia [136]. In some part of Nigeria leaves' decoction used for treating iron deficiency, folic acid deficiency, as well as treatment of anaemia. Leaves also act as blood purifier [138] and the leaf twigs is used against heart troubles [139] while cold leaf infusion is taken to restore appetite and strength, leaves used for ascites, pains, piles, tumours, gonorrhoea and fever [140]

The hepatoprotective effect of the ethanolic etract of ewedu amongst other vegetables against CCl_4 induced hepatic damage in rats was studied [141]. Ethanolic extracts of *Corchorus olitorious* was shown to produce a significant hepatoprotective effect by decreasing serum and liver levels of ALT, AST, and total protein at dose of 250 and 500mgkg^{-1} in carbon tetrachloride induced hepatotoxic rats [141]. Their result also shows a significant inhibition of lipid peroxidation as illustrated by the decreased value on the MDA Values.

The phenolic antioxidants in the leaves of *Corchorus olitorious* was identified to include phenolic [5-caffeoylquinic acid (chlorogenic acid), 3, 5-dicaffeoylquinic acid, quercetin 3-galactoside, quercetin 3-glucoside, quercetin 3-(6-malonylglucoside), and quercetin 3-(6-malonylgalactoside) (tentative)] were identified from the leaves of *Corchorus olitorious L.* by NMR and FAB-MS. The contents of these phenolic compounds, ascorbic acid, and alpha-tocopherol in *C. olitorius* leaves were determined, and their antioxidative activities were measured using the radical generator-initiated peroxidation of linoleic acid. The results obtained showed that 5-caffeoylquinic acid was a predominant phenolic antioxidant in C. olitorius leaves (phenolic antioxidants from the leaves of *Corchorus olitorius L.* None of these phenolic compounds was detected in recent study on the chemical composition and invitro antioxidant properties of some selected vegetables [69]. Only caffeic acid acid was present to significance in the vegetable by the GC-MS analysis. Caffeic acid is a phenolic compound widely present among many plants which has been studied extensively and known to share a spectrum of physiological activities including anti-inflammatory anti-allergic and anti tumour [142-144] They further investigated the peroxidation inhibitory capacity of corchorus oliotorius among other vegetables and they resolved that though all vegetables evaluated were able to inhibit lipid peroxidation, the consumption of the vegetables especially *Vernonia amygdalina* and *Corchorus olitorious* may afford a better cytoprotective effects. Further results from these study showed that the ethanolic extract of *Corchorus olitorious* and other evaluated vegetables has high superoxide and hydrogen peroxide scavenging ability of *Corchorus olitorious* which could possibly be due to the presence of caffeic acid, flavonoids and in general the high total antioxidants.

Oboh *et al* [145] carried out a comparative study of the antioxidant properties of hydrophilic extract (HE) and lipophilic extract (LE) constituents of the *Corchorious olitorius*. HE and LE of the leaf were prepared using water and hexane, respectively and their antioxidant properties were determined. HE showed a significantly higher (1,1-diphenyl-2-picrylhydrazyl radical-scavenging ability ,reducing power ,trolox equivalent antioxidant capacity than LE. conversely, LE showed a significantly higher hydroxyl scavenging activity than HE while there was no significant difference in their Fe(II) chelating ability. The higher 1,1-diphenyl-2-picrylhydrazyl radical-scavenging ability, reducing power and trolox equivalent antioxidant capacity of the hydrophilic extract may be due to its significantly higher total phenol (630.8 mg/100 g), total flavonoid (227.8 mg/100 g) and non-flavonoid polyphenols (403.0 mg/100 g), and its high ascorbic acid content (32.6 mg/100 g). While the higher OH. Scavenging ability of LE may be due to its high total carotenoid content (42.5 mg/100 g). Therefore, the synergistic antioxidant activities of the hydrophilic and lipophilic constituents may contribute to the medicinal properties of *C. olitorius* leaf [145].

Further study illustrated the the protective effect of aqueous extract of *Corchorus olitorius* leaves (AECO) against sodium arsenite-induced toxicity in experimental rats [146]. A significant inhibition of hepatic and renal antioxidant enzymes such as superoxide dismutase, catalase, glutathione-S-transferase, and glutathione peroxidase and glutathione reductase were observed. The level of reduced glutathione decreased while the levels of oxidized glutathione and thiobarbituric acid reactive substances in the selected tissues were increased following arsenic intoxication. Treatment with AECO at doses of 50 and 100mg/kg body weight p.o. for 15days after arsenic intoxication significantly improved hepatic and renal antioxidant markers in a dose dependant manner. AECO treatment also significantly reduced the arsenic-induced DNA fragmentation of hepatic and renal tissues. Histological studies on the ultrastructural changes of liver and kidney supported the protective activity of the AECO [146]. Thus aqueous extract of *Corchorus olitorius* leaves is significant in protecting animals from arsenic induced hepatic and renal toxicity.

2.6. *Gongronema latifolium*

Gongronema latifolium belongs to the family of Asclepiadaceae family. The plant common name is amaranth globe. The parts commonly used are leaves, stem and root. The origin of the plant is traced to Nigeria in West Africa. *Gongronema latifolium is* called *madumaro* by Yoruba ethnic group in Nigeria commonly called 'utazi' by the Ibo of south eastern part if Nigeria. It is a tropical rainforest plant primarily used as spice and vegetable in traditional folk medicine [147,148]. They are sharp-bitter, sweet and widely used as a leafy vegetable and as a spice for sauces, soups and salads. *Gongronema latifolium* is widely used in West Africa for medicinal and nutritional purposes. An infusion of the aerial parts is taken to treat cough, intestinal worms, dysentery, dyspepsia and malaria. It is also taken as a tonic to treat loss of appetite. In Sierra Leone an infusion or decoction of the stems with lime juice is taken as a purge to treat colic and stomach-ache. In Senegal and Ghana the leaves are rubbed on the joints of small children to help them walk. The boiled fruits in soup are eaten as a laxative. In Nigeria a leafy stem infusion is taken as a cleansing purge by Muslims during Ramadan. A decoction of leaves or leafy stems is commonly taken to treat diabetes and high blood pressure. The latex is applied to teeth affected by caries. It is also taken for controlling weight gain in lactating women and overall health management. Asthma patients chew fresh leaves to relieve wheezing. A cold maceration of the roots is also taken as a remedy for asthma [149]. A decoction of the roots, combined with other plant species, is taken to treat sickle cell anaemia. A maceration of the leaves in alcohol is taken to treat bilharzia, viral hepatitis and as a general antimicrobial agent [150].The leaves are used to spice locally brewed beer. In Sierra Leone the pliable stems are used as chew sticks. The bark contains much latex and has been tested for exploitation.

Phytochemical screening of Gongronema latifolium vegetable showed the presence of alkaloids, tannnis, glycosides, polyphenols, saponins and flavonoids [151, 152]. Other chemical analyses on the leaves revealed several 17β-marsdenin derivatives (pregnane glycosides) as well as β-sitosterol, lupenyl cinnamate, lupenyl acetate, lupeol, essential oils and saponins. The essential oil from the leaves contains as main components linalool (19.5%), (E)-phytol (15.3%) and aromadendrene hydrate (9.8%) [151, 153-154].

Hepatoxicity induced by carbon tetrachloride in albino rats was found to be relieved by the ethanolic extract of *Gongronema latifolium* GLE [155]. Carbon tetrachloride induction in the rats resulted in hepatic injuries hence the marker of liver damage AST and ALT was reported to be significantly high in carbon tetrachloride induced rats however ALP was not siginificantly increased. It is well documented from histological studies on the liver that necrosis in the centrilobular zone is a major cause of carbon tetrachloride induced acute liver injury [156]. Treatment with the ethanol extract of *Gongronema latifolium* was shown to reduce the AST and ALT concentration significantly. Reduced levels of ALT and AST in rats treated with the extract could be attributed to the ability of the GLE to prevent the metabolism of carbon tetrachloride into more toxic metabolite and minimized the production of free radicals and also boost the activities of the scavengers of free radicals [157] thus minimizing hepatocellular injury produced. No evident increase or decrease in the level of ALP was observed. Absence of any concomitant increase of decrease on the ALP levels, under experimental conditions, was attributed to the fact that the single dose, intraperitioneal injection of the carbon tetrachloride at the pre-stated concentration/dosage, may not have caused any significant ($P<0.05$) billiary tract obstruction or disease [158] while causing acute hepatocellular injury [159]. Also the protective role of *Gongronema latifolium* in acetaminophen induced hepatic toxicity in Wistar rats was elucidated by [160]. Serum enzyme activities such as AST, ALTand ALP were increased following acetaminophen and caffeine administration in their study. The increase in liver enzymes following acetaminophen administration has earlier been reported by [39,161]. It has been reported that acetaminophen could be bioactivated enzymatically by cytochrome P4502EI in both liver and kidney. The metabolic activation by reactive intermediate N-acetyl parabenzoquinoneimine is believed to play an important role in acetaminophen mediated toxicity [162]. The proinflammatory cytokines such as tumor necrosis factor (TNF-a) and interleukin-la, that are released in response to acetaminophen intoxication are thought to be responsible for some pathological manifestations of acetaminophen induced toxicity [161]. However, the simultaneous administration of acetaminophen, caffeine and extract of *G. latifolium* significantly lowered AST, ALT and ALP concentrations when compared with those that received acetaminophen only and acetaminophen and caffeine. This is in line with the work of [155, 163].The mechanism by which *G. latifolium* lowered liver enzymes may be attributed to their ability to maintain liver cell integrity. It can therefore be concluded that acetaminophen offer protection against acetaminophen and caffeine induced hepatoxicity.

Earlier the oral administration of aqueous and ethanolic extract of *Gonogronema latifolium* was shown to possess' antidiabetic properties on streptozotocin-induced diabetic [147]. Also both extracts were shown to significantly increase the activity of superoxide dismutase and the level of reduced glutathione. The aqueous extract further increased the activity of glutathione reductase while the ethanolic extract caused a significant increase in the activity of glutathione peroxidase and glucose-6-phosphate dehydrogenase and a significant decrease in lipid peroxidation.

Gongronema Latifolium has also been shown to possess antiplasmodal activity; this supports the traditional use of the leaf extract of the plant for local treatment of malaria. Akuodor [164] and his team in their review stated that *Gongronema Latifolium* (madumaro) is used in South Eastern Nigeria to treat various ailments such as cough, loss of appetite, malaria and stomach disorders.The liquor usually obtained after the plant is sliced and boiled with lime juice or infused with water over three days is usually taken as a purge for colic and stomach pains. Various parts of the plant, particularly the stems and leaves are used as chewing sticks or liquor in Sierra Leone. It is also used to treat symptoms related to worm infections. *Gongronema Latifolium* is good for maintaining healthy blood glucose level and has antibacterial activity.

It was also reported that the ethanol extract of *Gongronema Latifolium* leaves when evaluated were found to possess anti-ulcer, analgesic and antipyretic activities. The plant enjoys reputation as a remedy for inflammation, bacteria, ulcer, malaria, diabetes and analgesic [164].

Other researches show its antimalarial effect, anti-inflammatory properties, and antisickling properties [165, 166]. This vegetable is reservoir of many antioxidants capable of preventing and treating different diseases.

2.7. *Gnetnum africanum*

Gnetum africanum is one of the most popular leafy vegetable in Nigeria which is gaining popularity as a delicious food leaf in other African countries such as Cameroon, Gabon, Congo and Angola [167]. It is called with different Local names: 'fumbwa' (DRCongo), 'okok', 'eru' (Cameroon), 'afang', 'okazi' (Nigeria). G. africanum, a lone genus belonging to the family Gnataceae is a dioecious wild undestorey liana that grows on trees in the humid forest of Africa [168].

The leaves of *G africanum* are elliptic in shape and are lined with reticulate veins comparable to those of a dicotyledonous angiosperm [169]. Its leaves are eaten as a vegetable, either raw or finely chopped and cooked; they are also widely used as an ingredient in soups and stews and are much in demand for their nutritional and therapeutic properties. It is traditionally used in the treatment of enlarged spleen, sore throat and as as a cathartic [170]. It is also used to relief nausea and neutralizes poison in Congo as well as been applied externally to manage boils, warts and used to reduce child birth pain. The leaves of *A. Gnetum* species are also used as a disinfectant for wounds treat heamorrhoid and increase blood production in the human organism [171].

In Nigeria, the leaf of *G. africanum* is used in the treatment of an enlarged spleen, sore throats and as a cathartic [171]. In Ubangi (DR Congo), it is used to treat nausea and is considered to be an antidote to some forms of poison [171. In Congo-Brazzaville, the leaves of both species are used as a dressing for warts and boils and a tisane of the cut-up stem is taken to reduce the pain of childbirth [172].*Gnetum africanum* is also reported to be used for medicinal purposes in Mozambique [173].

The leaves have very high nutritional value and constitute an important source of protein, essential amino acids and mineral elements [168]. Flavonoids, phenols anthocyanins have been shown to be present in the leaves of *Gnetum africanum* [174]. As is already know flavonoids is a class of secondary plant phenolics with powerful antioxidant properties. Phenols are regarded as the most important oxidative components of plants, hence correlation between the concentration of total plant phenolics and total antioxidant capacities have been reported [175]. The presence of these phytochemicals agrees with previous work of Iweala et al [176] who elucidated the presence of phenolic substances, flavonoids, anthocyanidins, phytosterols, tannins, saponins, alkaloids, glycosides, cyanogenic and cardiac glycosides ingnetum africanum leaves. Long term feeding of *Gnetum africanum* supplemented diet caused significant increase in weight, haemoglobin and white blood cells [176]. Glutathione s transferase and superoxide dismutase where increased significantly while lipid peroxidation and serum protein was reduced significantly with supplementation of Gnetum africanum supplemented diet. The gain in weight was explained o be due to the presence of high quality nutrient present in this leafy vegetable while reduction in protein may be a consequence of indigestibility and unavalaibilty of protein content of *Gnetum africanum*. The presence of invitro antioxidants lile flavonoids and phenolic substance was reported to be responsible for the decrease in lipid peroxidation and increase in GST and SOD as well as increase in haemoglobin and white blood cells [176]. Also a recent study on the biochemical and histological changes in paracetamol induced hepatoxic rats showed that consumption of *Gnetum africanum* supplemented diet reduced liver necrosis caused by paracetamol induction [177]. They also reported that lipid peroxidation was significantly reduced in the diet supplemented group. Although the precise mechanism for this protective role was not reported, it may be associated to presence of flavonoids and phenolic compounds in the vegetable. In a more recent study [174] as earlier reported also evaluated the invitro antioxidant properties of the methanolic extract of two leafy vegetables telfaira occidenatalis and *Gnetum africanum*. They revealed that both vegetable extracts had strong DPHH radical and hydroxyl radical scavenging ractivities compared to the water soluble natural antioxidant ascorbic acid. Howevever *Telfaira occidentalis* extract was concluded to posses more scavenging activities than *Gnetum africanum*. The potent antioxidant activity of the two methanolic extracts might result from their high content of polyphenolic compound.

3. Antioxidant properties of selected fruits in African

Africa is blessed with several varieties of fruits which are either consumed for their nutrients or for their medicinal values. They are known to be rich with antioxidants that help in lowering incidence of degenerative diseases such as cancer, arthritis, arteriosclerosis, heart disease, inflammation, brain dysfunction and acceleration of the ageing process [6,178,179]. Antioxidants are substances which when present at low concentration are capable of preventing or delaying oxidative damage of lipids, proteins and nucleic acids by reactive oxygen species. These reactive oxygen species include reactive free radicals such as superoxide, hydroxyl, peroxyl, alkoxyl and non- radicals such as hydrogen peroxide, hypochlorous, etc. They scavenge radicals by inhibiting initiation and breaking chain propagation or suppressing formation of free radicals by binding to the metal ions, reducing hydrogen peroxide, and quenching superoxide and singlet oxygen [180]. The most abundant antioxidants in fruits are polyphenols, Vitamin C, Vitamins A, B and E while carotenoids are present to a lesser extent in some fruits. These polyphenols, most of which are flavonoids, are present mainly in ester and glycoside forms [181]. The defensive effects of the natural antioxidants in fruits and vegetables are related to the three major groups: vitamins, especially vitamin C; phenolics; and carotenoids, especially β-carotene [182]. Vitamin C and phenolics are known as hydrophilic antioxidants, while carotenoids are known as lipophilic antioxidants. The antioxidant properties of a number of tropical fruits have been investigated on an individual basis using different analytical methods [183-185].

3.1. *Psidium guajava L.*

One of the most gregarious of fruit trees, the guava, *Psidium guajava* L belongs to the myrtle family (Myrtaceae), is almost universally known by its common English name or its equivalent in other languages. In Africa the names are: *gwaabaa* (Hausa); *woba* (Efik); *ugwoba* (Igbo); *guafa* (Yoruba) *ugwaba* in Efik [186]. Guava fruit, usually 4 to 12 centimetres (1.6 to 4.7 in) long, are round or oval depending on the species [187]. The outer skin may be rough, often with a bitter taste, or soft and sweet. Varying between species, the skin can be any thickness, is usually green before maturity, but becomes yellow, maroon, or green when ripe. Guava fruit generally have a pronounced and typical fragrance, similar to lemon rind but less sharp. Guava pulp may be sweet or sour, tasting something between pear and strawberry, off-white ("white" guavas) to deep pink ("red" guavas), with the seeds in the central pulp of variable number and hardness, depending on species.

Guava is a good source of minerals like iron, calcium, and phosphorus as well as many vitamins like ascorbic acid, pantothenic acid, vitamin A, carotenoids such as B- carotene and lycopene, and niacin [188]. Single common guava (P. guajava) fruit contains about four times the amount of vitamin C as an orange [189]. The fruit has also been shown to contain saponin combined with oleanolic acid. Morin-3-O-α-L-lyxopyranoside and morin-3-O-α-L-arabopyranoside and flavonoids, phenolic compounds such as ellagic acid, anthocyanin, guaijavarin, and quercetin are also reported [189]. chemical analysis of guava plant extract have revealed the presence of anti-microbial compounds [190], tannins, phenol triterpenes, flavonoids, guajivolic acid, guajavanoic acid, linolenic acid, linoleic acid, guavacoumaric acid, galaturonic acid, asphaltic acid, benzaldehyde, essential oils, saponins, carofenoid, cectin, fibre ,fatty acids and a high content of vitamins C and A in its fruit [191].

The hydrophilic and lipophilic antioxidant properties of guava fruits were reported by Thaipong [192]. They concluded from their investigation that both white and pink flesh guavas fruits showed high hydrophilic antioxidant activity and compounds for phenolic and vitamin C indicated that regular consumption of guava might be beneficial to health. Also hydrophilic antioxidant activity, the major activity, had high correlations with both total phenolic and vitamin C indicating that the use of the total phenolic or vitamin C content to determine antioxidant activity level in guava fruit was feasible. Phenolic and vitamin C are the major contributors to the antioxidant activity of guava fruits, while the contribution of carotenoid is negligible.

A comparative study of the antioxidant properties of several tropical fruits showed that guava possess primary antioxidant potential, as measured by scavenging DPPH and iron (III) reducing assays [193]. Primary antioxidants scavenge radicals to inhibit chain initiation and break chain propagations. This characteristic of guava is attributed to its high total phenolic compounds. This result is in agreement with the report of a study which enumerated the antioxidant activity of guava fruits [194] thus the fruit of guava can be harnessed either for protective or preventive roles against diseases arising from oxidative stress

3.2. *Carica papaya*

The papaya is the fruit of *Carica papaya* which belongs to the genus Carica in the myrtle family (Caricaceae). The papaya is one of native plants of Central America but is wide spread throughout tropical Africa. It is a berry developing from syncarpous superior ovary with parietal plancentation [195]. It is popularly called pawpaw. Pawpaw fruit is one of the most nutritional fruits grown and consumed in Africa. A green papaya fruit has been reported to provides 26 calories, 92.1 g H2O, 1.0 g protein, 0.1 g fat, 6.2 g total carbohydrate, 0.9 g fiber and 0.6 g ash{ [196]. USDA National Nutrient database recorded an orange-freshed papaya (per 100 g) contained 39 calories, 88.8 g H2O, 0.61 g protein, 0.14 g fat, 9.81 g total carbohydrate, 1.8 g fiber, 0.61 g ash. Additionally, Oyoyede [197] tested the chemical profile of unripe pulp of *carica papaya* and reported papaya fruit was very rich in carbohydrate (42.28% starch, 15.15% sugar) but low levels of fat. Papaya fruit also contains high levels of vitamin C (51.2 mg/100g), vitamin A precursors including β-carotene (232.3 μg/100g), and β-cryptoxanthin (594.3 μg/100g), as well as magnesium (19.2-32.7 mg/100g), which has been reported by Wall [198] Papaya fruit also contains papain which is a major component of papaya latex and widely applied for meat tenderisation.In recent years, papain and other endopeptidases have been proven to have several medical benefits, such as defibrinating wounds and treatment of edemas [199]. In some African countries, such as Gambia, tropical papaya is used to treat paediatric burns due to its proteolytic enzymes. Exception of papain, other endopeptidases, such as leukopapain and chymopapain, is also able to facilitate wound cleaning, promoting growth and improving the quality of the scar. Some physical behavious (such as color and size) of papaya fruit are various due to various cultivars.

Though *C. papaya* is an edible and flavorful fruit, it has been used throughout Africa for its medicinal benefits since it was introduced from the Americas. *C. papaya* has been used as treatment for numerous maladies, ranging from gastrointestinal disorders to asthma and sexually transmitted diseases. Perhaps the most common use of *C. papaya* is that of its been an antihelmintic. Often, the plant is boiled along with herbal adjuvants in order to expel worms [200]. A decoction made from the seeds of *C. papaya* has been used to much the same effect. The leaves have also been used in infusions to treat internal parasites [201].

Along with its use as an antihelmintic, *C. papaya* has been used to treat numerous gastrointestinal disorders. The whole fruit of *C. papaya* has also been boiled and used as an infusion in order to treat stomach ulcers In Madagascar, a tea made of from *C. papaya* leaves has also been used in order to treat gastric ulcers as well as general gastric discomfort [202]. In the Congolese region of Africa, a decoction made of the ripe seeds is said to be a very effective treatment of dysentery [203]. *C. papaya* is also thought to be effective in treatment of malaria. Along with the leaves of *Azadirachta indica*, *C. papaya* has been used as a steam treatment for malaria [201]. The fruit of *C. papaya* has also been used as a popular hepatoprotective agent. In cases of jaundice and hepatitis, immature fruit is either eaten or used in a decoction [200]. Most studies reported that papaya fruits and its leaves had high antioxidant capacity due to their high contents of vitamin B (in leaves), vitamin C, E (in fruits), and carotenoids [193, 203,204].

Recently Oloyede *et al* [205] reported the antioxidative properties of ethyl acetate fraction of unripe pulp of carica papaya in mice. Quercetin and β-sitosterol were isolated from the methanolic extract and later liquid-liquid extract of unripe carica papaya fruits using soxhlet apparatus. They further investigated the invitro antioxidant properties of this fruit in mice and the result showed a significant increase ($p<0.05$) in the activities of Gluthaione reductase, Glutathione peroxidase, Gluthathione, and Glucose-6-phosphate dehydrogenase with a slight reduction in catalase activity in the ethyl acetate fraction in the liver. On the other hand No significant change in activities of GR, GST and CAT were observed in groups of animals administered ethyl acetate (100mg/kg) or Aqueous extract when compared to control that received distilled water only, but renal GPx activity decreased following administration of ethyl acetate fraction. It is likely that quercetin and β-sitosterol may be responsible for the antioxidant potential demonstrated by the ethyl acetate fraction from unripe fruit. Therefore it was suggested that carica papaya unripe fruit may be useful in the management of diseases such as diabetes, sickle cell anaemia and cardiovascular diseases where free radicals are often generated

3.3. *Citrullus lanatus*

Watermelon (*Citrullus lanatus*) which belong to the family of is a vine-like flowering plant originally from southern Africa [206] . The watermelon fruits loosely considered a type of melon has a smooth exterior rind(green, yellow and sometimes white) and a juicy, sweet interior flesh usually deep red to pink but sometimes orange, yellow and even green if not ripe. [206].water melon rinds are also edibles but most people avoid eating them due their unpleasant flavor.

C. lanatus is an annual herb with long (up to 10 m) stems lying or creeping on the ground, with curly tendrils. Leaves are 5-20 by 3-19 cm, and hairy, usually deeply palmate with 3-5 lobes, on 2-19 cm long petioles. Fruits vary considerably in morphology, size range from about 7cm in diameter to over 20cm. In addition, they vary in colour from pale yellow or light green (wild form) to dark green (cultivars), and with or without stripes; the pulp varies from yellow or green (wild forms) to dark red (cultivars). The flesh amounts to about 65% of the whole fruit, and of this 95% is water. The plant has become naturalized in many drier parts of West Africa [207, 208].

Water melon fruit is a good source of, amino acid citrulline, vitamin A, vitamin C, the antioxidant lycopene, Beta carotene and potassium. Cucurbitacin the bitter principle in some species has diuretic and purgative properties. The fruit has but few medicinal uses in West Africa; Bitter forms are used in Senegal as a drastic purge and are considered poisonous [209]. Some other ethno-medicinal uses of the fruit include diuretic, purgative, remedy for urinary conditions suggestive of gravel and stone in the bladder, gonorrhoea and leucorrhoea in women [210,211].

lycopene and citrulline have been shown to be present in this fruit and are helpful in preventing some chronic diseases[212]. The amount of lycopene in watermelon is highly variable, but generally exceeds that of tomato.Citrulline is present in all parts of the fruit [213]. Lycopene was found to be relatively stable in fresh cut watermelon, and could increase slightly in whole fruit held at room temperature [214]. Seedless watermelon generally had more lycopene than seeded types, and lycopene was present in red fleshed fruit, with small amounts in orange fleshed watermelon, and none in yellow fleshed types. Lycopene has been extensively studied for its antioxidant and cancer-preventing properties, in contrast to many other food phytonutrients, whose effects have only been studied in animals, lycopene has been repeatedly studied in humans and found to be protective against a growing list of cancers, these cancers now include prostate cancer, breast cancer, endometrial cancer, lung cancer and colorectal cancers [215,216]. The antioxidant function of lycopene lies in its ability to help protect cells and other structures in the body from oxygen damage. Protection of DNA (our genetic material) inside of white blood cells has also been shown to be an antioxidant role of lycopene [217]. The amino acid citrulline in watermelon is a known stimulator of nitric oxide. Nitric oxide is known to relax and expand blood vessels much like the erectilw dysfunction drug Viagra and may increase libido [218]. The health benefit of watermelon fruit is associated with its status as a powerful antioxidants found in vit A, lycopene and beta carotene. These helps to neutralize free radicals hence can be use in the the prevention of diseases associated with oxidative stress such as diabetes, asthma, artherosclerosis and so on.

3.4. *Persea Americana*

Persea americana belongs to the family *Lauraceae*a along with cinnamon, camphor, and bay laurel. . Avocados are commercially valuable and are cultivated in tropical and Mediterranean climate throughout the world. They are a green skinned, fleshy body that may be pear shaped egg shaped or spherical and ripens after harvesting. It is commonly called in English as avocado, in Yoruba "igba", ibo "Ube-beke" and Swahili "mparachichi, mpea, mwembe mafuta".

Avocado has been shown to possess valuable phytochemicals. These compound classes may be divided into alkanols (also sometimes termed "aliphatic acetogenins"), terpenoid glycosides, various furan ring-containing derivatives, flavonoids, and a coumarin. The highly functionalized alkanols [218,219-221] of avocado have exhibited quite diverse biological properties thus far. For example, Oberlies *et al* isolated 1, 2, 4-trihydroxyheptadec-16-ene, 1, 2, 4-trihydroxyheptadec-16-yne , and 1, 2, 4 -trihydroxynonadecane from the unripe fruits of *P. americana,* and found these substances to be moderately cytotoxic when evaluated against a small panel of cancer cell lines [219].Kawagishi *et al* isolated 5 alkanols from avocado fruits with "liver suppressing activity" (as determined by the changes in plasma levels of alanine aminotransferase and aspartate aminotransferase), including compounds 9-11[221]

Avocado has sometimes received the reputation as a fruit too high in fat. While it is true that avocado is a high-fat food (about 85% of its calories come from fat), the fat contained in avocado is unusual and provides research-based health benefits. The unusual nature of avocado fat is threefold. First are the phytosterols that account for a major portion of avocado fats. These phytosterols include beta-sitosterol, campesterol, and stigmasterol and they are key supporters of our inflammatory system that help keep inflammation under control [222]. The anti-inflammatory benefits of these avocado fats are particularly well-documented with problems involving arthritis. Second are avocado's polyhydroxylated fatty alcohols (PFAs). PFAs are widely present in ocean plants but fairly unique among land plants—making the avocado tree (and its fruit) unusual in this regard. Like the avocado's phytosterols, its PFAs also provide us with anti-inflammatory benefits [223]. Third is the unusually high amount of a fatty acid called oleic acid in avocado. Over half of the total fat in avocado is provided in the form of oleic acid—a situation very similar to the fat composition of olives and olive oil. Oleic acid helps our digestive tract form transport molecules for fat that can increase our absorption of fat-soluble nutrients like carotenoids [224]. As a monounsaturated fatty acid, it has also been shown to help lower our risk of heart disease [225]. Hence its reputation as a fruit high in fat is of great importance in maintain the the integrity of the heard. Like other high-fat plant foods (for example, walnuts and flaxseeds), avocado provides unique health benefits precisely because of its unusual fat composition.

Avocados are also good source of Vitamin K, dietary fiber, Vitamin B6, Vitamin C, Folate and copper. Avocados are also a good source of potassium: they are higher in potassium than a medium banana. They also contains essential nutrients such as carbohydrates, sugar, soluble and insoluble fiber, It is also good source of oil containing monounsaturated fat its oil contents varies depending on its varieties and the period of extraction of oil by cold-press process. Avocado is a rich source of mineral [226]. The presence of the above mentioned phtytochemicals and vitamins makes avocado fruit a rich source of antioxidants hence capable of preventing quite a large number of diseases which are usually as a result of excessive free radical generation. For instance avocado has the ability to help prevent the occurrence of cancers in the mouth, skin, and prostate gland. This has been studied at a preliminary level by health researchers, mostly through the use of cancer cells or lab studies involving animals and their consumption of avocado extracts. But even though this anti-cancer research has been limited with respect to humans and diet, it is believed that the preliminary results are impressive. The anti-cancer properties of avocado are definitely related to its unusual mix of anti-inflammatory and antioxidant nutrients [227]. That relationship is to be expected since cancer risk factors almost always include excessive inflammation (related to lack of anti-inflammatory nutrients) and oxidative stress (related to lack of antioxidants). But here is where the avocado story gets especially interesting. In healthy cells, avocado works to improve inflammatory and oxidative stress levels. But in cancer cells, avocado works to increase oxidative stress and shift the cancer cells over into a programmed cell death cycle (apoptosis), lessening the cancer cell numbers [228]. In other words, avocado appears to selectively push cancer cells "over the brink" in terms of oxidative stress and increase their likelihood of dying, while at the same time actively supporting the health of non-cancerous cells by increasing their supply antioxidant and anti-inflammatory nutrients.

4. Antioxidant properties of mushrooms

Mushrooms have been used for many years as nutritional food and food flavouring materials as well as medicines [229]. Because of their flavour and aroma, mushrooms are greatly appreciated in many countries. According to the definition of Chang and Miles [230], a mushroom is 'a macrofungus with a distinctive fruiting body, which can be hypogeous or epigeous, large enough to be seen with the naked eye and to be picked by hand'. They constitute at least 14 000 and perhaps as many as 22 000 known species. The number of mushroom species on the earth is estimated to be 140 000, suggesting that only 10% are known [231]. Research indicates mushrooms have potential antiviral, antimicrobial, anticancer, antihyperglycemic, cardioprotective, and anti-inflammatory, activities.

A number of bioactive molecules, including antitumor substances, have been identified in many mushroom species. Polysaccharides are the best known and most potent mushroom derived substances with antitumor and immunomodulating properties [232,233]. Historically, hot-water-soluble fractions (decoctions and essences) from medicinal mushrooms, i.e., mostly polysaccharides, were used as medicine in the Far East, where knowledge and practice of mushroom use primarily originated [234). Mushrooms such as *Ganoderma lucidum* (Reishi), *Lentinus edodes* (Shiitake), *Inonotus obliquus* (Chaga) and many others have been collected and used for hundreds of years in Korea, China, Japan, and eastern Russia. Those practices still form the basis of modern scientific studies of fungal medical activities, especially in the field of stomach, prostate, and lung cancers. It is notable and remarkable how reliable the facts collected by traditional eastern medicine are in the study of medicinal mushrooms [235].

They are reputed to possess anti-allergic and anticholesterol activities. Aqueous extracts from *Pleurotus sajor caju* have been proven good in renal failure [236] showed mushrooms cure epilepsy, wounds, skin diseases, heart ailments, rheumatoid arthritis, cholera besides intermittent fevers, diaphoretic, diarrhea, dysentery, cold, anesthesia, liver disease, gall bladder diseases and used as vermicides.

Ganoderma lucidum are known to lower blood pressure and serum cholesterol concentration of hypertensive rats [237]. *Lentinus tigrinus* and *G. lucidium* are proved anticholesterolmic

[238]. *Lentinus edodus* has been used to enhance vigour, sexuality, energy and as an anti aging agent [239]. Lentinan sulphate obtained from *Lentinus* species inhibits HIV [239]. Jong et al. [240] reported that mushrooms cause regression of the disease state. Puffballs have been used in urinary infections [241]. Maitake extract has been shown to kill HIV and enhance the activity of T-helper cells [242,243] *Ganoderma* nutriceuticals have also exhibited promising antiviral effects like, anti-hepatitis B [243]Kino et al., 1989), anti-HIV [245,246]Kim et al., 1993; Liu and Chang, 1995). Dreyfuss and Chapela ([247] reported hundreds of secondary metabolites of fungal origin possessing biological activity. Mushrooms act as biological response modifiers by promoting the positive factors and eliminating the negative factors from the human body and thus regarded as the fourth principal form of the conventional cancer treatment.

Karst is believed to act as an anti-inflammatory and antidiabetic agent [248]. It is also used by Indian tribals for treating joint pain [249] Various reported medicinal uses of mushrooms like *reishi, cordyceps, enoki, maitake, lion's mane* and *splitgill* have been reported for cancer treatment; *shiitake, blazei, reishi, enoki, cordyceps, maitake, mesima* and oyster were found effective against cholesterol reduction. Reishi, cordyceps, shiitake and maitake is used for reducing stress. Lion's mane has been used for memory improvement; reishi for inducing sleep cordyceps for physical endurance and sexual performance, reishi, cordyceps, chaga and lion's mane for asthma and allergy treatment. They are also believed to be a good health elevator [250]. Auricularia species were used since times for treating hemorrhoids and various stomach ailments [251]. Pleurotus tuber-regium mushroom have been used for curing headache, high blood pressure, smallpox, asthma, colds and stomach ailments [252,253]. It has been reported *that P. ostreatus* lowers the serum cholesterol concentration in rats [254]. Puffballs (*Clavatia, Lycoperdon*) have been used for healing wounds [255]. Fresh mushrooms are known to contain both soluble and insoluble fibres; the soluble fibre is mainly beta-glucans polysaccharides and chitosans which are components of the cell walls [256]. Soluble fibre present in mushrooms prevents and manages cardiovascular diseases [257]. Wasser [258] reported that mushroom health supplements are marketed in the form of powders, capsules or tablets made of dried fruiting bodies, extracts of mycelium with substrate, biomass or extract from liquid fermentation. *P. sajor-caju* has been found to be inductive for growth of probiotic bacteria [259]. *Cordyceps sinensis* also treated as half caterpillar and half mushroom has been known and used for many centuries in traditional Chinese medicine. *Cordyceps* has been used to induce restful sleep, acts as anticancer, antiaging, and antiasthama agents besides proved effective for memory improvement and as sexual rejuvenator [260].

The antioxidant properties of mushroom have been reported. They are regarded as organisms which possess naturally occurring antioxidants. This is correlated with their phenolic and polysaccharide compounds [261]). Mau et al. [262] found antioxidant properties of several ear mushrooms. Tyrosinase from *A. bisporus* is antioxidant [180]. Lakshmi et al. [263] determined antioxidant activity of *P. sajor caju*. [264] observed that triterpenoides are the main chemical compounds in *G. lucidium.*

Three species of *Pleurotus florida, P. pulmonarius and P. citrinopileatus* were examined for their antioxidant potentialities with a view to popularize medicinal mushrooms among common middle class people at low-cost instead of administering costly medicines. Reducing power, chelating activity of Fe^{2+} and total phenol were observed to be higher in *P. florida* than in *P. pulmonarius* and *P. citrinopileatus* respectively. Among antioxidative enzymes, *P. florida* exhibited highest peroxidase and superoxide dismutase (SOD) where as catalase activity was found to be highest in *P. pulmonarius* [265]. The alcohol and aqueous extracts of *G. lucidum* and *C. sinensis* showed a high anti-oxidative activity by giving protection against oxidative DNA damage[266]. The reducing power and chelating activity of Fe^{2+} of *G. lucidum* and *C. sinensis* ethanol extract has been shown to increase with increase in concentration. The *G. lucidum* ethanol extract showed higher anti-oxidative properties than *C. sinensis*, probably due to differences in the compounds present in the fruiting bodies [267]. Previous workers obtained 6.001+0.04 μmg-1, 7.501+0.10 μmg^{-1} and 6.72+0.05 μmg^{-1} of phenol components in ethanol extract of *P. sajor-caju, P. florida* and *P. aureovillosus* respectively [268, 269]. It is showed that antioxidant activity of *Phellinus rimosus* seems to be more effective than the *Pleurotus florida, P. sajour-caju* and *G. lucidum* [263,270]. Fruiting bodies of medicinal mushroom (*G. lucidum*) contain polysaccharides, triterpenoids, adenosine, germanium, protein (L2-8), amino acids which have been found to have antitumor and immuno-modulating affect [271]. Methanol extract of *P. rimosus* have been shown to effectively reduce ferric ion in FRAP assay and scavenged DPPH radicals [272].

Extracts from fruiting bodies and mycelia of *G. lucidum* occurring in South India were found to possess *in vitro* antioxidant activity [266] and antimutagenic activities [263]. Antioxidant assays of the ethyl acetate, methanol and aqueous extract of *G. lucidum* effectively scavenged the O_2 and OH radicals [272]. However the aqueous extract was not effective to inhibit the ferrous ion induced lipid peroxidation [266] The extract showed significant reducing power and radical scavenging property as evident from FRAP assay [272] and DPPH radical scavenging assay [263,272]. The antioxidant potential of *L. edodes* methanol extract was investigated in the search for new bioactive compounds from natural resources. The measured DPPH radical scavenging activity is depicted by Sasidharan et al. [273]. The free radical scavenging activities were 39.0%, 41.0% and 66.00% for the *L. edodes* extract, vitamin E and BHT, respectively. The EC50 value is 4.4 mg/mL ($y = 11.7x - 1.693$, $R2 = 0.988$) which is the concentration of the crude extract that decreases the initial DPPH radical concentration by 50%. Effectiveness of antioxidant properties was found to be inversely correlated with EC50 values. Cheung and Cheung [274] also reported the antioxidant activity of *L. edodes* against lipid peroxidation. They found that the low molecular weight sub-fraction of the water extract of *L. edodes* had the highest antioxidant activity against lipid peroxidation of rat brain homogenate, with IC50 values of 1.05 mg/mL. In addition, other mushrooms have also been reported to possess antioxidant activity. Wong and Chye [275] reported the antioxidant activity of *Pleurotus porrigens, Hygrocybe conica, Xerula furfuracea (Rooted oude), Schizophyllum commune, Polyporus tenuiculus (Pore fungus)* and *Pleurotus florida*. Petroleum ether (PE) and methanolic extracts from these edible wild mushrooms were effective in DPPH radical scavenging and metal chelating ability. PE extracts were more effective than methanolic extracts in antioxidant activity using the DPPH, whereas methanolic extracts were more effective in reducing power and metal chelating ability.

5. Chemoprotective effects of African vegetables, fruits and mushrooms against mycotoxin induced oxidative stress and diseases

There are compelling evidences to show that mycotoxins are amongst the dietary factors that contribute to the risk of several types of diseases. The toxicologist and Nutritionist are particularly interested in mycoxins such as aflatoxins, ochratoxin A, fumonisins, Zeralenone and deoxynivalenol as they are attributed to the implication of several disease conditions.

Aflatoxin BI is the commonest form of Aflatoxin which is produced by *Apergillus flavus*. It is has been implicated in quite a number of diseases including, kwarshiorkhor, hepatitis, lung cancer, and liver cancer. It can either cause cancer alone or in synergy with hepatitis [276]. Cancer is induced by Aflaxoxin BI via metabolic activation by CYP3A4, CYP3A5 and/ or CYP1A2 [277, 278] to exo-8,9-epoxide which can form adduct with DNA leading to guanine nucleotide substitutions [279] specifically to codon 249 of the p53 gene [280]. Epidemiological studies have shown increased codon- 249 p53 mutations in areas of high aflatoxin B1 exposure [281]. Since hepatitis B virus and aflatoxin exposure have also been linked to hepatocellular carcinoma, recent studies have shown the interactive effect of increasing p53 mutation in persons with hepatitis B and coexposure to aflatoxin [282].

Ochratoxin A, a toxin produced by *Aspergillus ochraceus, Aspergillus carbonarius* and *Penicillium verrucosum,* is one of the most abundant food-contaminating mycotoxins [283]. It is found as contaminant in human foods, including various cereals, coffee, cocoa, wines and dried fruits. Depending on the dose, OTA may be carcinogenic, genotoxic, immunotoxic or teratogenic and even neurotoxic [284]. Exposure to OTA has been associated with the incidence of a kidney disease in humans, involving chronic interstitial nephritis as well as tumours of the urinary tract termed Baslkan Endemic Nephropathy (BEN) because of its geographical distribution [285]. It has been reported that occurrence of OTA with aflatoxin B1 in the same crop potentiates the mutagenic ability of the latter [286].

Zearalenone (ZEA) is a mycotoxin produced mainly by fungi belonging to the genus Fusarium in foods and feeds. It is frequently implicated in reproductive disorders of farm animals and occasionally in hyperoestrogenic syndromes in humans. It is found worldwide in a number of cereal crops such as maize, barley, wheat, oats and sorghum [287]. A wide variety of clinical effects attributed to zearalenone have been described in the literature. Decreased fertility, abnormal estrus cycles, swollen vulvas, vaginitis, reduced milk production and mammary gland enlargement are the most common findings reported in cattle and swine. ZEA binds to estrogen receptors influencing estrogen dependent transcription in the nucleus [288]. Receptor binded by ZEA has been shown to inhibit the binding estrogenic hormones in rat mammary tissues [289]. It was reported also by Hagler [290] that zearalenone causes hyperoestrogenism in swine. The potential for Zearelenon to stimulate growth of human breast cancer cells has also been demonstrated [291].

Fumonisins are a family of toxic and carcinogenic mycotoxins produced by *Fusarium verticillioides* (formerly *Fusarium moniliforme*), a common fungal contaminant of maize [292] Studies have shown the implication of fumonisins in the aetiology of a number of diseases such as rat liver cancer and haemorrhage in the brain of rabbits [293]. It has been reported that Fumonisin induce apoptosis in cultured human cells [294] and nephrotoxicity in certain animals [295].

Although fumonisin contaminated food has not been conclusively linked to human health harzards however a few studies have associated consumption of maize contaminated with fuminisins to human oesophageal carcinoma in some parts of South Africa and China [296]. Recently fumonisin toxicity has been linked reactive oxygen species (ROS) damage. For Instance It was reported that there was increase in lipid peroxidation, production of ROS, increase in caspase-3- like protease activity, internucleosomal DNA fragmentation and intracellular reduction of glutathione in human U-118MG glioblastoma cells treated with fumonisin B1 [297].

Deoxynivalenol (also called DON or vomitoxin) is one of an array of trichothecene mycotoxins produced by *Fusarium graminearum* and several other species of Fusarium that cause Fusarium head blight (also called FHB or scab) of wheat, barley, and other grasses and ear and stalk rot of corn. DON does not constitute a significant threat to public health. In a few cases short-term nausea and vomiting have been recorded [298].

The protective effect of various extract of *Vernonia amygdalina* on breast and prostate cancer has earlier been reported above. Mycotoxins such as Aflatoxin B1 are potent causative agent of several forms of cancer and this result from oxidative damage on macromolecules like DNA, proteins, lipids and carbohydrates. Vegetables, fruits and mushrooms have been reported to be reservoirs of antioxidants capable of scavenging and chelating reactive oxygen species thus preventing and protecting against such diseases arising from mycotoxin induced oxidative damage. For instance It was shown in a study that a diet incorporated with VA protected weanling albino rats against aflatoxin B1-induced hepatotoxicity [299]

Recent findings on the cause of cancer reveal that the damage caused by free radical to DNA is one of the reasons for carcinogenesis. The *Ocimum sanctum* has been well known for its antioxidant property with active ingredient such as eugenol and hence the plant has been studied for its anticancer activity. The protective effect of alcoholic extract of the leaves of

Ocimum sanctum on 3-methylcholanthrene (MCA), 7,12-dimethyl-benzanthracene (DMBA) and aflatoxin B, (AFB(1)) induced skin tumorigenesis in a mouse model was reported[300]. The extract of *Ocimum sanctum* leaf was shown to provide protection against chemical carcinogenesis in one or more of the following mechanisms: (i) by acting as an antioxidant; (ii) by modulating phase I and II enzymes; (iii) by exhibiting antiproliferative activity [300].

Treatment with aqueous and ethanolic extracts of *Ocimum sanctum* at 50μg/ml in mice bearing Sarcoma-180 solid tumors mediated a significant reduction in tumor volume and an increase in lifespan.These findings conclude *Ocimum sanctum* extracts possess anticancer activity [301].

Several studies have been reported to show that different types of fruits and vegetables are valuable sources of nutraceuticals. According to several studies as noted above these fruits and vegetables have high values of important nutrients and phytochemicals which exhibit antioxidant functions hence many form of diseases arising from the consumption of mycotoxin contaminated food can be protected. Lycopene, a carotenoid is present in many fruits and vegetables; such as grapefruit, guava, watermelon ansd pawpaw however, tomatoes and processed tomato products constitute the major source of lycopene [302]. Several studies have indicated that lycopene is an effective antioxidant and free radical scavenger. Lycopene, because of its high number of conjugated double bonds, exhibits higher singlet oxygen quenching ability compared to β-carotene or α-tocopherol [303]. In *in vitro* systems, lycopene was found to inactivate hydrogen peroxide and nitrogen dioxide [304, 305]. Using pulse radiolysis techniques, Mortesen *et al.* [306] demonstrated its ability to scavenge nitrogen dioxide ($NO_2^·$), thiyl ($RS^·$) and sulphonyl ($RSO_2^·$) radicals. Lycopene is highly lipophilic and is most commonly located within cell membranes and other lipid components. It is therefore expected that in the lipophylic environment lycopene will have maximum ROS scavenging effects. Hsiao et al. [307] showed the scavenging activity of lycopene on DPPH radical in rat brain homogenates and its ability to inhibit nitric oxide formation in cultured microglia stimulated by lipopolysaccharide. They further reported the protective effect of lycopene on ischemic brain injury *in vivo.*Epidemiological data strongly imply that lycopene consumption and tomato products contribute to prostate cancer risk reduction via different mechanisms which cooperate in reducing the proliferation of normal and cancerous prostate epithelial cells thereby reducing DNA damage and improving oxidative stress defense from free radicals arising from mycotoxins. . The mechanisms include inhibition of prostatic IGF-I signaling, IL-6 expression, and androgen signaling ([308] Moreover, lycopene improves gap-junctional communication and induces phase II drug metabolizing enzymes as well asoxidative defense genes. Lycopene was also demonstrated to inhibit mitogen-activated protein kinases, such as ERK1/2, p38 and JNK, and the transcription factor, nuclear factor-kappaB [309]

Mushrooms have been reported as useful in preventing diseases such are hypertension, hypercholesterolemia, cancer and other diseases linked to reactive oxygen species damage their extracts may act as biological response modifiers with anticancer activities. Though the mechanism of their antitumor actions is still not completely understood, stimulation and modulation of key host immune responses by these mushroom polymers appears central.

A study on the protective effect of some edible mushrooms on aflatoxin B1 induction revealed that mushroom at low doses of 100mg/Kg and 200mg/Kg body weight significantly reduced aflatoxin B1 toxicity [310]. The Liver function enzymes, AST. ALT and marker of kidney function, uric acid and creatine was shown to be reduced significantly on treatment with the extract of mushroom species while the antioxidant superoxide dismustase was significantly increased when compared to the aflatoxin B1 induced rats.

6. Conclusion

This chapter has reviewed only few vegetables, fruits and mushrooms with chemopreventive and antioxidant properties in African which validates some of the acclaimed traditional use. There is still a great deal of vegetables, fruits and mushrooms in African whose antioxidant studies has been carried out both at the preliminary and advanced stage. The consumption of these vegetables, fruits and mushrooms is capable of preventing and protecting against some of the diseases arising from the ingestion of mycotoxin contaminated foods in both humans and livestock.

Author details

R.U. Hamzah, A.A. Jigam, H.A. Makun, and E.C. Egwim
Department of Biochemistry, Federal University of Technology, Minna, Niger State, Nigeria

7. References

[1] Halliwell, B. and Gutteridge., J.M. Free radicals in biology and medicine. Clarendon press, Oxford. Press: Oxford; 1989.

[2] Aruoma O. I. Methodological considerations for characterizing potential antioxidant actions of bioactive components in food plants. Mut. Res. 2003; 523 – 524:9-2.

[3] Knekt, P.; Kumpulainen, J.; Järvinen, R.; Rissanen, H.; Heliövaara, M.; Raunanen, A.; Hakulinen, T.; Aromaa, A.. Flavonoid intake and risk of chronic diseases. Am. J. Clin. Nutr., 2002; 75: 560-568

[4] Amin, I, Zamaliah, M. M, and Chin, W. F. (2004)Total Antioxidnat activity and phenolic contented of selected vegetables. *Food Chem*: 87: 581-586.

[5] Sahlin, E., Savage, G.P. and Lister, C.E. Investigation of the antioxidant properties of tomatoes after processing. Journal of Food composition and Analysis. 2004; 17: 635-647.

[6] Halliwell B, Gutteridge JMC. Free Radicals in Biology and Medicine. Fourth Edition, Oxford University Press, Oxford, UK, 2007.

[7] Miller, R.A., Britigan, B.E. Role of oxidants in microbial pathophysiology. *Clin. Microbiol. Rev.* 1997;1 0 ;1 – 18..

[8] Ames BN, Shigenaga MK, Hagen TM Oxidants, antioxidants, and the degenerative diseases of aging. Proc Natl Acad Sci 1993; 90:7915-22.

[9] Atiqur, Rahman, Mizanur, Rahman M, Md Mominul *et al.*, 2008. Free radical scavenging activity and phenolic content of *Cassia sophera*. L: *Afr. J. Biotechnol.* 7 (10):1591-1593.

[10] Dragland S, Senoo H, Wake K. et al. Several culinary and medicinal herbs are important sources of dietary antioxidants. Nutr. 2003; 133(5):1286-1290.

[11] Odukoya, O.A., A.E. Thomas and A. Adepoju-Bello, 2001. Tannic acid equivalent and cytotoxic activity of selected medicinal plants. West Afr. J. Pharm., 15: 43-45.

[12] Atawodi SE (2005). Antioxidant potential of African medicinal plants. Afr. J. Biotechnol. 4(2):128-133.

[13] Amin I, Zamaliah MM, Chin WF. (2004)Total antioxidant activity and phenolic content in selected vegetables. *Food Chem.*; 87:581–586.

[14] Breene, W. (1990). Nutritional and medicinal value of speciality mushrooms. Journal of Food Production 53, 883-894.

[15] Fasidi IO Studies on *Volvariella esculenta* mass singer, Cultivation on Agricultural Wastes and Proximate Composition of Stored Mushrooms, *Food Chemistry*, 1996; 55:161 – 163.

[16] Okwulehie IC and Odunze ET Evaluation of the Myco-chemical and Mineral Composition of Some Tropical Edible Mushroom. *Journal of Sustainable Agriculture and Environment*, 2004 6:1; 63-70.

[17] Bano ZS and Rajarathnam.(1981). Studies on the Cultivation of Pleurotus Species. *Mushroom J.*, 101:243 – 245.

[18] Kurasawa S L, Sugahana J and Hayashi J Studies on Dietary Fibre of Mushroom and Edible Wild Mushroom and Plants. *Nut. Rep. Int.*1982; 26:167-173.

[19] Ola, F.L. and G. Oboh, 2000. Nutritional Evaluation of Cassia siamea Leaves. J. Technosci., 4: 1-3.

[20] Adejumo, T. O. and Awosanya, O. B. 2005. Proximate and mineral composition of four ediblemushroom species from South Western Nigeria. African Journal of Biotechnology 4 (10): 1084-1088.S

[21] Akpaso, M. I., Atangwho, I J., Akpantah, A., Fischer1, V. A. Igiri, A. O and Ebong, P. E. Effect of Combined Leaf Extracts of *Vernonia amygdalina* (Bitter Leaf) and *Gongronema latifolium* (Utazi) on the Pancreatic β-Cells of Streptozotocin- *British Journal of Medicine & Medical Research* 2011 *1(1): 24-34.*

[22] Yeap, S. K. ,.Ho, W Y. Beh, , B. K., Liang, W. S., Ky, H., Yousr1 A. N and Alitheen, B. *Vernonia amygdalina*, an ethnoveterinary and ethnomedical used green vegetable with multiple bioactivities. Journal of Medicinal Plants Research 2010; 4(25): 2787-2812

[23] Huffman MA, Seifu M . Observation on the illness and consumption of a possibly medicinal plant Vernonia amygdalina (Del.), by a wild chimpanzee in the Mahale Mountains National Park, Tanzania. Primates 1989; 30: 51-63.

[24] Ijeh, I. I. and Ejike. C.E. C. C. Current perspectives on the medicinal potentials of Vernonia amygdalina Del Journal of Medicinal Plants Research 2011; 5(7): 1051-1061.

[25] Igile, G. O., Olezek, W., Jurzysata, M., Burda, S., Fafunso, M., Fasanmade, A.A. Flavonoids from Vernonia amygdalina and their antioxidant activities. Journal of Agricultrual and Food Chemistry 1994; 42 (11): 2445 –2448.

[26] Iwu MM .Empirical investigation of dietary plants used in Igbo- Ethnomedicine. In: Iwu MM. Plants in indigenous medicine and diet. Nina Etkined Redgrove Publishers Co, New York, 1986: 131-50.

[27] Farombi, E. O. and Owoeye, O.Antioxidative and Chemopreventive Properties of Vernonia amygdalina and Garcinia biflavonoid Int. J. Environ. Res. Public Health 2011 8; 2533-2555.

[28] Ayoola GA, Coker HAB, Adesegun SA, Adepoju-Bello AA, Obaweva K, Ezennia EC, Atangbayila TO (2008). Phytochemical screening and antioxidant activities of some selected medicinal plants used for malaria therapy in Southwestern Nigeria. Trop. J. Pharm. Res., 7: 1019-1024.

[29] Owolabi MA, Jaja SI, Oyekanmi OO, Olatunji J Evaluation of the Antioxidant Activity and Lipid Peroxidation of the Leaves of *Vernonia amygdalina*. J. Compl. Integr. Med. 2008; 5: 21.

[30] Erasto P, Grierson DS, Afolayan AJ. Evaluation of antioxidant activity and the fatty acid profile of the leaves of *Vernonia amygdalina* growing in South Africa. Food Chem.2007b; 104: 636-642.

[31] Adesanoye, O.A.; Farombi, E.O. Hepatoprotective effects of *Vernonia amygdalina* (astereaceae) in rats treated with carbon tetrachloride. *Exp. Toxicol. Pathol.* 2010, *62*, 197-206.

[32] Iwalokun BA, Efedede BU, Alabi-Sofunde JA, Oduala T, Magbagbeola OA, Akinwande A. Hepatoprotective and antioxidant activities of *Vernonia amygdalina* on acetaminophen-induced hepatic damage in mice. J. Med. Food 2006; 9: 524-539.

[33] Oloyede, G.Kand Ajila J. M . Vernonia Amygdalina Leaf Extracts: A Source Of Noncytotoxic Antioxidant Agents. EJEAFChe 2012; 11 (4): 339-350.

[34] Aruoma OI (1993). Experimental tools in free radical Biochemistry in: O:I. Aruoma (ed) free radical in tropical disease. Harwood Academic Publishers, U.S.A pp 233 – 267.

[35] *Genestra M (2007).* Oxyl radicals, redox-sensitive signalling cascades and antioxidants. *Cell Signal 19, 1807–1819.*

[36] Nwanjo HU (2005). Efficacy of aqueous leaf extract of *Vernoniaamygdalina* on plasma lipoprotein and oxidative status in diabetic rat models. Nig. J. Physiol. Sci., 20: 39-42.

[37] Gutpa, S., Shukla, R., Prabhu, K.M., Agarwal, S., Rusia, U. and Murthy, P.S. (2002). Acute and chronic toxicitystudies on partially purified hypoglycemic preparation from water extract of bark of Ficus bengalensis Ind. J.Cli. Biochem., 17: 56-63

[38] Atangwho IJ, Ebong PE, Egbung GE, Eteng MU, Eyong EU (2007a).Effect of *Vernonia amygdalina* Del. on liver function in alloxaninduced hyperglycaemic rats. Journal of Pharmacy and Bioresources,4, R Retrieved January 13, 110, from http://ajol.info/index.php/jpb/article/view/32107.

[39] Ebong PE, Atangwho IJ, Eyong EU, Egbung GE (2008) The antidiabetic efficacy of combined extracts from two continental plants: *Azadirachta indica* (A. Juss) (Neem) and *Vernonia amygdalina* (Del.) (African bitter leaf). Am. J. Biochem. Biotechnol., 4: 239-244.

[40] Jisaka M, Ohigashi H, Takegawa K, Hirota M, Irie R, Huffman MA, Koshmizu K (1993a). Steroid gluccosides from *Vernonia amygdalina,* a possible chimpanzee medicinal plant. Phytochem., 34: 409-413

[41] Osinubi AAA (2007). Effects of Vernonia amygdalina and chlorpropamide on blood glucose. Med.J. Islam. World Acad. Sci., 16: 115-119.

[42] American Cancer Society (ACS) (2010). Cancer facts and letters. Atlanta GA, pp. 9-11.

[43] Parkin OM, Bray FI, Devesa SS (2001) Cancer burden in the year 2000: the global picture. Eur. J. Cancer, 37(8): 54-66.

[44] Jisaka M, Ohigashi H, Takagaki T, Nozaki H, Tada T, Hiroto M, Irie R, Huffman MA, Nishida T, Kagi M, Koshimizu K (1992). Bitter steroid glucosides, vernoniosides A1, A2, A3 and related B1 from a possible medicinal plant - *Vernonia amygdalina* used by wild chimpanzees.Tetrahedron, 48: 625-632.

[45] Wall ME, Wani MC, Manikumar G, Abraham P, Taylor H, Hughes TJ, Warner J, MacGivney R (1998). Plant antimutagenic agents,flavonoids. J. Nat. Prod., 51: 1084-1089.

[46] Izevbigie EB (2003). Discovery of water-soluble anticancer agents (edotides) from a vegetable found in Benin City, Nigeria. Exp. Biol. Med., 228: 293-298.

[47] Oyugi DA, Luo X, Lee KS, Hill B, Izevbigie EB (2009). Activity markers of the anti-breast carcinoma cell growth fractions of Vernonia amygdalina extracts. Exp. Biol. Med., 234: 410-417.

[48] Khalafalla MM, Abdellatef E, Daffalla HD, Nassrallah AA, Aboul-Enein KM, Lightfoot DA, Cocchetto A, El-Shemy HA (2009). Antileukemia activity from root cultures of *Vernonia amygdalina.* J. Med. Plants Res., 3: 556-562.

[49] Froelich S, Onegi B, Kakooko A, Schubert C, Jenette-Siems K (2006). In vitro antiplasmodial activity and cytotoxicity of ethnobotanically selected east African plants used for the treatment of malaria. Planta Medica, 72: https://www.thiemeconnect.de/ejournals/abstract/plantamedica/doi/10.1055/s-2006- 949815.

[50] Izevbigie EB, Byrant JL, Walker A (2004). A novel natural inhibitor of extracellular signal-regulated kinases and human breast cancer cell growth. Exp. Biol. Med., 229: 163-169.

[51] A.A.A. Kayode and O.T. Kayode, 2011. Some Medicinal Values of *Telfairia occidentalis*: A Review. *American Journal of Biochemistry and Molecular Biology, 1: 30-38.*

[52] FAO. Some medicinal plants of Africa and Latin America. FAO Forestry Paper, 67. Rome 1989.

[53] Akoroda, M.O., 1990. Ethnobotany of *Telfairia occidentalis* (cucurbitaceae) among Igbos of Nigeria. Econ. Bot., 44: 29-39.

[54] Gbile, Z.O., 1986. Ethnobotany, Taxonomy and Conservation of Medicinal Plants. In: The State of Medicinal Plants Research in Nigeria, Sofowora, A. (Ed.). University of Ibadan Press, Ibadan, Nigeria.

[55] Oboh, G., 2005. Hepatoprotective property of ethanolic and aqueous extracts of *Telfairia occidentalis* (Fluted Pumpkin) leaves against garlic-induced oxidative stress. J. Med. Food, 8: 560-563.

[56] Oboh, G. and A.A. Akindahunsi, 2004. Change in the ascorbic acid, total phenol and antioxidant activity of sun-dried commonly consumed green leafy vegetables in Nigeria. Nutr. Health, 18: 29-36.

[57] Oboh, G., E.E. Nwanna and C.A. Elusiyan, 2006. Antioxidant and antimicrobial properties of *Telfairia occidentalis* (Fluted pumpkin) leaf extracts. J. Pharmacol. Toxicol., 1: 167-175.

[58] Nwanna, E.E. and G. Oboh, 2007. Antioxidant and hepatoprotective properties of polyphenol extracts from *Telfairia occidentalis* (Fluted Pumpkin) leaves on acetaminophen induced liver damage. Pak. J. Biol. Sci., 10: 2682-2687.

[59] Adaramoye, O.A., J. Achem, O.O. Akintayo and M.A. Fafunso, 2007. Hypolipidemic effect of *Telfairia occidentalis* (fluted pumpkin) in rats fed a cholesterol-rich diet. J. Med. Food, 10: 330-336.

[60] Emeka, E.J.I. and O. Obidoa, 2009. Some biochemical, haematological and histological responses to a long term consumption of *Telfairia occidentalis*-supplemented diet in rats. Pak. J. Nutr., 8: 1199-1203.

[61] Kayode, O.T., A.A. Kayode and A.A. Odetola, 2009. Therapeutic effect of telfairia occidentalis on protein energy malnutrition-induced liver damage. Res. J. Med. Plant, 3: 80-92.

[62] Kayode, A.A.A., O.T. Kayode and A.A. Odetola, 2010. *Telfairia occidentalis* ameliorates oxidative brain damage in malnorished rats. Int. J. Biol. Chem., 4: 10-18.

[63] Oboh, G., 2005. Hepatoprotective property of ethanolic and aqueous extracts of *Telfairia occidentalis* (Fluted Pumpkin) leaves against garlic-induced oxidative stress. J. Med. Food, 8: 560-563.

[64] Oboh, G. and A.A. Akindahunsi, 2004. Change in the ascorbic acid, total phenol and antioxidant activity of sun-dried commonly consumed green leafy vegetables in Nigeria. Nutr. Health, 18: 29-36.

[65] Oboh, G., 2004. Prevention of garlic-induced hemolytic aneamia by some tropical green leafy vegetables. Biomed. Res., 15: 134-137.

[66] Baynes, J.W., 1991. Perspective in diabetes: Role of oxidative stress in development complications in diabetes. Diabetes, 40: 405-412.

[67] Amic, D., D. Davidovic-Amic, D. Beslo and N. Trinajstic, 2003. Structure-radical scavenging activity relationship pf flavonoids. Croatia Chem. Acta, 76: 55-61.

[68] Blazovics, A., A. Lugasi, K. Szentmihalyi and A. Kery, 2003. Reducing power of the natural polyphenols of *Sempervivum tectorum in vitro* and *in vivo*. Acta Biol. Szeg., 47: 99-102

[69] Salawu O. S, Akindahunsi, A.A. and Comuzzo, P. chemical composition and invitro antioxidant Activities of some Nigerian vegetables. Journal of Pharmacology and Toxicology 2006(1)5: 429-437

[70] Duke, J.A., 1992. Handbook of Biological Active Phytochemicals and Their Activity. 1st Edn., CRC Press, New York, ISBN-10: 0849336708.

[71] Moreira, A. S., V. Spitzer, E.E. Schapoval and E.P. Schenkel. Anti-inflammatory activity of extracts and fractions from the leaves of Gochnatia polymorpha. Phytother. Res., 2000;14:638-640.

[72] Hudson, E. A., P. A. Dinh, T. Kokubun, M.S. Simmonds and A. Gescher, 2000. Characterization of potentially chemopreventive phenols in extracts of brown rice that inhibit the growth of human breast and colon cancer cells. Cancer Epidemiol. Biomark. Prev., 9: 1163-1170.

[73] Soleas, G.J., Grass, P. D. Josphy, D.M. Goldberg and E.P. Diamandis. A comparison of the anticarcinogenic properties of four red wine polyphenols. Clin. Biochem;35: 119-124

[74] Sun J, Chu YF, Wu X and Liu RH (2002). Antioxidant and antiproliferative activities of common fruits. J. Agric. Food Chem., 50: 7449-7454.I

[75] Chu YF, Sun J, Wu X and Liu RH (2002). Antioxidant and antiproliferative activities of common vegetables. *J. Agric. Food Chem.*, 50: 6910-6916.

[76] Eseyin, O.A., A.C. Igboasoiyi, E. Oforah, P. Ching and B.C. Okoli, 2005. Effects of leaf extract of *Telfairia occidentalis* on some biochemical parameters in rats. Global J. Pure Applied Sci., 11: 77-79.

[77] Kayode, A.A.A. and Kayode, O.T. . Some Medicinal Values of *Telfairia occidentalis*: A Review. American Journal of Biochemistry and Molecular Biology, 2011; 1: 30-38.

[78] Salman,T.M, Olayaki, L. A. and. Oyeyemi, W. A. Aqueous extract of Telfairia occidentalis leaves reduces blood sugar and increases haematological and reproductive indices in male ratsAfrican Journal of Biotechnology . 2008; 7 (14:) 2299-2303.

[79] Alada, A.R.A., 2000. The haematological effect of *Telfairia occidentalis* diet preparation. Afr. J. Biomed. Res., 3: 185-186.

[80] Fasuyi, A.O., 2006. Nutritional potentials of some tropical vegetable leaf meals chemical characterization and functional properties. Afri. J. Biotechnol., 5: 49-53.

[81] Ganong WF (2005). A review of medical physiology. Appleton and Lange; p. 496.

[82] Fasuyi AO, Nonyerem AD . Biochemical, nutritional and haematological implications of *Telfairia Occidentalis* leaf meal as protein supplement in broiler starter diets. Afr. J. Biotechnol.2007; 6(8): 1055-1063.

[83] Eseyin O. A. Ebong, P., Eyong , E. U., Umoh,E Awofisayo, O. Comparative Hypoglycaemic Effects of Ethanolic and Aqueous Extracts of the Leaf and Seed of *Telfairia Occidentalis. Turk J. Pharm. Sci 2010;. 7 (1),:29-34, 2010.*

[84] Tikkiwal M, Ajmera RL, Mathur NK . Effect of zinc administration on seminal zinc and fertility of oligospermic males. Indian. J. Physiol. Pharmacol. 1987;31; 30-34.

[85] Dawson EB, Harris WA, Rankin WE, Charpentier LA, McGanity WJ.Effect of ascorbic acid on male fertility. Ann. N. Y. Acad. Sci. 1987; 498: 312-323.

[86] Vezina D, Mauffette F, Roberts KD, Bleau G . Selenium-vitamin E supplementation in infertile men. Effects on semen parameters and micronutrient levels and distribution. Biol. Trace. Elem. Res. 1996; 53: 65- 83.

[87] Scibona M, Meschini P, Capparelli S, Pecori C, Rossi P, Menchini Fabris GF . L-arginine and male infertility. Minerva. Urol. Nefrol, 1994;. 46: 251-253.

[88] Ogbe, R. J.,, Adoga, G. I. and Abu, A. H. Antianaemic potentials of some plant extracts on phenyl hydrazine-induced anaemia in rabbit. Journal of Medicinal Plants Research 2010; 4(8): 680-684.

[89] Okochi, V.I., J. Okpuzor and L.A. Alli, . Comparision of an african herbal formula with commercially available haematinics. Afr. J. Biotechnol.,2003; 2: 237-240.

[90] Diallo, A., M. Gbeassor, A. Vovor, K. Eklu-Gadegbeku and K. Aklikokou *et al*.,. Effects of *Tectona grandis* on phenylhydrazine induced anaemia in rats. Fitoterapia, 2008;` 79: 332-336.

[91] Okoli, B.E. and C.M. Mgbeogu, 1983. Fluted Pumpkin, *Telfairia occidentalis*: West African vegetable crop. Econ. Bot.,1983; 37: 145-149.

[92] Mindel E. H, Herb Bible. Simon and Schuster, New York (1992) pp. 55-59. 2. J.

[93] Dalziel, J. M. Useful Plant of West Tropical Africa, Crowns Agents for Overseas Government, London, (1956).

[94] F. El-Said, E. A. Sofowora, S. A Malcolm and A. Hofer, An Investigation into the Efficacy of Ocimum Gratissimum (Linn) as Used in Nigerian Native Medicine. Planta Medica., 17, 195 (1969).

[95] F. D. Onajobi, Smooth Muscle Contracting Lipid Soluble Principles in Chromatographic Fractions of Ocimum Gratissimum, J. Ethnopharmacol., 18, 3-11(1986).

[96] Wome B. Febrifuge and antimalarial plants from Kisangani, upper Zaire. Bulletin de la Societe Royale de botanique de Belgique, 115, 1982:243–250.

[97] Giron LM, Freire V, Alonzo A and Vaceres A.Ethnobotanical survey of the medicinal flora used by the cribs of Guatemala. J. Ethnopharmacol., 34, 1991:173– 187.

[98] Omale J., Olajide J. E. and Okafor P.N. Comparative Evaluation Of Antioxidant Capacity And Cytotoxicity Of Two Nigerian *Ocimum* Species Int. J. Chem. Sci.: 6(4), 2008, 1742-1751

[99] Viorica H. Polyphenols of *Ocimum basilicum* L.Chujul Med., 60, 1987:340–344.

[100] Fatope MO and Takeda Y. The constituents of the leaves of *Ocimum basilicum.* Planta Medica,54, 1988: p-190.

[101] Akinmoladun, A C. Ibukun, E. O., Afor, E., Obuotor E. M., and Farombi E.O. Phytochemical constituent and antioxidant activity of extract from the leaves of *Ocimum gratissimum*. Scientific Research and Essay Vol. 2 (5), pp. 163-166, May 2007.

[102] Dubey NK Tiwari TN Mandin D Andriamboavonjy H Chaumont JP Antifungal properties of *Ocimum gratissimum* essential oil (ethyl cinnamate chemotype). Fitoterapia 2000; 7(15): 567-569.

[103] Sulistiarini D, Oyen LPA, Nguyen Xuan Dung *Ocimum gratissimum* L. In: Plant Resources of South-East Asia. No. 19: Essentialoils Plants. Prosea Foundation, Bogor, Indonesia. 1999;. 140-142.

[104] Holets FB, Ueda-Nakamura T, Filho BPD, Cortez DAG, Morgado-Diaz JA, Nakamura CV (2003). Effect of essential oil of *Ocimum gratissimum* on the trypanosomatid *Herpetomonas samuelpessoai.* Act. Protonzool 42: 269-276.

[105] Awah F. M. and Verla,A. W. Antioxidant activity, nitric oxide scavenging activity and phenolic contents of Ocimum gratissimum leaf extract. Journal of Medicinal Plants Research 2010;4(24), pp. 2479-2487

[106] Uhegbu, F.O. Elekwa,I., Akubugwo, E. I. Godwin C. C. and Iweala, E E.J. Analgesic and Hepatoprotective Activity of Methanolic Leaf Extract of Ocimum gratissimum (L.) Research journal of medicinal plant 2012; 6[1]:108-115.

[107] Wickens GE, Lowe P .The Baobabs: Pachycauls of Africa, Madagascar and Australia, Springer; 2008.

[108] Venter F, Venter J (1996). Baobab In Making the most of indigenous trees. Briza publications, Pretoria, South Africa, 196; 26-27.

[109] Sibibe M, Williams JT .Baobab – *Adansonia digitata*. Fruits for the future. Int. Centre Underutil. Crops, Southampton, UK, 2002;

[110] Yazzie D.; VanderJagt D. J.; Pastuszyn A.; Okolo A.; Glew R. H., (1994), The amino acid and mineral content of baobab (Adansonia digitata L.) leaves. Journal of Food Composition and Analysis, 7, (3), 189-193

[111] Gebauer J, El-Siddig K, Ebert G (2002). Baobab (Adansonia digitata L.): A review on a multipurpose tree with promising future in the Sudan. Gartenbauwissenschaft, 67: 155-160.

[112] Sidibe, M., Scheuring, J.F., Tembely, D., Sidibé, M.M., Hofman, P., Frigg, M. (1996). *Baobab – Homegrown Vitamin C for Africa.* Agroforestry Today, 8 (2), 13-15.

[113] Wickens, G.E. Chapter 15: *The uses of the baobab (Adansonia digitata* L.) *in Africa.* In: *Taxonomic aspects of African economic botany,* editor, Kunkel, G., 1979.

[114] Vertuani S, Braccioli E, Buzzoni V, Manfredini S (2002). Antioxidant capacity of Adansonia digitata fruit pulp and leaves. Acta Phytotherapeutica, 86: 2

[115] Vimalanathan S, Hudson JB (2009). Multiple inflammatory and antiviral activities in Adansonia digitata (Baobab) leaves, fruits and seeds. J. Med. Plants Res., 3: 576-582.

[116] Masola SN, Mosha RD, Wambura PN (2009). Assessment of antimicrobial activity of crude extracts of stem and root barks from *Adansonia digitata* (Bombacaceae) (African baobab). Afr. J. Biotechnol., 8: 5076-5083.

[117] Anani K, Hudson JB, de Souzal C, Akpagana K, Tower GHN, Amason JT, Gbeassor M (2000). Investigation of medicinal plants of Togo for antiviral and antimicrobial activities. Pharm. Biol., 38: 40-45.

[118] Shri V T, Ramprasath. D, Karunambigai.K. Nagavalli. D, Hemalatha. S . Studies of Pharmacognostical Profiles of *Adansonia digitata* Linn.Ancient Science of Life 2004; 24(2).

[119] Scheuring J.F., Sidibé M. and Frigg M. (1999). Malian agronomic research identifies local baobab tree as source of vitamin A and vitamin C. *In Sight of Life Newsletter* pp 21-24.

[120] Sena L.P., Vanderjagt D.J., Rivera C., Tsin A.T.C., Muhamadu I., Mahamadou O., Millson M., Pastuszyn A. and Glew R.H. (1998). Analysis of nutritional components of eight famine foods of the Republic of Niger. *Plant Foods for Human Nutrition* 52 (1), 17-30.

[121] Nordeide M.B., Hatloy A., Folling M., Lied E. and Oshaug A. (1996). Nutrient composition and nutritional importance of green leaves and wild food resources in an agricultural district, K outiala, in Southern Mali. *International Journal of Food Sciences and Nutrition* 47 (6), 455-468.

[122] Chadare, F.J., Linnemann, A.R., Hounhouigan, J.D., Nout, M.J.R., Van Boekel, M.A.J.S. (2009). Baobab Food Products: A Review on their Composition and Nutritional Value. Critical Reviews in Food Science and Nutrition, 49, 254-274.

[123] Cook J.A., Vanderjagt D.J., Dasgupta A., Mounkaila G., Glew R.S., Blackwell W. and Glew R.H. (1998). Use of the Trolox assay to estimate the antioxidant content of seventeen edible wild plants of Niger. *Life sciences* 63, 105-110.

[124] Tarwadi K. and Agte V. (2005). Antioxidant and micronutrient quality of fruit and root vegetables from the Indian subcontinent and their comparative performance with green leafy vegetables and fruits. *Journal of the Science of Food and Agriculture* 85, 1469-1476.

[125] Karumi Y, Augustine AI, Umar IA (2008). Gastroprotective effects of aqueous extract of Adansonia digitata leaf on ethanol-induced ulceration in rats. J. Biol. Sci. 8: 225-228.

[126] Hirokawa, T., Boon-Chieng, S. and Mitaku, S. (1998) SOSUI: Classification and Secondary Structure Prediction System for Membrane Proteins. Bioinformatics (formerly CABIOS), 14(4), 378-379.

[127] Hernandez, J.A., A. Jimenez, P. Mullineaux and F. Sevilla, 2000. Tolerance of pea (*Pisum sativum* L.) to long term salt stress is associated with induction of antioxidant defences. Plant Cell Environ., 23: 853-862.

[128] Penisi, A., Piezzi, R., 1999. Effect of dehydroelucidine on mucus production. A quantitative study. Digestion Disease Sciences 44, 708–712.

[129] Bagchi D., Carry, O., Tran, W., Krolin, T.,Bagchi, D. J.,Garry, A., Bagchi, M.,Mitra, S., and Stohs, S. Stresss, diet and alcohol induced oxidation gastrointestinal mucosal injury in rats and protection by bismuth and subsalicylate. J.Applied Toxicol.,1998;18(1): 3-13.

[130] Arrigori, O. and De Tullio, M. C. Ascorbic acid: Much more than just an antioxidant. Biochem. Biophys. Acta, 2002;1569(1-3): 1-9.

[131] Nwafor, P. A., K. D. Effraim and T. W. Jacks.Gastroprotecitve effects of Aqueous extract of Kaya sinegalensis on indomethecin induced ulceration in rats. West Afri. J. Pharmacol.Drug Res.,1996; 12:45-50.

[132] Samra, I., Piliz, S., Ferdag ,C.(2007):Antibacterial and antifungal activity of *Corchorus olitorius* L. (Molekhia extracts) *international Journal of natural and Engineering Sci.* 1 (3) 39-61.

[133] Tindall, H.D. (1983.) Vegetables in the tropics. Macmillan, London. Pp. 325-379

[134] Oke,O.I.(1968): Chemical changes in some Nigerian vegetables during growth. *ExperimentalAgriculture* 4: 345-349.

[135] Zakaria, Z.A., Somchit, M.N., Zaiton, H., Mat-Jais, A.M., Suleiman, M.R., Farah, W.,Nazaratul- Marawana, R. and Fatimah, C.A.(2006): The invitro antibacterial activity of *Corchorous olitorius* extracts. *Int. J . of Pharmacology* 2(2) 213-215.

[136] Ndlovu, J. and Afolayan, A.J.(2008): Nutritional analysis of the south African wild vegetable *Corchorus olitorius* L. *Asian J of Plant Science* 7 (6) 615-618.

[137] Zeghichi, S.S., Kallithkara and Simopoulos, A.P. (2003): Nutritional composition of molehiya (*Corchorus olitorius*) and Stamnagathi (*Cichorium spinosum*) in: plants in human health and nutrition policy (eds. Simopoulus A.P. and C. Gopalan). Karger, Basel pp 1-22.

[138] Aiyeloja AA, Bello OA (2006). Ethnobotanical potentials of common herbs in Nigeria: A case study of Enugu state. Educ. Res. Rev., 1 (1): 16-22.

[139] Fondio L, Grubben GJH (2004). Corchorus olitorius L. In: Grubben GJH, Denton OA (Editors). PROTA 2: Vegetables/Légumes. [CD-Rom].PROTA, Wageningen, Netherlands.

[140] .Fasinmirin JT, Olufayo AA (2009). Yield and water use efficiency of jute mallow *Corchorus olitorius* under varying soil water management strategies. J. Med. Plants Res., 3(4): 186-191.

[141] S.O. Salawu and A.A. Akindahunsi. Protective Effect of Some Tropical Vegetables Against CCl_4 -Induced Hepatic Damage Journal of Medicinal Food. June 2007, 10(2): 350-355.

[142] Soleas, G. J., Grass, L.,Josphy, P. D., Goldberg, D. M. and Diamandis, E. P. A comparison of the anticarcinogenic properties of four red wine polyphenols. Clin. Biochem, 35: 119-124.

[143] Moreira, A. S, Spitzer, V.,Schapoval, E. E. and Schenkel, E. P. Anti-inflammatory activity of extractsand fractions from the leaves of Gochnatia polymorpha. Phytother. Res. 2000;14: 638-640.

[144] Kimata, M. , Inagaki, N and Nagai. Effect of luteolin and other flavonoids on IGE-mediated allergic reactions. Planta Med., 2000; 66: 25-29.

[145] Oboh, G · Raddatz, H · Henle, T Characterization of the antioxidant properties of hydrophilic and lipophilic extracts of Jute (Corchorus olitorius) leaf. Epub 2009;60 (2):124-34.

[146] Das AK, Bag S, Sahu R, Dua TK, Sinha MK, Gangopadhyay M, Zaman K, Dewanjee S. Protective effect of Corchorus olitorius leaves on sodium arsenite-induced toxicity in experimental rats. Food Chem Toxicol. 2010 ;48(1):326-35.

[147] Ugochukwu NH, Babady NE. Antihyperglycemic effect of aqueous and ethanolic extracts of *Gongronema latifolium* leaves on glucose and glycogen metabolism in livers of normal and streptozotocin-induced diabetic rats. Life Sci. 2003;73(15):1925–1938. doi: 10.1016/S0024-3205(03)00543-5.

[148] Ugochukwu NH, Babady NE, Cobourne M, Gasset SR. The effect of *Gongronema latifolium* leaf extract on serum lipid profile and oxidative stress of hepatocytes of diabetic rats. J Biosci. 2003;28:1–5.

[149] Sonibare, M.A. & Gbile, Z.O. Ethnobotanical survey of anti-asthmatic plants in south western Nigeria. African Journal of Traditional, Complementary and Alternative Medicine 2008; 5(4): 340–345.

[150] Burkill, H.N., The useful Plants of West Tropical Africa, Kew, published by Royal Botanic Gardens. 2nd Edition,1985; 456-596.

[151] Morebise, O., Fafunso, M.A., Makinde, J.M., Olajide, O.A. & Awe, E.O. Antiinflammatory property of the leaves of Gongronema latifolium. Phytotherapy Research 2002; 16(1): 75–77.

[152] Atangwho IJ, Ebong PE, Eyong EU, Williams IO, Eteng MU, Egbung GE (2009b). Comparative chemical composition of leaves of some antidiabetic medicinal plants: Azadirachta indica, Vernonia amygdalina and Gongronema latifolium Afr. J. Biotech., 8: 4685- 4689.

[153] Schneider C, Rotscheidt K, Breitmaier E. 4 new pregnane glycosides from *Gongronema latifolium* (Asckepiadaceae) Liebigs Annalen Der Chemie. 1993;10:1057–1062.

[154] Morebise O, Fafunso MA. Antimicrobial and phytotoxic activities of saponin extracts from two Nigerian edible medicinal plants. Biokemistri. 1998;8(2):69–7.

[155] Etim, O.E., Akpan, E.J. & Usoh, I.F. Hepatotoxicity of carbon tetrachloride: protective effect of Gongronema latifolium. Pakistan Journal of Pharmaceutical Sciences. 2008; 21(3): 269–274.

[156] Shi J, Asiaki K, Ikawa Y and Wake K.. Evidence of hepatocyte apoptosis in rat liver after the administration of carbontetrachloride. *J. Med. Res.2003;* 4: 1-8.

[157] Chung HS, Chong LC, Lee SK, Shamon LA, Breemen RBV, Mehta RG, Farnsworth NR, Pezzuto JN and Kinghorn AD Flavonoids constituents of chlorinzan diffused with potential cancer chemopreventive activity. J. Agric. Food Chem.,1999; 47:35-4.

[158] Wettstern M, Gerol W and Hausinger D.Hypoxia and CCl4-induced liver injury, but not acidosis, impair metabolism cysteinyl. Hepatol.,1990; 11: 866-873

[159] Recknagel RO. Carbon tetrachloride hepatotoxicity. Pharmacol. Rev., 1987;19: 145-195

[160] Ita SO, Akpanyung EO, Umoh BI, Ben EE, Ukafia SO. Acetaminophen induced hepatic toxicity: protective role of Ageratum conyzoides. Pak J Nutr 2009; 8(7): 928-932. .

[161] Nnodim J. Emejulu A. The protective role of Gongronema latifolium in acetaminophen induced hepatic toxicity in Wistar rats. Asian Pacific Journal of Tropical Biomedicine 201); 5151-5154.

[162] Raucy JL, Lasker JM, Lieber CS, Black M. Apap activation by human liver cytochromes P4502EI and P4501A2. Arch Biochem Biophys 1989; 271: 270-283.

[163] Kumarappan C, Vijayakumar M, Thilagam E, Balamurugan M, Thiagarajan M, Senthil S, et al. Protective and curative effects of polyphenolic extracts from Ichnocarpus frutescense leaves on experimental hepatotoxicity by carbon tetrachloride and tamoxifen. Ann Hepatol 2011; 10(1): 63-72.

[164] Akuodor, G.C., M.S. Idris-Usman, C.C. Mbah, U.A. Megwas and J.L. Akpan *et al.* Studies on anti-ulcer, analgesic and antipyretic properties of the ethanolic leaf extract of *Gongronema latifolium* in rodents. Afr. J. Biotechnol.2010; 9: 2316-2321.

[165] Eguyoni, A., Moody, J.O. & Eletu, O.M., 2009. Anti-sickling activies of two ethnomedicinal plant recipes used for the management of sickle cell anaemia in Ibadan, Nigeria. African Journal of Biotechnology 8(1): 20–25.

[166] Etetim, E.N., Useh, M.F. & Okokon, J.E., 2008. Pharmacological screening and evaluation of antiplasmodial activity of Gongronema latifolium (utazi) against Plasmodium berghei berghei infection in mice. Nigerian Journal of Health and Biomedical Sciences 7(2): 51–55.

[167] Eyo E and Abel U (1983): Chemical composition of amino – acid content of Gnetum Africanum leaves, *Nig J. Nutr. Sci*, 4, 52 – 57.

[168] Mialoundama, F. 1993. Nutritional and socio-economic value of *Gnetum* leaves in Central African forest. *In* Hladik, C.M. *et al., Tropical forests, people and food: Biocultural interactions and applications to development*. Carnforth, UK: Parthenon Publishing Group.

[169] Doyle, J. A. Molecules, morphology, fossils and the relationship of Angiosperms and Gnetales. Mol. Phylogenet, Evol., 448-462.

[170] Burkill, H.M. *The Useful Plants of West Tropical Africa. Volume 2: Families E-I.* Kew. Royal Botanic Gardens, Kew. 1194;90-94.

[171] Ndam M,J.P Nkefor and P. Blackmore(2000): Domestication of Gnetum africanum and G.buchholzianum, an over exploited wild forests vegetable of the Equato – Congolian Region. In press XVIth AETFAT proceeding.

[172] Bouguet, A. 1969. *Féticheurs et medicines traditionnelles du Congo (Brazzaville),*Paris: ORSTOM.

[173] Watt, J.M.A & M.G. Breyer-Brandwijk. 1962. *The medicinal and poisonous plants of Southern and Eastern Africa*. Edinburgh: E & S Livingstone.

[174] Akintola A. O, Ayoola P.B, and Ibikunle, G.J Antioxidant Activity of Two Nigerian Green Leafy Vegetables. Journal Of Pharmaceutical and Biomedical Sciences 2012.;14: 15 1-5.

[175] Moskotivz J, Yim K.A, Choke P.B (2002): Free radicals and disease. Arch Biochem. Biophys, volume 397, pp: 354-59.

[176] Iweala, E.E.J., F.O. Uhegbu and O. Obidoa, 2009. Biochemical and histological changes associated with long term consumption of *Gnetum africanum* Welw. Leaves in Rats. Asian J. Biochem., 4: 125-132.

[177] Iweala, E. J. and Osundiya O. A. (2010).). Biochemical, Haematological and Histological Effects of Dietary supplementation with leaves of Gnetum africanum welw on paracetamol induced Hepatotoxicity in Rats. International Journal of pharmacology (6): 872-879.

[178] Feskanich, D., Ziegler, R. G., Michaud, D. S., Giovannucci, E. L., Speizer, F. E., Willett, W. C., et al. Prospective study of fruit and vegetable consumption and risk of lung cancer among men and women. Journal of the National Cancer Institute, 2000;92:1812–1823.

[179] Gordon, M. H. (1996). Dietary antioxidants in disease prevention. Natural Product Reports, 265–273.

[180] Shi, H. L., Noguchi, N., & Niki, E. Introducing natural antioxidants. In J. Pokorny et al. (Eds.), Antioxidants in food: practical applications. Woodhead Publishing Ltd. and CRC Press.2001.

[181] Fleuriet, A., & Macheix, J. J.. Phenolic acids in fruits and vegetables. In C. A. Rice-Evans & L. Packer (Eds.), Flavonoids in health and disease. Marcel Dekker Inc..2003.

[182] Klein, B. P., & Kurilich, A. C. Processing effects on dietary antioxidants from plant foods. HortScience,2000; 35(4): 580-584.

[183] Jimenez-Escrig, A., Rincon, M., Pulido, R., & Saura-Calixto, F. Guava fruit (Psidium guajava L.) as a new source of antioxidant dietary fiber. Journal of Agricultural and Food Chemistry 2001; 49: 5489–5493.

[184] Leong, L. P., & Shui, G. (2002). An investigation of antioxidant capacity of fruits in Singapore markets. Food Chemistry, 76, 69–75.

[185] Someya, S., Yoshiki, Y., & Okubo, K. (2002). Antioxidant compounds from bananas (Musa Cavendish). Food Chemistry, 79, 351–354.

[186] Okujagu, T. F., Etatuvie Sam O., Ifeyinwa E., Jimoh B., Nwokeke. Book of abstract of published Research finding on Nigerian Medicinal plant and traditional medicine practice. 2005; 1: 90.

[187] Dey, Kanny Lall: The indigenous drugs of India - short descriptive notices of the principal medicinal plants met with in British India. 2nd edition. Thacker, Spink & Co. 1896. Calcutta.

[188] Mercadante AZ, Steck Z, Pfander H. Carotenoids from guava (*Psidium guajava* L.): isolation and structure elucidation. *J Agric Food Chem* 1999;47:145-51.

[189] Misra K, Seshadri TR. Chemical components of the fruits of *Psidium guajava*. *Phytochemistry* 1968; 7:641-45.

[190] Arima, H.; Danno, G.: Isolation of antimicrobial compounds from guava (*Psidium guajava* L.) and their structural elucidation. Bioscience, Biotechnology and Biochemistry. 2002;66(8) 1727-1730.

[191] Suntornsuk, L. Quantitation of vitamin C content in herbal juice using direct titration. *J. Pharm. Biomed. Anal*. 2002;28(5) : 849 -855.

[192] Thaipong K, Boonprakob U, Crosby K, Cisneros-Zevallos L, Byrne D (2006). Comparison of ABTS, DPPH, FRAP, and ORAC assays for estimating antioxidant activity from guava fruit extracts. J. Food Compos. Anal. 19: 669-675.

[193] Lim Y.Y., Lim, T.T., and Tee J.J.. Antioxidant properties of several tropical fruits: A comparative study. Food Chemistry 2007); 103:1003–1008.

[194] Jimenez-Escrig, A.. Guava fruit (Psidium Guajava L.) as a new source of antioxidant Dietary fiber. J. Agric. Food. Chem. 2002;49(11): 5489-93.

[195] Rice RP, Rice LW, Tindall HD (1987). Pawpaw. In: Fruits and vegetable production in Africa. A Textbook. Macmillan publishers ltd, London.1987, p170.

[196] Dukes, J.O., (1992). Handbook of medicinal herbs, CRC Press, N.Y., pp: 11-30, 102.

[197] Oyoyede, O. L. Chemical profile of unripe pulp of carica papaya. Pak. J. Nutri. 2005; 496: 379-381.

[198] Wall.,M .M. Ascorbic acid, vitamin A, and mineral composition of banana (Musa sp.) and papaya (Carica papaya) cultivars grown in Hawaii.Journal of Food Composition and Analysis; 2006(19); 434–445.

[199] Nitsawang S, Hatti-Kaul R, Kanasawuda P 2006. Purification of papain from *Carica papaya* latex: aqueous two-phase extraction versus two-step salt precipitation. *Enzyme Microb Technol 39*: 1103-1107.

[200] Neuwinger HD. African Traditional Medicine: A Dictionary of Plant Use and Applications. Stuttgart, Germany: Medpharm Gmbh Scientific Publishers; 2000

[201] Iwu, Maurice. Handbook of African Medicinal Plants. Boca Raton, FL: CRC Press; 1993.

[202] Novy JW. Medicinal plants of the eastern region of Madagascar. J Ethnopharmacol. Jan 1997;55(2):119-126

[203] Tona L, Kambu K, Ngimbi N, Cimanga K, Vlietinck AJ. Antiamoebic and phytochemical screening of some Congolese medicinal plants. J Ethnopharmacol. May1998;61(1):57-65.

[204] Setiawan, B., Sulaeman, A., Giraud, D. W., & Driskell, J. A. (2001). Carotenoid content of selected Indonesian fruits. Journal of Food Composition Analysis, 14, 169–196..

[205] Oloyede O., Franco, J., Roos Dl, Rocha, J., Athayde, M. Boligon A. Antioxidative Properties of Ethyl Acetate Fraction of Unripe Pulp of Carica Papaya In Mice 2011; 1 (3): 409-425.

[206] Koocheki, A., S.M.A. Razavi, E. Milani, T.M. Monghadam, S. Alamatiyan and S. Izadkhah..Physical properties of watermelon seed as a function of moisture content and variety. *Int. Agrophysics, 2007;* 21: 349-359.

[207] Vaughan JG, Geissler C. The new Oxford book of food plant (second edition), Oxford University press. 2009; Pp 348.

[208] Janiene E . Citrullus lanatus (Thunb.)Matsun. & Nakai. http://www.FAO/Watermelon citan 2010

[209] Florabase. Flora of western Australia, Plant description by Amanda Spooner, James Carpenter, GillianSmith and Kim Spence 2007, http://florabase.calm.wa.gov.au/browse/profile/7370. Accessed on 15/12/2011.

[210] Plants for a future. http://www.ptaf.org/database/plants.php/Citrullus+lanatus Accessed on 06/12/2011.

[211] Schaefer H, Renner SS. Phylogenetic relationships in order cucurbitales and a new classification of the gourd family cucurbitaceae. *Taxon*. 2011; 60(1): 122-138

[212] Edwards AJ, Vinyard BT, Wiley ER et al. Consumption of watermelon juice increases plasma concentrations of lycopene and beta-carotene in humans. J Nutr 2003;133(4):1043-50.

[213] Collins JK, Wu G, Perkins-Veazie P, Spears K, Claypool PL, Baker RA, Clevidence BA. Watermelon consumption increases plasma arginine concentrations in adults. Nutrition. 2007;23(3):261-6.

[214] Perkins-Veazie P, Collins JK. Carotenoid changes of intact watermelons after storage. *J Agric Food Chem*. 2006;54(16):5868-74.

[215] Jian L, Lee AH, Binns CW. Tea and lycopene protect against prostate cancer. Asia Pac J Clin Nutr. 2007; 1:453-7.

[216] Erhardt JG, Meisner C, Bode JC, Bode C. Lycopene, beta-carotene, and colorectal adenomas. *Am J Clin Nutr*. 2003 ;78(6):1219-24.

[217] Wood, Rebecca. The Whole Foods Encyclopedia. New York, NY: Prentice-Hall Press; 1988.

[218] Kashman Y, Neeman I, Lifshitz A. New compounds from avocado pear. Tetrahedron 1969;25:461731.

[219] Oberlies NH, Rogers LL, Martin JM, McLaughlin JL. Cytotoxic and insecticidal constituents of the unripe fruit of *Persea americana*. J Nat Prod 1998;61:781-5.

[220] Rodriguez-Saona C, Millar JG, Trumble JT. Isolation, identification, and biological activity of isopersin: a new compound from avocado idioblast oil cells. J Nat Prod 1998;61:1168-70.

[221] Kawagishi H, Fukumoto Y, Hatakeyama M, He P, Arimoto H, Matsuzawa T, *et al.* Liver injury suppressing compounds from avocado (*Persea americana*). J Agric Food Chem 2001;49:2215-21.

[222] Ojewole JA, Kamadyaapa DR, Gondwe MM et al. Cardiovascular effects of Persea americana Mill (Lauraceae) (avocado) aqueous leaf extract in experimental animals. Cardiovasc J Afr. 2007;18(2):69-76.

[223] Rosenblat G, Meretski S, Segal J et al. Polyhydroxylated fatty alcohols derived from avocado suppresses inflammatory response and provides non-sunscreen protection against UV-induced damage in skin cells. Arch Dermatol Res. 2010

[224] Naveh E, Werman MJ, Sabo E et al. Defatted Avocado Pulp Reduces Body Weight and Total Hepatic Fat But Increases Plasma Cholesterol in Male Rats Fed Diets with Cholesterol. J. Nutr., 2002; 132: 2015 - 2018.

[225] Guzmán-Gerónimo RI and Dorantes L. Fatty acids profile and microstructure of avocado puree after microwave heating. Arch Latinoam Nutr. 2008;58(3):298-302.

[226] Batista Cadeno, A., Cerezal Mezquita, P. and Funglay, V. (1993). E.I. Aguacate (persea Americana) Nutritional Composition of Avocado Pear, (63):63-69

[227] Donnarumma G, Paoletti I, Buommino E et al. AV119, a Natural Sugar from Avocado gratissima, Modulates the LPS-Induced Proinflammatory Response in Human Keratinocytes. Inflammation. 2010

[228] Ding H, Han C, Guo D et al. Selective induction of apoptosis of human oral cancer cell lines by avocado extracts via a ROS-mediated mechanism. Nutr Cancer. 2009;61(3):348-56.

[229] Tel G, Apaydın M, Duru ME, Öztürk M. Antioxidant and Cholinesterase Inhibition Activities of Three *Tricholoma* Species with Total Phenolic and Flavonoid Contents: The Edible Mushrooms from Anatolia. Food Anal. Methods 2012;5:495–504.

[230] Chang ST, Miles PG. Mushrooms biology—a new discipline. Mycologist 1992;6:64–5.

[231] Lindequist U, Niedermeyer THJ, Julich W. The Pharmacological Potential of Mushrooms. eCAM 2005;2(3)285–299.

[232] Tzianabos Ao: Polysaccharide immunomodulators as therapeutic agents: structural aspects and biologic function. Clin Microbiol Rev 2000; 13: 523-533,.

[233] Reshetnikov SV, Wasser SP, Tan KK Higher Basidiomycota as a source of antitumor and immunostimulating polysaccharides. Int J Med Mushrooms 2001;3:361–394.

[234] Hobbs C.Medicinal value of Lentinus edodes (Berk.) Sing. (Agaricomycetideae). A literature review. Int J Med Mushrooms 200; 2:287–302.

[235] Stamets P .Growing gourmet and medicinal mushrooms, 3rd edn. Ten Speed Press, Berkeley, Calif 2000.

[236] Bahl N. Medicinal value of edible fungi. In: Proceeding of the International Conference on Science and Cultivation Technology of Edible Fungi. Indian Mushroom Science II, 1983; 203-209.

[237] Kabir Y, Kimura S, Tamura T. Dietary effect of *Ganoderma lucidum* mushroom on blood pressure and lipid levels in spontaneously hypertensive rats (SHR). J. Nutr. Sci. Vitaminol., 1988;34: 433-438.

[238] Ren L, Visitev AV, Grekhov AN, Tertov VV, Tutelyan VA. Antiatherosclerotic properties of macrofungi. *Voprosy Pictaniya*, 1989;1: 16- 19.

[239] Gareth JEB Edible Mushrooms in Singapore and other South East Asian countries. The Mycologist, 1990; 4: 119-124.

[240] Jong SC, Birmingham JM Medicinal benefits of the mushroom Ganoderma. Adv. Appl. Microbiol., 1991; 37: 101-134.

[241] Buswell JA, Chang ST (1993). Edible mushrooms attributes and applications. In: *Genetics and breeding of edible mushrooms* (Chang, S.T.J. Buswell, J.A and Miles PG (Eds). Gordon and Breach, Philadelphia, pp. 297-394.

[242] Nanba H (1993). Maitake mushroom the king mushroom. Mushroom News, 41: 22-25.

[243] King TA (1993). Mushrooms, the ultimate health food but little research in U. S to prove it. Mushroom News, 41: 29-46.

[244] Kino KY, Yamaoka K., Watanabe J, Kotk SK, Tsunoo H (1989). Isolation and characterization of a new immunomodulatory protein Zhi-8 (LZ-8) from *Ganoderma lucidum*. J. Biol. Chem., 264: 472- 478.

[245] Kim BK, Kim HW, Choi EC (1993). Anti-HIV activity of *Ganoderma lucidum*. J. Biol. Chem., 264: 472-478.

[246] Liu FO, Chang ST (1995). Antitumor components of culture filtrates from *Tricholoma sp*. World J. Microbiol. Biotechnol., 11: 486-490.

[247] Dreyfuss MM, Chapela IH (1994). Potential of fungi in the discovery of natural products with therapeutic potential (Gull, V.P. ed.) Bulterworth- Heinemann, Boston MA, pp. 49-80.

[248] Teow SS (1997). The effective application of *Ganoderma* nutriceuticals. In: Recent progress in *Ganoderma lecidum* research (Kim BK, Moon CK, Kim TS eds.). Seoul Korea. Pharm. Soc. Korea, pp. 21-39.

[249] Harsh NSK, Rai BK, Tiwari DP (1993). Use of *Ganoderma lucidum* in folk medicine. J. Trop. Biodivers., 1: 324-326

[250] Mizuno T (1996). Oriental medicinal tradition of Ganoderma lucidum (Reishi) in India. In: Ganoderma lucidum (Mizuno,T and Kim,B.K eds.). Li Yang Pharm. Co. Ltd., Seoul, Korea, pp. 101-106.

[251] Chang ST, Buswell JA (1996). Mushroom Nutriceuticals. World J. Microbiol. Biotechnol., 12: 473-476.

[252] Oso BA (1997). *Pleurotus tuber-regium* from Nigeria. *Mycologia* 69: 271-279.

[253] Fasidi IA, Olorunmaiye KS (1994). Studies on the requirements for vegetative growth of *Pleurotus tuber regium* (Fr) Singer. Mushroom Food Chem., 50: 397-401.

[254] Bobek P, Ozdin L, Kuniak L (1996). Effect of oyster mushroom (*Pleurotus ostreatus*) and its ethanolic extract in diet on absorption and turnover of cholesterol in hypercholesterolemic rat. Nahrung, 40: 222-224.

[255] Delena T (1999). Edible and useful plants of Texas and South west –A practical guide university of Texas press, pp. 542.

[256] Sadler M (2003). Nutritional properties of edible fungi. Br. Nutr. Found. Nutr. Bull. 28: 305-308.

[257] Chandalia M, Garg A, Lutjohann D, von Bergmann K, Grundy SM, Brinkley LJ (2000). Beneficial effects of high dietary fiber intake in patients with type 2 diabetes mellitus. N. Eng. J. Med., 342:1392-1398

[258] Wasser SP (2005). Reishi or Lingzhi (*Ganoderma lucidum*). Encyclopedia of Dietary Supplements, Marcel Dekker, Germany, pp. 603-622.

[259] Oyetayo VO, Oyetayo FL (2005). Preliminary investigation of health promoting potentials of *Lactobacillus fermentum* OVL and *Plerotus sajor caju* administered to rats. Pakistan J. Nutr., 4: 73-77.

[260] Sharma TK (2008). Vegetable caterpillar, Science Reporter. 5th May ISBN 0036-8512. National institute of science communication and information resources (NISCAIR), CSIR, pp. 33-35.

[261] Mau, J. L., Tsai, S. Y., Tseng, Y. H., & Huang, S. J. (2005). Antioxidant properties of hot water extracts from Ganoderma tsugae Murrill. LWT Food Science and Technology, 38, 589-597.

[262] Mau CN, Huang SJ, Chen CC (2004). Antioxidant properties of methanolic extract from *Grifola frondosa, Morchella esculenta* and *Termitomyces albuminosus* mycelia. Food Chem., 87: 111-118.

[263] Lakshmi, B., Tilak, J.C., Adhikari, S., Devasagayam, T.P.A., Janardhanan, K.K. (2004). Evaluation of antioxidant activity of selected Indian mushrooms. Pharmaceutical Biol., 42, 179-185.

[264] Russell R, Paterson M (2006). *Ganoderma* – A therapeutic fungal factory Phytochemistry. J. Phytochem., 67: 1985-2001

[265] Khatun, S., Bandopadhyay, S., Mitra, S., Roy, P., Chaudhuri, S.K., Dasgupta, A., Chattopadhyay, N.C. (2009). Nutraceutical and antioxidative properties of three species of *Pleurotus* mushrooms. Proc. 5th Int. Medicinal Mushroom Conference, Mycological Society of China, Nantong, China. pp. 234-241.

[266] Jones, S., Janardhanan, K.K. (2000). Antioxidant and antitumor activity of *Ganoderma lucidum* (Cart. Fr.) P.Karst.-Reishi (Aphyllophoromycetidae) from South India. Int. J. Med. Mushroom, 2, 195-200

[267] Singh, R.P., Mishra, K.K., Singh, M. (2006). Biodiversity and utilization of medicinal mushrooms. J. Mycol. Pl. Pathol., 3, 446-448.

[268] Laganathan, K.J., Gunasundari, D., Hemalatha, M., Shenbhagaraman, R., Kaviyarasan, V. (2010). Antioxidant and phytochemical potential of wild edible mushroom *Termitomyces reticulatus*: Individual cap and stipe collected from South Eastern Part of India. Int. J. Pharm. Sci., 1(7), 62-72.

[269] Laganathan, K.J., Ramalingam, S., Venkatasubbu, V., Venketesan, K. (2008). Studies on the phytochemical, antioxidant and antimicrobial properties of three indigenous *Pleurotus* species. Journal of Molecular Biology & Biotechnology, 1, 20-29.

[270] Ajith, T.A., Janardhanan, K.K. (2003). Cytotoxic and antitumor activities of a polypore macrofungus *Phellinus rimosus* (Berk) Pilat, J. Ethnopharmacol. 84, 157-162.

[271] Singh, R.P., Pachauri, V., Verma, R.C., Mishra, K.K. (2008). Catepillar fungus (*Cordyceps sinensis*). A review. J. Eco-Friendly Agric., 3(1), 1-15.

[272] Ajith, T.A., Janardhanan, K.K. (2007). Indian Medicinal Mushrooms as a Source of Antioxidant and Antitumor Agents. J. Clin. Biochem. Nutr., 40, 157-162.

[273] Sasidharan, S., Aravindran, S., Lachimanan, Y.L., Ratnasamy, V., Saravanan, D., Santhanam, A. (2010). *In vitro* antioxidant activity and hepatoprotective effects of *Lentinula edodes* against paracetamol-induced hepatotoxicity. Molecules., 15, 4478- 4489.

[274] Cheung, L.M., Cheung, P.C.K. (2005). Mushroom extracts with antioxidant activity against lipid oxidation. Food Chem., 89, 403-409.

[275] Wong, J.Y., Chye, F.Y. (2009). Antioxidant properties of selected tropical wild edible mushrooms. J. Food Compos. Anal., 22, 269-277.

[276] Groopman JD, Kensler TW The light at the end of the tunnel for Chemical specific biomarkers: daylight or headlight? Carcinogenesis 1999; 20:1-11.

[277] Ueng YF, Shimada T, Yamazaki H, Guengerich FP. Oxidation of aflatoxin B1 by bacteria recombinant human cytochrome P450 enzymes. Chem. Res. Toxicol. 1995;. 8: 218-225.

[278] Wang H, Dick R, Yin H, Licad-Coles E, Kroetz DL, Szklarz G, Harlow G, Halpert JR, Correia MA . Structure-function relationships of human liver cytochrome P450 3A: Aflatoxin B1 metabolism as a probe. Biochemistry 1998; 37: 12536-12545

[279] Lilleberg SL, Cabonce MA, Raju NR, Wagner LM, Kier LD. Alterations in the p53 tumor suppressor gene in rat liver tumors induced by afatoxin B1. Prog. Clin. Biol. Res. 1992; 376:203-222.

[280] Aguilar F, Hussdain SP, Cerutti P. Aflatoxin B1 induces the transversion of GT in codon 249 of the p. 53 tumor suppressor gene in human hepatocytes. Proc. Natl. Acad. Sci. USA. 1993; 90: 8586-8590.

[281] Greenblatt MS, Bennett WP, Hollsten M, Harris CC . Mutations in the p53 tumor suppressor gene: clues to cancer etiology and molecular pathogenesis. Cancer Res. 1994; 54: 4855-4878.

[282] Lunn RM, Zhang YJ, Wang LY, Chen CJ, Lee PH, Lee CS, Tsai WY, Santella RM. p.53 Mutations, chronic hepatitis B virus infection, and aflatoxin exposure in hepatocellular carcinoma in Taiwan. Int. J. cancer 1997; 54: 931-934

[283] Al-Anati L, Petzinger E (2006). "Immunotoxic activity of ochratoxin A". *J. Vet. Pharmacol. Ther.*2006; 29 (2): 79–90.

[284] Neal GE, Judah DJ (2000). Genetic implications in the metabolism and toxicity of mycotoxins. In Molecular Drug Metabolism and Toxicology (eds) Williams GM, Aruoma OI, OICA Intl.(UK) Limited Lond. pp. 1- 15.

[285] Petkova-Bocharova T, Castegnaro M, Michelon J, Maru V. Ochratoxin A and other mycotoxin in cereals from an area of Balkan endemic nephropathy and urinary tract tumors in Bulgaria In Mycotoxins, Endemic Nephropathy and Urinary Tract Tumors (eds) Castegnaro M, Plestina R, Dirheimer G, Chemozensky IN, Barsch H.1991; 245-253. IARC Scientific Publications: Lyon.

[286] Sedmikova M, Resinerora H, Dufkova Z, Burta I, Jilek F .Potential harzard of simulataneous occurrence of aflatoxin B1 and ochratoxin A. Vet Med. 2001; 46:169-174.

[287] D'Mello, J. P. F., and A. M. C. Macdonald. Mycotoxins. Animal Feed Sciences Technology.1997; 69: 155-166.

[288] Kolb, E. Recent knowledge on the mechanism of action and metabolism of mycotoxins. Zeitschrift Gesamte Innovation in Medicine. 1984; 39: 353-358.

[289] Boyd, P. A. and Wittliff, J. L. Mechanism of Fusarium mycotoxin action in mammary gland. Journal of Toxicology Environment of Health. 1978; 4:1-8.

[290] Hagler, W. M. Jr., N. R. Towers, C. J. Mirocha, R. M. Eppley, and W. L. Bryden. Zearalenone: Mycotoxin or mycoestrogen? In B. A. Summerell, J. F. Leslie, D. Backhouse, W. L. Bryden and L. W. Burgess (Eds). Fusarium: Paul E. Nelson Memorial Symposium. APS Press, St. Paul, Minnesota 2001; 321–331.

[291] Ahamed, S. Foster, J. S., Bukovsky, A and Wimalasena, J. Signal transduction through the ras/ERK pathway is essential for the mycoestrogen zearelenone –induced cell cycle progression in MCF-7 cells. Molecular carcinogenesis, 2001; 30:88-98.

[292] Marasas WF, Riley RT, Hendricks KA, Stevens VL, Sadler TW, Gelineau-van Waes J, Missmer SA, Cabrera J, Torres O, GelderblomWC, Allegood J, Martinez C, Maddox.Fumonisins disrupt sphingolipid metabolism, folate transport, and neural tube development in embryo culture and in vivo: a potential risk factor for human neural tube defects among populations consuming fumonisin contaminated maize. J.Nutr.2004; 134 (4):711-716.

[293] Marasas WFO Fumonisins: their implications for human and animal health. Nat. Toxins. 1995; 3: 193-198.

[294] Tollenson WH, Dooley KL, Sheldon WC, Thurman JD, Bucci TJ, Howard PC. The mycotoxin fumonisin induces apoptosis in cultured human cells and in livers and kidneys of rats. In: Jackson LS et al.,(eds) Fumonisins in food, Advances in Experimental Med. And Biol. Plenum Press, New York. 1996; 237-250.

[295] Howard PC, Eppley RM, Stack ME, Warbritton A, Voss KA, Lorentzen RJ, Kovach RM, Bucci TJ. Fumonisin b1 carcinogenicity in a two-year feeding study using F344 rats and B6C3F1 mice. Environ Health Perspect. 2001; 109 (2):277–282.

[296] IPCS. (International Program on Chemical Safety) Environ. Health Criteria 219-Fumonisin B1 WHO, Geneva. 2000; 1-150.

[297] Stockmann-Juvala H, Mikkola J, Naarala J, Loikkanen J, Elovaara E, Savolainen K. Fumonisin B1-induced toxicity and oxidative damage in U-118MG glioblastoma cells. Toxicology 2004; 202(3): 173-83.

[298] Perkowski J, Chelkowski J, Wakulinski W. Deoxynivalenol and 3-acetyl-deoxynivalenol in wheat kernels and chaff with head fusariosis symptoms. Nahr Food. 1990; 34:325–328.

[299] Ijeh II, Obidoa O Effect of dietary incorporation of Vernonia amygdalina Del. on AFB1-induced hepatotoxicity in weanling albino rats. Jamaican J. Sci. Tech., 2004; 15: 32-36.

[300] Rastogi, Shipra; Shukla, Yogeshwer; Paul, Bhola N.; Chowdhuri, D. Kar; Khanna, Subhash K.; Das, Mukul. Protective effect *of* Ocimum sanctum on 3-methylcholanthrene, 7, 12-dimethylbenz(a)anthracene and aflatoxin *B1* induced skin tumorigenesis in mice. Toxicology and Applied Pharmacology 2007; 224(3):228-240.

[301] Karthikeyan K, Gunasekaran P, Ramamurthy N, Govindasamy S. Anticancer activity of *Ocimum sanctum*, Pharm. Biol., 1999; 37(4):285-290.

[302] Nguyen ML, Schwartz SJ. Lycopene: chemical and biological properties. Food Technol. 1999; 53: 38-45.

[303] DiMascio P, Kaiser S, Sies H: Lycopene as the most effective biological carotenoid singlet oxygen quencher. Arch Biochem Biophys 1989; 274: 532–538.

[304] Bohm F, Tinkler JH, Truscott TG: Carotenoids protect against cell membrane damage by the nitrogen dioxide radical. Nature Med 1995;1: 98–99.

[305] 305. Lu Y, Etoh H, Watanabe N: A new carotenoid, hydrogen peroxide oxidation products from lycopene. Biosci Biotech Biochem 1995;59: 2153–2155.

[306] Mortensen A, Skibsted LH: Relative stability of carotenoid radical cations and homologue tocopheroxyl radicals. A real time kinetic study of antioxidant hierarchy. FEBS Lett1997; 417: 261–266.

[307] Hsiao G, Fong TH, Tzu NH, Lin KH, Chou DS, Sheu JR . A potent antioxidant, lycopene, affords neuroprotection against microglia activation and focal cerebral ischemia in rats. In Vivo 2004; 18(3):351-6.

[308] Wertz K, Siler U, Goralczyk R. Lycopene: modes of action to promote prostate health.Arch Biochem Biophys. 2004; 430(1):127-34.

[309] Kim GY, Kim JH, Ahn SC, Lee HJ, Moon DO, Lee CM, Park YM. Lycopene suppresses the lipopoly-saccharide-induced phenotypic and functional maturation of murine dendritic cells through inhibition of mitogen-activated protein kinases and nuclear factor-kappaB. Immunology 2004; 113(2): 203-11.

[310] Q.A. Nogaim, H.A.S. Amra and S.A. Nada. The Medical Effects of Edible Mushroom Extract on Aflatoxin B_1. Journal of Biological Sciences, 2011; 11: 481-486.

Chapter 10

Regulation and Enforcement of Legislation on Food Safety in Nigeria

Jane Omojokun

Additional information is available at the end of the chapter

http://dx.doi.org/10.5772/54423

1. Introduction

Many health problems encountered today arising from consumption of unsafe food are not new as they date far back in history. Contamination of food and feeds arising from naturally occurring toxicants, microbiological contaminants, chemical contaminants such as additives used above the permitted levels, pesticide and veterinary residues in food or as toxic components from food processing could have deleterious effects in humans and animals. Naturally occurring toxicants are of both plant and animal origin. Examples of toxicants of plant origin include alkaloids (pyrrolizidine and solanum alkaloids), allergens, cyanogens, phytooestrogen, glucosinolates, lectins, oxalates, phytates and phenolics. Also included are toxic lipids, peptides and amino acids. The sources of toxicants in foods of animal origin are mostly marine e.g. saxitoxin, neosaxitoxin and gonyautoxins in shellfish poisoning and tetrodoxin in pufferfish poisoning.

Bacterial contamination, fungal toxins, pesticides and toxic metals are the food contaminants of major health concerns. Bacterial food-borne diseases caused by species of *Salmonella, Clostridium, Campylobacter and Escherichia* are of major health concerns in Nigeria contributing to the morbidity and mortality rates of the country. The presence of mycotoxins produced by toxigenic fungi in food and feed exacerbates endemic diseases such as malaria, hepatitis, HIV with consequent acute and chronic effects. Mycotoxins of significant effects in agriculture and public health are aflatoxins, fumonisins, ochratoxins, zearalenone, deoxynivalenol, T-2 toxin, patulins and citrinin. The greatest concern about these mycotoxins particularly aflatoxins and fumonisins is their carcinogenicity. Recently in Africa, fatal aflatoxin-poisoning outbreaks including the episodes in Kenya and Nigeria were reported.

The lack of or inadequate application of Good Agricultural Practices (GAP) and the abuse or misuse of agrochemicals by farmers and during storage in developing countries had serious health effects on the population. Other unsafe common practices include the use of pesticides for fishing, inappropriate application of pesticides to stored products such as beans and grains to prevent insect infestation, inappropriate application of chemicals to fruits such as bananas to ripen them or to vegetables such as carrots and cabbages to control insect infestation. The recent lead poisoning in Zamfara state of Nigeria which caused the death of dozens of infants and children shows the poor attention given to toxic metals in food consumed in Sub Saharan Africa. Similarly, improper use of food additives such as artificial sweeteners, butylated hydroxyl anisole (BHA), nitrates, nitrites, food colours etc could result in various ailments ranging from gastrointestinal disorders to carcinogenesis and death. Some packaging materials with toxic degradable components that are no longer in use in developed countries are still used in rural Africa. Of concern also is the partial or complete destruction or removal of nutrients during food processing. Inferior digestibility or utilization of nutrients and generation of new potentially harmful chemicals arising from bad manufacturing and handling practices are another source of health concern.

The issue of food safety and food – borne toxicants in Sub Saharan Africa, including Nigeria, is exacerbated by public ignorance on the subject, uncoordinated approach to food control, lack of technical expertise and adequately equipped laboratories in some cases, poor enforcement of legislations and regulatory limits. Other factors include introduction of contaminated food into the food chain which has become inevitable due to shortage of food supply caused by drought, wars and other socioeconomic and political insecurity (Wagacha et al. 2008) among others. The occurrence of foodborne disease remains a significant health issue in developed and developing countries despite the efforts being made by governments all over the world to improve the safety of the food supply.

In view of the serious and negative public health and economic impact of unsafe food which is more pronounced in Sub Saharan Africa, this chapter will examine the roles of relevant bodies in assuring food safety all along the farm to table continuum, legislations, food control systems, structures and strategies with particular focus on the Nigerian context. To do this, the following outline would be used for the proposed book chapter.

Keywords: Food, Food Safety, Food Control, Contaminants, Registration, Regulation, Health, Nigeria

2. National food control

National food control systems are designed to address specific needs and priorities of countries. They may differ from country to country but to be effective, they should contain key components such as food legislation and regulations, policy and institutional frameworks, food inspection and monitoring, food laboratory services, involvement of all stakeholders and dissemination of information to them.

There are a number of principles that underscore food control activities and these include:

a. recognizing that food control is a widely shared responsibility and requires interaction between all stakeholders in the farm-to- table continuum,
b. establishing a holistic, integrated and preventive approach to reduce risks of contamination all along the food chain which is the most effective way to produce safe food,
c. developing science-based control strategies,
d. prioritizing activities based on risk analysis and effectiveness of risk management strategies,
e. establishing emergency procedures for dealing with specific hazards or failures (e.g. product recalls) etc.

The roles of the private sector and consumers are important therefore their views and capacity should be taken into account. Communication between the public sector (government), private sector (industry) and consumers is also crucial to food control.

2.1. Objectives

The main objectives of a national food control system are: i) to protect public health by reducing food borne illnesses, ii) to protect consumers from insanitary, contaminated, unwholesome, mislabeled or adulterated food and iii) to maintain consumer confidence in the food system which will give rise to economic development due to increased domestic and international trade in safe food.

2.2. Scope

The scope of food control systems should cover all food from the farm-to-table continuum including imported food i.e. food produced, prepared, processed, imported, exported, stored, transported, distributed and marketed within a country. Such a system should have a statutory basis and be mandatory.

3. National food safety policy

A co-ordinated approach to food control could be achieved by establishing a national food safety policy that will amongst other things assign roles and responsibilities to all stakeholders and co-ordinate all food safety activities. This would reduce the lack of co-ordination and co-operation at national levels and conflict arising from the overlap of functions of the food regulatory bodies which results in ineffective control and inefficient performance.

The National Council on Health of Nigeria at its 40th meeting in November, 1995, directed that a National Policy on Food Hygiene and Safety be put in place. The policy which was formulated with inputs from relevant stakeholders and finally approved by the National Council on Health at its 44th Meeting in 1999 is currently being reviewed.

The National Policy on Food Safety is intended to assign roles and responsibilities and provide official guidelines on the minimum food safety practices which must be adhered to and also assure consumers about the safety of food and food products meant for human consumption in Nigeria. It is an integral part of the Nigerian National Health Policy.

The National Food Safety Policy provides for the establishment of a National Committee on Food Safety which shall draw its membership from the public and private sectors relevant to the production, storage, processing/preparation, distribution, transportation, and sale of food intended for consumption.

i. The Public Sector includes:
   a. Federal Government Ministries
   b. Federal Government Food Control Agencies
   c. State Government Ministries of Health
   d. State Government Ministries of Agriculture
   e. Local Government Departments of Health
   f. Local Government Departments of Agriculture
ii. The Private Sector includes:
   a. Industry
   b. Non- Governmental Organizations (NGOs)
   c. International Development Partners
   d. Universities and Research Institutes
   e. Professional Bodies/Associations
   f. Consumer Associations.

3.1. Legal framework

From as far back as 1958, various laws and regulations had been promulgated over the years to ensure the safety and wholesomeness of the nation's food supply. Such legislations include the following:

a. Public Health Laws (1917) now known as Public Health Ordinance Cap 165 of 1958;
b. The Standards Organization of Nigeria Decree No. 56 of 1971;
c. The Food and Drug Act No 35 of 1974 (now Food and Drug Act Cap F32 Laws of the Federal Republic of Nigeria, 2004)
d. The Animal Disease Control Decree No. 10 of 1988;
e. The Marketing of Breast Milk Substitute Decree No. 41 of 1990 (now Marketing (Breast Milk) Act Cap M5 LFN 2004;
f. The National Agency for Food and Drugs Administration and Control Decree No 15 of 1993 (now NAFDAC Act CAP N1 Laws of the Federal Republic of Nigeria, 2004);
g. The Food, Drug and Related Products (Registration etc) Decree No 19 of 1993 [now Food, Drugs & Related Products (Registration etc) Act Cap F33 Laws of the Federal Republic of Nigeria (LFN), 2004];
h. The Counterfeit and Fake Drugs and Unwholesome Processed Food Act No 25 of 1999 (now Counterfeit & Fake Drugs and Unwholesome Processed Foods (Miscellaneous Provisions) Act Cap C34 LFN 2004;
i. Various bye-laws enacted by various LGAs in the country.

3.2. Goals

The overall goal of the National Policy on Food Safety is to establish a national institutional framework that will consolidate all existing food safety and control systems in the country and ensure the attainment of a high level of food safety standards that will achieve the following:

a. Promote the availability and consumption of safe, wholesome and nutritious foods;
b. Improve public health and reduce/eliminate incidences of food borne and related diseases throughout the country.
c. Protect the health of consumers by the reduction of exposure to hazards through producing, processing, and distributing safe food.
d. Meet consumers' needs and preferences in addition to facilitating international trade in food

The specific goals of the National Policy on Food Safety are as follows:

i. To review, update and promote all Government policies, laws and regulations concerned with the control of safety of food during its policy formulation, production, storage and handling, processing/preservation, trade, transportation and marketing, preparation and consumption.
ii. To improve the quality of healthcare delivery by ensuring that only foods that are safe, wholesome and of good quality are produced and/or marketed in Nigeria in accordance with prescribed food safety management systems such as but not limited to HACCP (Hazard Analysis and Critical Control Point) and are accessible to the consumer at affordable price.
iii. To update, strengthen, harmonize, integrate and publicize all existing laws/regulations, standards and codes of practice with respect to control and regulation of food safety practices; eliminate areas of duplication/conflict and make them more relevant to the needs of the country and also create a national data base needed for future planning.
iv. To establish a risk based food control system that will assist in setting appropriate level of protection for the consumers; prioritization of food safety programmes and monitoring safety trends in the national food supply

Food safety activities are sometimes fragmented and compounded by overlap of functions of the government regulatory bodies with roles along the farm-to-table continuum. The National Policy on Food Safety aims to integrate and harmonize all existing laws, standards and codes that regulate food safety practices in Nigeria, redefine and coordinate existing food control infrastructures at various levels of government and eliminate areas of overlap and conflict. Implementation of the National Policy on Food Safety (NPFS) would minimize the risk of outbreak of diseases arising from poor safety practices and reduce the prevalence of food-borne and related diseases. The principles and practice of Hazard Analysis and Critical Control Point (HACCP) system would be applied during the preparation, production, handling, storage, processing/preservation, transportation and distribution of foods.

4. Bodies with roles to play in food safety

4.1. Government bodies

4.1.1. The Federal Ministry of Health (FMOH)

The Federal Ministry of Health is responsible for the formulation of national policies, guidelines and regulations on food safety including monitoring and evaluation. It is also responsible for the assessment of the nutritive value of food, environmental sanitation, food environment and handlers, control of food borne disease, quality of public water from taps, as well as national and international matters relating to food.

4.2. The National Agency For Food And Drug Administration and Control (NAFDAC)

The National Agency for Food and Drug Administration and Control (NAFDAC) is responsible for the regulation and control of the importation, exportation, manufacture, advertisement, distribution, sale and use of food, drug, cosmetics, medical devices, chemicals, packaged water and detergent at Federal and State levels in Nigeria. Appropriate tests are conducted and compliance with standard specifications for the effective control of the quality of food, bottled water and the raw materials as well as their production processes in factories and other establishments is ensured. The Agency undertakes appropriate investigations into production premises and raw materials for food and establishes relevant quality assurance systems including certification of the production sites and the regulated products and pronounces on the quality and safety of food, bottled water and chemicals. The role of the Agency also includes the inspection of imported food facilities to ascertain relevant quality assurance systems necessary for certification of the imported food product.

4.3. The Standards Organization of Nigeria (SON)

The Standards Organisation of Nigeria is responsible for the formulation and enforcement of set standards on the composition of imported and locally manufactured food.

4.4. The Federal Ministry of Agriculture and Rural Development (FMA&RD)

The Federal Ministry of Agriculture and Rural Development is responsible for formulating policies on primary agricultural production and practices which cover plants, animals, pests and diseases etc.; supervising and overseeing its departments and parastatals i.e. research institutes, colleges of agriculture, colleges of fisheries etc.

4.5. The Federal Department of Fisheries

The Federal Department of Fisheries has the responsibility for ensuring that fish and fishery products produced, imported into or exported from Nigeria conform to international quality standards of wholesomeness as stipulated in the Sea Fisheries (Fish Inspection and Quality Assurance) Regulation of 1995. The aim of all of which is to ensure compliance with the Fish Quality and Quarantine Services Regulation of 1995.

4.6. Nigeria Plant Quarantine Service (NPQS)

The NPQS was established in 1960 with an Act of Parliament "The Agriculture (Control of Importation) Act No.28 of 1959" which gave the Division the mandate to put in place quarantine regulations, infrastructural facilities, trained personnel and scientific equipment and regulations that would enable her to meet the objective of preventing the introduction of dangerous and destructive foreign plant pests (insects, fungi, bacteria, virus, nematodes and weeds) of plants and plant products into the country and prevent the establishment and spread where introduction occurs despite all preventive measures. This mandate is in line with the text of the International Plant Protection Convention (IPPC) of the Food and Agriculture Organization (FAO) of 1959, and revised in 1979 which Nigeria is a signatory. There has been a review of the NPQS enabling laws and drafting of the Nigeria Plant Protection Act also known as The Agricultural Control of Importation and Exportation Act Amendment 2003 to conform with international standards. Nigeria is one of the founding members of Inter-African Phytosanitary Commission and is being represented by Nigeria Plant Quarantine Service.

4.7. Consumer Protection Council

Consumer Protection Council is the government agency responsible for protecting consumers from unwholesome practices and assisting them seek redress for unscrupulous practices and exploitation. The agency encourages trade, industry and professional associations to develop and enforce quality standards designed to safeguard the interest of the consumer.

4.8. Federal Ministry of Environment

The Federal Ministry of Environment has a role to play in the control of environmental food contaminants, persistent organic pollutants, environmental pollution, waste disposal, etc.

4.9. Federal Ministry of Trade and Investment

The Federal Ministry of Trade and Investment is the Notification Authority on World Trade Organization (WTO) Sanitary and Phytosantary rules in Nigeria and therefore has a role to play in international trade in safe food.

4.10. Federal Ministry of Education

Federal Ministry of Education has a role to play through enlightenment and manpower development by incorporating subjects on safe food handling in the school curriculum and courses on Food Safety Management Systems i.e. Good Agricultural Practices (GAP), Good Hygienic Practices (GHP), Good Manufacturing Practices (GMP), Hazard Analysis Critical Control Points (HACCP) etc in tertiary institutions necessary for manpower development.

4.11. Local Government Areas (LGAs)

The Local Government Areas are responsible for Street Vended Foods, Bukaterias, Catering establishments, local abattoirs and traditional markets.

4.12. Universities and Research Institutes

Tertiary and Research Institutes are responsible for research and will provide scientific basis for policy development and programme design in addition to relevant training programmes for capacity building and manpower development.

4.13. Private sector

The food processing/service industry applies the various standards, regulations and guidelines to ensure that food manufactured, imported, exported, distributed and sold for human consumption comply with the relevant food safety laws/regulations. They should maintain appropriate internal Quality Assurance based on the Hazard Analysis Critical Control Point (HACCP) principles to ensure product safety and consumer protection. The private sector is also expected to collaborate and complement government efforts in specific areas of education and awareness creation on the need to adopt and cultivate safe food handling habits by all categories of employees. It is recommended that small and medium scale entrepreneurs complement the efforts of the regulatory bodies by forming umbrella associations (e.g. packaged water producers, cocoa farmers association etc) that will employ self regulation of their practices. This enables the group to easily arrange consultative meetings with the regulatory bodies during which their views, issues of concerns and capacities are discussed and taken into account during decision making. Forming such associations also enables the regulatory bodies organize targeted capacity building training programmes for the group.

Various bodies are involved in food safety activities all along the food chain therefore proper co-ordination of their activities is crucial for an effective food control system. Poor or lack of co-ordination of activities sometimes leads to duplication of efforts, higher cost of doing business, discouragement of entrepreneurs etc and an ineffective food control system.

The global trend in food safety control emphasizes a multifaceted and multidisciplinary approach with effective co-ordination and collaboration between the regulatory bodies, the industry, academia, research institutes, professional bodies, consumer associations and the general public. A national food safety policy which spells out the roles and responsibilities of all stakeholders is essential for achieving an effective food safety control system.

5. National food control systems

An effective national food control system takes into account current situations and develops a national food control strategy to enable the country develop an integrated, coherent, dynamic and effective control. Situations differ from country to country therefore the programmes to achieve the objectives of the food control strategy are country specific. Official food control systems provide the possibility for implementation of the regulatory activities of government bodies aimed at ensuring that all foods are safe, wholesome and fit for human consumption, and are honestly and accurately labelled. Important components of a food control system include: policy and institutional frameworks; food legislation and regulations; food inspection and monitoring; laboratory services and dissemination of information to all stakeholders. The private sector and consumers should be fully carried along and their views and capacities taken into account, because they play a crucial role in ensuring that the overall goals of the food control systems are achieved. It is essential for adequate communication between government, private sector and consumers to be active and sustained.

The widely accepted principles of food control systems include: the role of scientific evidence and use of the risk analysis framework to make food safety decisions, structures to achieve prevention and control along the entire food value chain and ensuring that food chain operators realize that the primary responsibility to ensure safe and good quality foods rests on them. A well planned and structured food control system should give rise to a suitable national system developed in line with international best practices and harmonized with Codex Alimentarius Commission standards and World Trade Organization (WTO) requirements.

There are various organizational structures for national food control systems; however the three main types that are considered suitable are as follows:

- A single agency system which involves a unified, single agency being responsible for national food control;
- A multiple agency system where multiple agencies are responsible for national food control;
- An integrated system based on a national integrated approach.

The type of system does not matter as much as its fitness for the intended purpose. Whatever system is in place, adequate communication and coordination among different institutions are crucial. The system that would facilitate regulatory action for food safety should be based on the principles of transparency, inclusiveness, integrity; clarity of roles and rules; accountability, science/risk-based approach and equivalence as the benchmarks against which it would be measured.

5.1. Single agency system

The single agency system puts the responsibility for food safety and public health protection in a single Food Control Agency. The relevant bodies responsible for food control along the value chain are domiciled in one agency and under the same management therefore the system is coordinated and makes for quicker response and effectiveness. This kind of system shows that Government places high priority on food safety and reduction of food-borne illness. The advantages of a single agency system include:

- Coordinated and uniform approach to food safety and public health protection
- Reduction or elimination of overlap of functions, duplication of efforts, delays, increased cost of doing business and wastage
- Improved efficiency, cost effectiveness and better use of resources and expertise
- Increased ability to respond quickly to emerging challenges (e.g. emerging pests and diseases) and food safety emergencies (e.g. melamine, dioxin, nucleotide etc contamination of food)
- Delivering more efficient service that facilitates the growth of industry and promotes trade.

5.2. Multiple agency system

Food control systems serve the primary purpose of ensuring food safety and protection of the health of consumers although there are other important objectives such as ensuring fair practices in trade, facilitating food export trade, developing the food sector to operate in a professional and scientific manner and economic benefits.

The systems that specifically deal with these objectives can be sectoral i.e. based on the need to develop a particular sector such as roots and tubers; fisheries; meat and meat products etc. It could be mandatory or voluntary. It is put in effect through a general food law or a sectoral regulation. For example, an export inspection law that requires certain foods to be mandatorily inspected before export; regulated systems for grading and marking fresh agricultural produce which are sold directly to the consumer; specific commodity inspection regulations such as for milk and milk products, fats and oils, meat and meat products etc. Sectoral initiatives may give rise to separate food control activities which leads to the creation of multiple agencies with responsibilities for food control. In this type of system, the food control responsibilities are usually shared between government ministries such as Health, Agriculture, Commerce, Environment, Trade, Industry and Tourism and government agencies such as the National Food Control Body or the Food Standards Body. The enabling laws specify the roles and responsibilities of the relevant government bodies which are different but sometimes overlap. This gives rise to challenges such as fragmentation, increased bureaucracy, increased cost of doing business, duplication of functions and lack of co-ordination between the various bodies with roles to play all along the farm to table continuum.

Food control systems may also be fragmented between national, state and local government bodies and the thoroughness of implementation depends on the competence and efficiency of the agency responsible at each level. Therefore consumers may not receive the same level of protection throughout the country and it may be difficult to properly evaluate the effectiveness of interventions at national, state and local government levels.

While the multiple agency system may be the most used, the serious drawbacks include:

- Difference in the level of expertise and resources resulting in uneven implementation
- Conflicts arising from overlap of functions and lack of cohesion between bodies with roles in food safety and consumer protection leading to over-regulation and undue delays
- Conflicts between public health objectives and facilitation of trade and industry development
- Limited capacity for appropriate scientific inputs in decision-making processes
- Lack of overall co-ordination at the national level
- Reduction of domestic consumer confidence and foreign partners in the credibility of the system.

It is often difficult to have a unified or integrated food control system in this kind of set up because of the various historical and political reasons therefore the national food control strategy should clearly identify and assign roles to each agency to avoid duplication of efforts and to enable some measure of coherence amongst them.

5.3. Integrated system

Integrated food control systems are operated where there is the desire and political will to achieve effective collaboration and coordination between agencies across the farm-to-table continuum. An integrated National Food Control Agency should address the entire food chain and have the mandate to move resources to high priority areas and to address important sources of risk. The system should be structured such as to have several levels of operation as follows:

Level 1: Formulation of policy, risk assessment and management and development of standards and regulations
Level 2: Coordination of food control activity, monitoring and auditing
Level 3: Inspection and enforcement
Level 4: Education and training.

This model calls for the establishment of an autonomous national food agency which is responsible for activities at levels 1 and 2 with existing multi-sectoral agencies retaining responsibility for level 3 and 4 activities. The advantages include:

- Politically more acceptable as it does not disturb the day to day inspection and enforcement roles of other agencies
- Separates risk assessment and risk management functions, hence objective consumer protection measures with resultant confidence among domestic consumers and credibility of foreign buyers;
- Provides coherence in the national food control system;
- Promotes uniform application of control measures across the food value chain throughout the country;

- Better equipped to deal with international dimensions such as participation in Codex work, Sanitary and Phytosanitary Measures/Technical Barriers to Trade (SPS/TBT) Agreements;
- Encourages transparency in decision-making processes and accountability in implementation; and
- Is more cost effective in the long term.

The role of such an agency is to establish national food control goals, put into effect the strategic and operational activities necessary to achieve the goals. It should also revise and update the national food control strategy as needed; advise on policy matters including determination of priorities and use of resources; draft regulations, standards and codes of practice and promote their implementation; coordinate the activities of the various inspection agencies and monitor performance; develop consumer education and community outreach programmes and promote implementation; support research and development and establish quality assurance schemes for industry and support their implementation. The agency should consider the role of private analytical, inspection and certification services particularly for export trade.

6. National Codex Committee (NCC)

Nigeria is a member of the Codex Alimentarius Commission, a Joint FAO/WHO Food Standards Programme. The National Codex Committee (NCC) was established in July 1973 by the approval of the Federal Executive Council and reconstituted in 2002 to incorporate all stakeholders to enable the committee function effectively towards providing relevant inputs and asserting the country's position at the Codex Alimentarius Commission in view of the implications for food safety and quality, protection of consumer health, fair practices in food trade as well as the enhancement of the national economy. The National Codex Committee (NCC) operates within the provisions of the NCC Procedural Manual that sets out the General Rules of the National Codex Committee (NCC) and the other internal procedures necessary to achieve the objectives of the National Codex Committee; lists out the core functions of the National Codex Committee Secretariat, the four (4) Technical Committees and their terms of reference; sets out the guidelines for meetings of the National Codex Committee and its technical committees and lists the membership of the National Codex Committee . The chair of the NCC is currently the Federal Ministry of Health but with the review of the NCC Procedural Manual, will become rotational between the Federal Ministry of Health and the Federal Ministry of Agriculture and Rural Development. The Secretariat of the NCC and Codex Contact Point (CCP) is the Standards Organisation of Nigeria (SON).

The membership of the NCC consists of the Federal Ministry of Health; Federal Ministry of Agriculture and Rural Development; Standards Organisation of Nigeria (SON); National Agency for Food and Drug Administration and Control (NAFDAC); Federal Ministry of Science and Technology; Federal Ministry of Trade and Investment; Federal Ministry of

Environment; Ministry of Foreign Affairs; Federal Ministry of Justice; National Planning Commission; Consumer Protection Council; Nigeria Customs Service; National Biotechnology Development Agency (NABDA); National Association of Small & Medium Scale Enterprises (NASME); Federal Department of Fisheries; Association of Food Beverages and Tobacco Employers (AFBTE); Institute of Public Analyst of Nigeria (IPAN); National Food Reserve Agency; Nigerian Institute of Food Science and Technology (NIFST); Nigeria Agricultural Quarantine Services (NAQS); National Association of Small Scale Industrialists (NASSI); Trawlers Owners Association; Vulnerable Empowerment Creative Network; Nigeria Institute of Oceanography and Marine Research (NIOMR); Nigeria Export Promotion Council (NEPC); and 2 (two) appointed Private Consultants.

6.1. Codex Contact Point

The Codex Contact Point is primarily a coordinator and focal point for Codex activities within the country, and is the link between the country and the Codex Alimentarius Commission (and its Secretariat). It receives all the correspondence from the Codex Secretariat and Codex Committees and also invitation letters to attend Codex Committee and Commission meetings and coordinates all the necessary activities to facilitate the desired response. The Codex Contact Point which also serves as the secretariat for the National Codex Committee in Nigeria is domiciled in the Standards Organization of Nigeria.

6.2. National Codex Committee Technical Committees

The National Codex Committee has 4 (four) technical committees that deliberate on Codex texts and Circular Letters received from the Codex Secretariat requiring government comments at steps 3 and 6 of the 8-step standard setting procedure of the Codex Alimentarius Commission. The technical committees meet to synthesize the national position and prepare the country delegation that would attend Codex Committee and Commission meetings. The recommended country positions are endorsed by the National Codex Committee and forwarded by the Codex Contact Point to the Codex Secretariat, respective Codex Committees and the Codex Commission as the case may be. The National Codex Committee also provides a technical forum for:

e. Articulating national guidelines for protecting the health of the consumers and ensuring fair practices in the trade of food.
f. Promoting co-ordination of all food standards work undertaken by national, international governmental and non-governmental organizations.
g. Determining priorities and initiating draft standards with the aid of the appropriate organizations.
h. Initiating review of published standards, after appropriate survey in the light of current developments.
i. Discussing issues relating to Codex and other regional standards on composition, safety, labeling, analysis and marketing of foods.

j. Initiating scientific and technical data, generating research or collaborative studies, collating and processing data to enhance and enrich national, Codex and regional standards and all aspects of food regulations and marketing.

The technical committees are responsible for work on the assigned Codex Committees as shown below:

1. General Purposes Technical Committee chaired by the National Agency for Food and Drug Administration and Control (NAFDAC) is responsible for Pesticide Residues in Food; Food Additives; Contaminants in Food; Food Labelling; Food Hygiene; Food Import and Export Inspection and Certification; Methods of Analysis and Sampling and General Principles.
2. Animal and Animal Products Technical Committee chaired by the Federal Ministry of Agriculture and Rural Development is responsible for Meat and Meat Products; Poultry and Poultry Products; Fish and Fisheries Products; Milk and Milk Products; Residues of Veterinary Drugs in Foods; Fats and Oils (animal origin) and Animal Feeding.
3. Plants and Plants Products Sub-Committee chaired by the Association of Food Beverages and Tobacco Employers is responsible for Cereals, Pulses and legumes; Vegetable Proteins; Fats and Oils (Plant Origin); Cocoa Products and Chocolate; Sugars and Honey; Fresh Fruits and Vegetables; Processed Fruits and Vegetables; Soups and Broths; Bouillon Cubes; Roots and Tubers; and Nuts.
4. Special Projects Technical Committee chaired by the Federal Ministry of Science and Technology (FMST) is responsible for Biotechnology; Food for Special Dietary Uses;
5. Mineral Waters; Food Supplements; Beverages (alcoholic and non alcoholic).

7. National Agency for Food & Drug Administration & Control (NAFDAC)

The National Agency for Food & Drug Administration & Control (NAFDAC) is the regulatory authority in Nigeria with the mandate to regulate and control the manufacture, importation, exportation, advertisement, distribution, sale and use of food, drug, cosmetics, medical devices, chemicals, detergents and packaged water often referred to as regulated products. NAFDAC is the lead Agency for food safety and quality.

7.1. Regulatory strategies

a. Product Registration

   The product registration process is one of the regulatory strategies of NAFDAC. The Agency uses product registration to establish and monitor the ownership and/or distributorship of the products it regulates, generally known as regulated products (i.e. food, drug, cosmetics, medical devices, chemicals, detergents and packaged water); their safety; quality; labeling; claims etc. NAFDAC employs a structured and systematic procedure for product registration at the end of which the product is assigned a NAFDAC Registration Number which is an attestation to the safety, quality and appropriateness for its intended use. The registration process involves:

- Documentation: Documents are required such as Power of Attorney from the manufacturer authorizing an applicant to speak for his principal on all matters relating to the latter's specialties; Certificate of Manufacture and Free Sale which is an evidence that the product is manufactured and freely sold in the country of origin; Certificate of Incorporation of the representative company in Nigeria; Evidence of Trade Mark registration; Comprehensive Certificate of Analysis of the batch of product to be registered. The permit to import samples for registration purposes is issued if documentation is satisfactory.
- Labeling: Labels should be informative, clear and accurate; indicate the name of product; name and address of the manufacturer, packer, distributor, importer, exporter, or vendor; make provision for NAFDAC Registration Number; batch number, manufacturing date and expiry or best before date; net content, ingredients list in metric weight in case of solids, semi solids and aerosols and metric volume in case of liquids.
- Inspection: Good Manufacturing Practice (GMP) inspection of the production facility is carried out prior to registration of the product.
- Product Approval Committee Meetings: A three (3) tier product approval meeting is held to consider the documentation, laboratory reports, GMP inspection reports, product labels etc. of a product prior to its registration.

Once a product is satisfactory, it is assigned a NAFDAC Registration Numbers and can be freely sold or marketed within the country.

b. Consultative Meetings

NAFDAC encourages sectoral groups, small and medium scale entrepreneurs etc to form umbrella associations (e.g. Association of Food, Beverage and Tobacco Employers (AFBTE); National Association of Small Scale Industrialists (NASSI); Association of Table Water Producers (ATWAP), Association of Fast Foods and Confectionaries Operators of Nigeria (AFFCON); All Farmers Association etc). These organizations are encouraged to self regulate their practices and can easily arrange for consultative meetings with the Agency where their views and concerns are addressed and taken into account when making regulatory decisions that concern them. Such an arrangement also enables NAFDAC to organize targeted and focused capacity building training programmes for the various groups.

Consultative meetings could also be at the instance of the Agency to give information and enlighten the public on NAFDAC requirements, discuss perceived regulatory challenges, inform on international best practices and regulatory trends etc.

c. Public Enlightenment Campaigns

The Agency organizes public enlightenment campaigns on topical and emerging issues using the electronic media, print media and physical presence at campaigns held at grassroots levels where the rural dwellers are invited with the cooperation and involvement of their local chiefs to inform and educate the populace. Programmes such as "NAFDAC and Your Health" are popular television and radio programmes where regulatory officers are invited to speak on issues such as food safety, Codex activities, food supplements, how to check food products for important information on the labels such as date markings, NAFDAC Registration Number etc. Some of the programmes are phone-in programmes where the public has the opportunity to ask questions and be further enlightened. The Agency also uses television advertisements and radio jingles to inform and educate the public.

d. Training and Publications
NAFDAC organizes international, national and in-house capacity building training programmes consistently for staff , the industry and the general public. There are also collaborations and exchange programmes with credible regulatory authorities and international bodies such as the United States Food and Drug Administration (USFDA), US Department of Agriculture (USDA), International Atomic Energy Agency (IAEA), World Health Organization (WHO), Directorate General for Health and Consumers (DG SANCO) of the European Commission, African Union/Interafrican Bureau for Animal Resources (AU/IBAR) etc.

The Agency produces informative news bulletins, pamphlets, magazines etc such as the "Consumer Safety" Magazine which not only offers technical information to the general public but also has a catch-them-young programme for schools through the Consumer Safety Club where NAFDAC educates members of the club on food safety issues and organizes annual essay competitions on selected food safety topics for member schools. The winners are celebrated in a NAFDAC organized national event where they receive awards and gifts for their schools and themselves. In addition to inculcating food safety and hygienic practices at an early age, the idea of the Consumer Safety Club also includes reaching out to the household or family level with food safety news and practices through the kids..

8. Challenges of regulatory control of food borne toxicants in Nigeria

The challenges of regulatory control of food borne toxicants range from variations in the quality of raw materials supplied to the food processors (because in many cases they are sourced separately and pooled together); having many food handlers and middlemen with the risk of practices that expose the food to contamination; inadequate infrastructure and laboratory capacity and expertise; insufficient number of regulatory officers, inadequate co-ordination of food safety activities along the value chain to insufficient knowledge by food handlers. Problems sometimes occur due to poor post harvest handling; inadequate storage facilities and cold stores or conditioned warehouses; inadequate infrastructure such as transport facilities; good road networks, absence or shortage of electricity supply and clean water. Lack of the requisite knowledge and expertise in good agricultural practices at the farm level, good hygienic practices/ good manufacturing practices at the production level and poor traceability also play a part.

Certain unwholesome practices such as improper use of agrochemicals by traders of food commodities e.g. application to unpackaged or bulk beans meant for sale in the open markets during their storage, have led to pesticide residues levels exceeding the maximum limits and emergency food safety concerns. Poor handling and storage of products such as melon seeds, groundnuts, rice etc lead to fungal growth and mycotoxin production with levels that exceed the acceptable limits.

Street vended foods are an important component of the food supply chain but unfortunately such foods are generally prepared in unhygienic conditions with poor food handling, unhygienic surroundings and limited water supply. These conditions expose the food to microbiological contamination and could be a source of illness for the consumer.

All these challenges could be addressed through public enlightenment, better coordination of roles along the food value and food supply chain, capacity building, improved infrastructure, training from the farm to the processing or preparation levels, adequately equipping the producers and regulators to perform their functions better through training and retraining in addition to providing the necessary working tools.

Author details

Jane Omojokun
National Agency For Food And Drug Administration and Control (NAFDAC), Nigeria

9. References

[1] Assuring Food Safety and Quality : Guidelines for Strengthening National Food Control Systems, FAO Food and Nutrition Paper 76, ISBN 92-5-104918-1 © FAO and WHO 2003

[2] Draft National Policy on Food Safety In Nigeria Produced by the Federal Ministry of Health, Abuja, Nigeria, 2011

[3] Enhancing Participation in Codex Activities : An FAO/WHO Training Package, © FAO/WHO , 2005

[4] FAO/WHO Global Forum of Food Safety Regulators Marrakesh, Morocco, 28 - 30 January 2002, "The Nigerian Experience on Food Safety Regulations" by R.K. Omotayo and S.A. Denloye

[5] Procedural Manual of the National Codex Committee (NCC), Federal Republic of Nigeria Produced by the National Codex Committee , 2nd Edition (2007) (under review, 2012)

[6] www.fao.org/food/food-safety-quality/food-control/en/ Food Control and Consumer Protection

For EU product safety concerns:
IN TECH d.o.o., Prolaz Marije Krucifikse Kozulić 3, 51000 Rijeka, Croatia,
info@intechopen.com or visit our website at intechopen.com.